Mark D. Hoover

D0858180

NANOTOXICOLOGY

NANOTOXICOLOGY

CHARACTERIZATION, DOSING AND HEALTH EFFECTS

EDITED BY

NANCY A. MONTEIRO-RIVIERE
North Carolina State University
Raleigh, North Carolina, USA

C. LANG TRAN
Institute of Occupational Medicine
Edinburgh, UK

2007

informa
healthcare

New York London

Informa Healthcare USA, Inc.
52 Vanderbilt Avenue
New York, NY 10017

© 2007 by Informa Healthcare USA, Inc.
Informa Healthcare is an Informa business

International Standard Book Number-10: 1-4200-4514-8 (Hardcover)
International Standard Book Number-13: 978-1-4200-4514-7 (Hardcover)

Library of Congress Cataloging-in-Publication Data

Nanotoxicology : characterization, dosing and health effects / edited
   by Nancy A. Monteiro-Riviere, C. Lang Tran.
      p. ; cm.
   Includes bibliographical references and index
   ISBN-13: 978-1-4200-4514-7 (hardcover : alk. paper)
   ISBN-10: 1-4200-4514-8 (hardcover : alk. paper) 1. Nanotechnology–Health aspects.
   2. Nanotechnology–Environmental aspects
I. Monteiro-Riviere, Nancy A.
II. Tran, C. L.
   [DNLM: 1. Nanostructures–toxicity. 2. Nanotechnology-methods.
   3. Nanostructures-therapeutic use. QT 36.5 N188 2007]

   R857.N34N37 2007
   610.28–dc22   2007018543

Visit the Informa web site at
www.informa.com

and the Informa Healthcare Web site at
www.informahealthcare.com

Preface

The field of nanoscience has experienced unprecedented growth during the last few years and as a result has received a great deal of attention from the public, regulatory agencies, and the science community. However, there are many challenges that must be overcome before we can apply nanotechnology to the field of nanomedicine or conduct science-based occupational or environmental exposure risk assessments. This resultant new field of nanotoxicology will continue to grow and emerge as new products are produced.

This is the first book to provide basic knowledge relative to nanomaterial safety and is intended for basic scientists, environmental scientists, toxicologists, chemists, engineers, risk assessors, federal regulators, and others involved in assessing the safety of manufactured nanomaterials for occupational and environmental health. Nomenclature standards, physicochemical characteristics of nanoparticles that determine their toxicity, characterization, and obstacles using in vitro and in vivo studies are presented. This includes techniques and the importance of working with well-characterized materials, estimating nanoparticle dose, agglomeration problems, biodistribution and kinetics and levels of exposure that could be used for risk assessment analysis. Methods used to assess nanoparticle toxicity including genomics, proteomics, electron microscopy, and dispersion of nanoparticles are addressed. Specific target organ systems that have been utilized to study the adverse effects in the eye, pulmonary, cardiovascular, integumentary, and nervous systems are covered.

Also, the environmental and ecological impacts regarding nanomaterial fate, occurrences, and characterization are presented. Knowledge of exposure and hazard are needed for understanding risks associated with nanomaterials. We need to understand the broad concepts that apply to pathways of dermal, oral, and inhalational exposures so that we can focus on hazard assessment. The general principles governing the safety of all particles scenarios need to be evaluated in order to establish specific nanotoxicology safety and testing guidelines following occupational exposure during manufacture, exposure in academic research laboratories, or environmental exposure, either from manufacturing waste or post-consumer use.

Nanomaterials are structures with characteristic dimensions between 1 and 100 nm; engineered appropriately, they exhibit a variety of unique and tunable chemical and physical properties. These characteristics have made engineered nanoparticles central components in an array of emerging technologies, and many new companies have been formed to commercialize products. Although they have widespread potential applications in material sciences, engineering, and medicine, the toxicology of these materials has not been thoroughly evaluated under likely environmental, occupational, and medicinal exposure scenarios. To date, insufficient data has been collected to allow for full interpretation or thorough understanding of the toxicological implications of occupational exposure or potential environmental impact of nanomaterials. In order to avoid past mistakes made when new technological innovations, chemicals, or drugs were released prior to a broad-based risk assessment, information is needed now regarding the potential toxicological impact of nanomaterials on human health and the environment.

Nancy A. Monteiro-Riviere
C. Lang Tran

Contents

Contributors

Andrew J. Alexander   School of Chemistry, University of Edinburgh, Edinburgh, U.K.

James R. Baker, Jr.   Department of Internal Medicine and Michigan Nanotechnology Institute for Medical and Biological Sciences, University of Michigan, Ann Arbor, Michigan, U.S.A.

T. Michelle Blickley   Integrated Toxicology Program and Division of Coastal Systems Science and Policy, Duke University Marine Laboratory, Beaufort, North Carolina, U.S.A.

Vincent Castranova   National Institute for Occupational Safety and Health, Morgantown, West Virginia, U.S.A.

Nic. Christofi   Centre for Health and the Environment, School of Life Sciences, Napier University, Edinburgh, U.K.

Mary Jane Cunningham   Houston Advanced Research Center, The Woodlands, Texas, U.S.A.

Gregory A. Day   National Institute for Occupational Safety and Health, Morgantown, West Virginia and Cincinnati, Ohio, U.S.A.

Ken Donaldson   ELEGI Colt Laboratory, Medical Research Council/ University of Edinburgh Centre for Inflammation Research, Queen's Medical Research Institute, Edinburgh, U.K.

Rodger Duffin   ELEGI Colt Laboratory, Medical Research Council/ University of Edinburgh Centre for Inflammation Research, Queen's Medical Research Institute, Edinburgh, U.K.

Aaron Erdely   Tissue Injury Team, Toxicology and Molecular Biology Branch, Health Effects Laboratory Division, National Institute for Occupational Safety and Health, Morgantown, West Virginia, U.S.A.

Ivana Fenoglio   Interdepartmental Center "G. Scansetti" for Studies on Asbestos and Other Toxic Particulates and Dipartimento di Chimica IFM, University of Torino, Torino, Italy

Theresa F. Fernandes   Centre for Health and the Environment, School of Life Sciences, Napier University, Edinburgh, U.K.

Bice Fubini   Interdepartmental Center "G. Scansetti" for Studies on Asbestos and Other Toxic Particulates and Dipartimento di Chimica IFM, University of Torino, Torino, Italy

Martin C. Garnett   School of Pharmacy, University of Nottingham, Nottingham, U.K.

Mridul Gautam   College of Engineering and Mineral Resources, West Virginia University, Morgantown, West Virginia, U.S.A.

Charles L. Geraci   National Institute for Occupational Safety and Health, Morgantown, West Virginia and Cincinnati, Ohio, U.S.A.

Rosemary M. Gibson   Health Effects Division, Health and Safety Laboratory, Derbyshire, U.K.

Mary L. Haasch   USEPA Mid-Continent Ecology Division, Molecular and Cellular Mechanisms Research Branch, Duluth, Minnesota, U.S.A.

Peter H.M. Hoet   Unit of Lung Toxicology, Laboratorium of Pneumology, K.U. Leuven, Leuven, Belgium

Mark M. Banaszak Holl   Department of Chemistry and Michigan Nanotechnology Institute for Medical and Biological Sciences, University of Michigan, Ann Arbor, Michigan, U.S.A.

Mark D. Hoover   National Institute for Occupational Safety and Health, Morgantown, West Virginia and Cincinnati, Ohio, U.S.A.

Marc Hoylaerts   Center for Molecular and Vascular Biology, K.U. Leuven, Leuven, Belgium

Alfred O. Inman   Center for Chemical Toxicology Research and Pharmacokinetics, North Carolina State University, Raleigh, North Carolina, U.S.A.

Barbara P. Karn   U.S. Environmental Protection Agency, Office of Research and Development, National Center for Environmental Research, Washington, D.C., U.S.A.

Michael J. Keane   Health Effects Laboratory Division, National Institute for Occupational Safety and Health, Morgantown, West Virginia, U.S.A.

Ian Kinloch   School of Materials, University of Manchester, Manchester, U.K.

Elena Kisin   National Institute for Occupational Safety and Health, Morgantown, West Virginia, U.S.A.

Eileen D. Kuempel   National Institute for Occupational Safety and Health, Cincinnati, Ohio, U.S.A.

Stephen S. Leonard   National Institute for Occupational Safety and Health, Morgantown, West Virginia, U.S.A.

Zheng Li   Tissue Injury Team, Toxicology and Molecular Biology Branch, Health Effects Laboratory Division, National Institute for Occupational Safety and Health, Morgantown, West Virginia, U.S.A.

Gregory V. Lowry   Department of Civil and Environmental Engineering, Carnegie Mellon University, Pittsburgh, Pennsylvania, U.S.A.

Andrew J. Lucking   Cardiovascular Research, Division of Medical and Radiological Sciences, University of Edinburgh, Edinburgh, U.K.

Gerard A. Lutty   Wilmer Ophthalmological Institute, Johns Hopkins Hospital, Baltimore, Maryland, U.S.A.

William MacNee   ELEGI Colt Laboratory, Medical Research Council/ University of Edinburgh Centre for Inflammation Research, Queen's Medical Research Institute, Edinburgh, U.K.

Antonio Marcomini   Venice Research Consortium and Department of Environmental Science, University Cà Foscari, Venice, Italy

Andrew D. Maynard   Project on Emerging Nanotechnologies, Woodrow Wilson International Center for Scholars, Washington, D.C., U.S.A.

Patricia D. McClellan-Green   Department of Environmental and Molecular Toxicology and Center for Marine Sciences and Technology, North Carolina State University, Raleigh, North Carolina, U.S.A.

Nicholas L. Mills   Cardiovascular Research, Division of Medical and Radiological Sciences, University of Edinburgh, Edinburgh, U.K.

Nancy A. Monteiro-Riviere   Center for Chemical Toxicology Research and Pharmacokinetics, North Carolina State University, Raleigh, North Carolina, U.S.A.

Ashley R. Murray   National Institute for Occupational Safety and Health, Morgantown, West Virginia, U.S.A.

David Murray   Health Effects Laboratory Division, National Institute for Occupational Safety and Health, Morgantown, West Virginia, U.S.A.

Benoit Nemery   Unit of Lung Toxicology, Laboratorium of Pneumology, K.U. Leuven, Leuven, Belgium

Abderrahim Nemmar   Department of Physiology, College of Medicine & Health, Sultan Qaboos University, Al-Khod, Sultanate of Oman

David E. Newby   Cardiovascular Research, Division of Medical and Radiological Sciences, University of Edinburgh, Edinburgh, U.K.

Eva Oberdörster   Department of Biology, Southern Methodist University, Dallas, Texas, U.S.A.

Tong-man Ong   Health Effects Laboratory Division, National Institute for Occupational Safety and Health, Morgantown, West Virginia, U.S.A.

Bradford G. Orr   Department of Physics and Michigan Nanotechnology Institute for Medical and Biological Sciences, University of Michigan, Ann Arbor, Michigan, U.S.A.

Giulio Pojana   Venice Research Consortium and Department of Environmental Science, University Cà Foscari, Venice, Italy

Dale W. Porter   National Institute for Occupational Safety and Health, Morgantown, West Virginia, U.S.A.

Tarl Prow   Wilmer Ophthalmological Institute, Johns Hopkins Hospital, Baltimore, Maryland, U.S.A.

Jim E. Riviere   Center for Chemical Toxicology Research and Pharmacokinetics, Biomathematics Program, North Carolina State University, Raleigh, North Carolina, U.S.A.

Victor A. Robinson   National Institute for Occupational Safety and Health, Morgantown, West Virginia, U.S.A.

Jessica P. Ryman-Rasmussen   Center for Chemical Toxicology Research and Pharmacokinetics, North Carolina State University, Raleigh, North Carolma, U.S.A.

Tina Sager   National Institute for Occupational Safety and Health, Morgantown, West Virginia, U.S.A.

Margaret Saunders   Biophysics Research Unit, Department of Medical Physics and Bioengineering, United Bristol Healthcare, National Health Service Trust, Bristol, U.K.

Diane Schwegler-Berry   National Institute for Occupational Safety and Health, Morgantown, West Virginia, U.S.A.

Xiao-Chun Shi   Health Effects Laboratory Division, National Institute for Occupational Safety and Health, Morgantown, West Virginia, U.S.A.

Anna A. Shvedova   National Institute for Occupational Safety and Health, Morgantown, West Virginia, U.S.A.

Petia P. Simeonova   Tissue Injury Team, Toxicology and Molecular Biology Branch, Health Effects Laboratory Division, National Institute for Occupational Safety and Health, Morgantown, West Virginia, U.S.A.

Aleksandr B. Stefaniak   National Institute for Occupational Safety and Health, Morgantown, West Virginia and Cincinnati, Ohio, U.S.A.

Vicki Stone   Centre for Health and the Environment, School of Life Sciences, Napier University, Edinburgh, U.K.

Maura Tomatis Interdepartmental Center "G. Scansetti" for Studies on Asbestos and Other Toxic Particulates and Dipartimento di Chimica IFM, University of Torino, Torino, Italy

C. Lang Tran Institute of Occupational Medicine, Edinburgh, U.K.

William E. Wallace Health Effects Laboratory Division, National Institute for Occupational Safety and Health and College of Engineering and Mineral Resources, University of West Virginia, Morgantown, West Virginia, U.S.A.

Mark R. Wiesner Department of Civil and Environmental Engineering, Duke University, Durham, North Carolina, U.S.A.

Frank A. Witzmann Department of Cellular and Integrative Physiology, Indiana University School of Medicine, Indianapolis, Indiana, U.S.A.

Shiqian Zhu Environmental Toxicology Research Program, National Center for Natural Products Research and Department of Pharmacology, School of Pharmacy, The University of Mississippi, University, Mississippi, U.S.A.

Stefano Zuin Venice Research Consortium and Department of Environmental Science, University Cà Foscari, Venice, Italy

1

Nanotoxicology: Laying a Firm Foundation for Sustainable Nanotechnologies

Andrew D. Maynard

Project on Emerging Nanotechnologies, Woodrow Wilson International Center for Scholars, Washington, D.C., U.S.A.

INTRODUCTION

In 2004, Donaldson and colleagues proposed a new idea to the world of toxicology—the idea that nanometer-scale particles behave so differently from their larger counterparts that a new subcategory of the field was needed (1). They named the new subcategory *nanotoxicology*—a term which found further support the following year in the review "Nanotoxicology: An emerging discipline evolving from studies of ultrafine particles" by Oberdörster et al. (2). Since Donaldson et al.'s original paper, nanotoxicology as a field of study has come into its own: Numerous meetings and conferences have been held around the world on the topic since 2004, and a casual search of the Web of Science shows the number of papers using the term to be increasing each year. The collection of chapters in this book is the latest step in the maturation of nanotoxicology from an idea to a recognized discipline, and represents a distillation of the knowledge and concepts that are defining the field. This collection is both an important milestone along the road to understanding and managing potential risks associated with nanoscale particles and a signpost to guiding future investigations. But there is still a long way to go before we can assess or predict the biological impact of nanoscale particles with confidence.

BACKGROUND

To understand the challenges being faced and the progress already made, it is worth stepping back a little. The danger of inhaling microscopically small fume or smoke particles has been recognized since ancient times (3). But it was not until the late 1980s that researchers started to systematically study the effect of particle size in the nanometer range (approximately 1–100 nm) on health impact (4,5). At about this time, a new form of carbon was discovered—carbon nanotubes—in which the atoms are arranged into tubelike structures of graphene sheets, with diameters as small as 1 nm and lengths that can be in excess of hundreds of nanometers (6). It did not take long for concerns to be raised over possible health issues associated with inhaling these nanoscale fibers (7), although only recently have results of systematic studies been published (8). The 1990s were also a period when epidemiology was beginning to uncover previously unexpected associations between fine particle inhalation and diseases of the respiratory and cardiovascular systems (9), with some speculation that it was the smallest particles in the nanometer size range that were responsible for some of the observed outcomes (10). However, it was a small band of toxicologists (many of them authors of the chapters in this book) that began systematic research to explore the associations between particle size, structure, and response in the lungs and thus lay the groundwork for understanding how particle size in the nanorange uniquely influences behavior in the body (11–14).

In 2004, the U.K. Royal Society and Royal Academy of Engineering published a seminal report on the opportunities and uncertainties of the emerging field of nanotechnology (or "nanotechnologies" as the authors preferred—reflecting the many different ways of exploiting our increasing ability to engineer matter at the nanoscale) (15). A key concern raised in the report was that "the lack of evidence about the risk posed by manufactured nanoparticles and nanotubes is resulting in considerable uncertainty" (15). Prior to 2004, there was a growing understanding of the size-specific biological behavior of nanoparticles, whether they arose from natural, incidental, or intentional processes; the Royal Society and Royal Academy of Engineering report shone the spotlight of concern clearly on those particles being developed and engineered as the precursors and components of nanotechnologies.

SIZE-SPECIFIC BEHAVIOR OF NANOMATERIALS

Nanotechnology depends in part on exploiting the size-specific properties of nanoscale materials, which in some cases includes an expression of quantum effects that are unique to nanoparticles. By the same token, these size-dependent properties also lead to the possibility of size-dependent biological activity. The concept of uniqueness is often used when discussing what makes "nano" different—usually in the context of physical or chemical properties. Yet research over the past two decades has demonstrated that nanoparticles may exhibit unique biological behavior, even when physical and chemical properties remain unaltered from those observed in larger particles. Perhaps the most striking examples are those in which particle size enables nanoscale particles to cross or circumvent barriers that are impenetrable to larger particles. Research showing the potential for nanoparticles to move up the olfactory nerves to the brain in rodents is a prime example of this unanticipated and size-unique behavior (16,17). But given that many biological processes occur at the nanoscale, there are numerous additional opportunities for precisely sized nanoparticles to interfere with normal biological functions. Just two recent examples: Zhao et al. have used computer models to predict that C_{60} molecules can damage DNA if intracellular exposure occurs (18) and Lynch et al. have hypothesized that adsorption of proteins onto nanoparticles could alter their shape to the extent that normally hidden amino acid residues are exposed as cryptic epitopes—triggering an immune response (19). In addition, interactions at the nanoscale may confound the interpretation of conventional assays, as was observed by Monteiro-Riviere and Inman in studies to assess the dermal impact of carbon nanomaterials (20).

It is these increasing indications and predictions of size-specific biological activity that underlie the special distinction of nanotoxicology from other branches of toxicology. These "unique" behaviors are requiring new tools and concepts within the field of toxicology to understand and predict how emerging engineered nanoparticles will interact with humans and environmental systems. But they are also fundamentally challenging established research and test methodologies. At the heart of these challenges is the role of particle form (or shape) in determining behavior. The properties of a nanoparticle are critically influenced by its form, and the arrangement of chemical components within this physical envelope. Both composition and form are dynamic, and may reflect the history and the local environment of a particle. This places a high premium on characterizing nanoparticles accurately in any study—not only before the particles have been prepared for administration, but also during administration, and after they have been introduced to the cell culture or animal model being used (see Chapters 2 through 4). In considering the elements of a nanomaterials toxicity screening strategy, Oberdörster et al. identified 17 particle attributes that should be considered when evaluating toxicity, including size, shape, surface area, surface chemistry, crystal structure, and many others (21). In a field where measured dose–response relationships are typically evaluated on the basis of chemical composition and mass concentration, this list was a radical departure from the norm. Moreover, many of the parameters listed can only be characterized using specialized techniques unfamiliar to toxicologists, and some are still beyond the capabilities of routine measurement methods.

NANOTOXICOLOGY CHALLENGES

Nanotoxicology requires its scientists to work with materials that behave in unconventional ways, and to collaborate with experts in unfamiliar fields. The challenges are significant, but will hopefully stimulate and energize researchers to make new advances in our understanding of nanoparticles in the biological environment. And it is clear that advances are needed, if we are to manage the tide of new engineered nanomaterials predicted to hit the market. In a recent paper in *Nature*, 14 scientists suggested that "the specter of possible harm—whether real or imagined—is threatening to slow the development of nanotechnology unless sound, independent and authoritative information is developed on what the risks are, and how to avoid them," and presented five "grand challenges" to the global research community to develop this information (22). Two of these grand challenges specifically targeted the need for new nanotoxicity testing strategies and predictive capabilities. Of the remaining three challenges, one dealt with exposure monitoring and another with life cycle assessment.

In meeting these challenges, the state of knowledge set out in the following chapters will be invaluable. Following a comprehensive grounding in nanotoxicology-relevant physicochemical properties and characterization in Chapters 2 through 4, Chapter 5 directly addresses the challenges of measuring exposure to engineered nanomaterials. Chapters 6 through 21 provide an extensive resource for understanding how nanoparticles behave in the body. The material presented will inform the development of toxicity tests that are relevant to target organs and systems—including the skin, cardiovascular system, pulmonary system, and central nervous system—and will help ensure that these tests are responsive to the potentially unique impacts of engineered nanomaterials. But these chapters also provide a basis on which models to predict the biological impact of existing and emerging nanomaterials might be developed and validated. Finally, Chapters 22 through 25 address the behavior and potential impact of nanoparticles in the environment. And so a compendium of current wisdom is offered, which addresses the possible impact of engineered nanomaterials from their generation to their disposal—through their life cycle.

The final grand challenge outlined by Maynard et al. was issued not to scientists, but to science policy makers. Nanotoxicology—as with other areas of research into the potential impact of nanotechnology—will not progress in any relevant way without strategic support that provides both funding and direction. And so the authors of the paper concluded by challenging policy makers in government and industry to develop and support strategic research programs that will result in information critical to the safe and successful development of nanotechnologies.

SUMMARY

Although the science of nanotoxicology may be complex, framing the issues and how to tackle them should not be so difficult. Already there are over 400 consumer products on the market allegedly based on nanotechnology (23), and the global market for nanotech-based products is projected to be worth US $2.6 trillion by 2014 (24). To understand the potential impact of the nanomaterials used in these products, we need to know about exposure potential, material characteristics, and hazard potential—at each point of the material and product life cycle. Nanotoxicology—understanding the size-specific behavior and impact of nanoparticles in particular—is a vital component of this information chain. The chapters in this book will provide an invaluable resource for understanding the challenges we face, and pointing toward the solutions we seek. This is just one step in a long journey toward understanding how nanoparticles behave in humans and the environment, but it is an important step. Donaldson et al. concluded their original nanotoxicology article by noting "A discipline of nanotoxicology would make an important contribution to the development of a sustainable and safe nanotechnology" (1). I am pleased to say that this book, and the research of the scientists contributing to it, demonstrates clearly that the new discipline of nanotoxicology is indeed *making* an important contribution to safe and sustainable nanotechnology. Let us hope that the impetus, support and enthusiasm for this global research continue, enabling the very real benefits of nanotechnology to be fully realized.

REFERENCES

1. Donaldson K, et al. Nanotoxicology. Occup Environ Med 2004; 61:727–8.
2. Oberdörster G, Oberdörster E, Oberdörster J. Nanotoxicology: an emerging discipline evolving from studies of ultrafine particles. Environ Health Perspect 2005; 13:823–40.
3. Maynard AD, Baron PA. Aerosols in the Industrial Environment. In: Ruzer LS, Harley NH, eds. Aerosols Handbook. Measurement, Dosimetry and Health Effects. Boca Raton, FL: CRC Press, 2004:225–64.
4. Oberdörster G, et al. Increased pulmonary toxicity of ultrafine particles. 2. Lung lavage studies. J Aerosol Sci 1990; 21:384–7.
5. Ferin J, et al. Increased pulmonary toxicity of ultrafine particles.1. Particle clearance, translocation, morphology. J Aerosol Sci 1990; 21:381–4.
6. Iijima S. Helical microtubules of graphitic carbon. Nature 1991; 354:56–8.
7. Coles GV. Occupational risks. Nature 1992; 359:99.
8. Lam CW, et al. A review of carbon nanotube toxicity and assessment of potential occupational and environmental health risk. Crit Rev Toxicol 2006; 36:189–217.
9. Dockery DW, et al. An association between air pollution and mortality in six U.S. cities. N Engl J Med1993; 329:1753–9.

10. Seaton A, et al. Particulate air pollution and acute health effects. Lancet1995; 345:176–8.
11. Lison D, et al. Influence of particle surface area on the toxicity of insoluble manganese dioxide dusts. Arch Toxicol 1997; 71:725–9.
12. Oberdörster G, et al. Association of particulate air pollution and acute mortality: involvement of ultrafine particles? Inhal Toxicol 1995; 7:111–24.
13. Fubini B. Surface chemistry and quartz hazard. Ann Occup Hyg 1998; 42:521–30.
14. Donaldson K, et al. Ultrafine particles: mechanisms of lung injury. Phil Trans R Soc Lond A 2000; 358:2741–9.
15. Royal Society and Royal Academy of Engineering. Nanoscience and Nanotechnologies: Opportunities and Uncertainties. London: 2004.
16. Oberdörster G, et al. Translocation of inhaled ultrafine particles to the brain. Inhal Toxicol 2004; 16:437–45.
17. Elder A, et al. Translocation of inhaled ultrafine manganese oxide particles to the central nervous system. Environ Health Perspect 2006; 114:1172–8.
18. Zhao X, Striolo A, Cummings PT. C_{60} binds to and deforms nucleotides. Biophys J 2005; 89:3856–62.
19. Lynch I, Dawson K, Linse S. Detecting cryptic epitopes created by nanoparticles. Sci STKE 2006; 327:pe14.
20. Monteiro-Riviere NA, Inman AO. Challenges for assessing carbon nanomaterial toxicity to the skin. Carbon 2006; 44:1070–8.
21. Oberdörster G, et al. Principles for characterizing the potential human health effects from exposure to nanomaterials: elements of a screening strategy. Part. Fiber Toxicol 2005; 2: doi:10.1186/1743-8977-2-8.
22. Maynard AD, et al. Safe handling of nanotechnology. Nature 2006; 444: 267–9.
23. PEN. Project on Emerging Nanotechnologies, Woodrow Wilson International Center for Scholars, Washington, D.C., 2006.
24. Lux Research. New York, NY: Lux Research Inc., 2006.

2

Carbon Nanotube Structures and Compositions: Implications for Toxicological Studies

Andrew J. Alexander

School of Chemistry, University of Edinburgh, Edinburgh, U.K.

INTRODUCTION

A substantial amount of money and effort has been funneled into research and development of carbon nanotubes (CNT), and they have been heralded as novel materials with unique properties and applications. Since 1991, the number of research papers published on the topic of CNT has increased exponentially, arriving at a current figure of 21,236 articles at a current rate of 100 per week (September 2006) (1). Global CNT production estimates vary, but are suggested to have been ∼100 tons in 2004, and ∼294 tons in 2005 (2). Underneath such statistics lies a trend that is seeing the Eastern and Asian markets taking the lead in the CNT research and production markets, with Korea predicted to be the world leader in CNT production in 2010 (2).

With such unprecedented levels of investment, it is no wonder that questions of potential toxicity have been raised and must be addressed (3). It will be important to anticipate outcomes of human exposure during processing, or from waste generated from consumer products that now contain these materials. Such consumer products have been slow in coming. Already, CNT are being used as fillers for plastic panels to dissipate charge during spray painting, in car manufacture for example. CNT are also being used in electrodes of lithium ion batteries. On the lighter side, it is possible to purchase tennis racquet and bicycle frames made from composites containing CNT. CNT also push the boundaries of past toxicological experience, e.g., there is debate as to whether they may be considered as fibers or as conventional nanoparticles (NP) (3).

At a glance, the structure of CNT looks uncomplicated: it may seem pedantic to devote more than a couple of lines to the details. Unfortunately, there are huge variances in the physical and chemical structures of CNT samples. There are some early indications that such variances are the cause of large disparities among some of the initial toxicological studies. CNT are manufactured by different companies and procedures, they contain differing amounts of impurities, and may have been subsequently processed by a vast array of possible methods. Homogeneity between batches of samples from the same source can also vary substantially. We look first at properties that are intrinsic to the tubes themselves (the "ideal" CNT), and then discuss features introduced in practice during synthesis, and finally in terms of postproduction processing.

INTRINSIC STRUCTURE

The simplest type of CNT is the single-walled CNT (SWCNT): this can be thought of as a single sheet of graphite rolled up to form a seamless cylinder (4). If a number of sheets are rolled up to form concentric tubes, we obtain multiwalled CNT (MWCNT) (Fig. 1). The spacing between cylinders in MWCNT is close to that of graphite (~0.34 nm). Double-walled tubes (DWCNT) are of particular interest recently, because the outer tube may be functionalized while the inner tube remains to all intents an intact SWCNT (5). The tube ends may be either uncapped, or capped with a curved shell of graphite. By contrast, carbon fibers are strands of graphite sheets that are layered, giving the overall fiber shape. The way that the hexagons tile gives rise to different structures, called the chirality of the tube.

Like graphite, CNT tend to aggregate to maximize contact between graphitic layers, and this is particularly the case for SWCNT. The resultant bundling contributes to the insolubility of CNT. CNT are seen as strongly resistant to chemical attack: they will burn in air at temperatures ~500°C (6). SWCNT are weaker, because the graphite of the wall is more highly curved, and therefore more strained (7). The end caps are also highly curved and will be weak points for attack, as will any uncapped ends. Along with the usual graphitic hexagonal rings, the end caps may contain pentagonal or heptagonal rings: these are chemically active points (Fig. 2) (8). Occasional defects can occur in the hexagonal tiling in the wall of an otherwise perfect tube, creating more reactive hotspots. Such defects can be stabilized on the tube as localized radicals, or by adsorbed oxygen (9). The relative amount of nongraphitic carbon can be determined by Raman spectroscopy, which has strong features for CNT. The G band is due to graphitic carbon, the D band

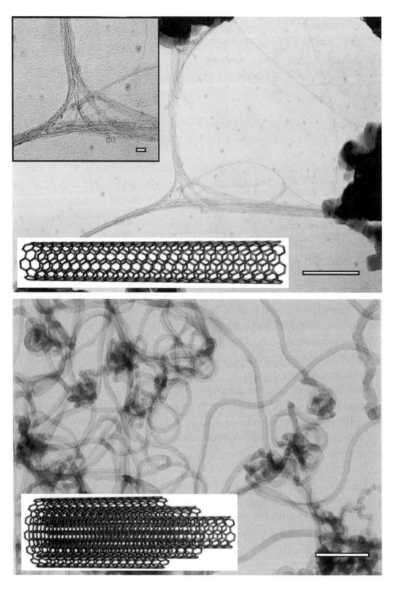

Figure 1 Schematic models and transmission electron microscope images of single-walled (*top*) and multiwalled (*bottom*) carbon nanotubes. Bundling is seen for the single-walled tubes, giving a nanotube bundle junction. Scale bars are: inset 10 nm, others 200 nm.

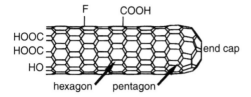

Figure 2 Schematic of a tube showing structural features, such as the end cap, pentagonal defects, and examples of chemical functional groups.

is a measure of nongraphitic carbon (either impurity materials, or defects in the tubes). So-called radial breathing modes indicate the presence of SWCNT (8).

CNT IN PRACTICE

The synthesis of CNT is critical in determining the practical features of the structure, side-products, impurities, and therefore potential toxic activity of any given sample. Tube widths are dependent on synthesis, but are generally found in the range 0.7 to 3 nm (SWCNT) (10) and 10 to 100 nm (MWNT) (11). Tube lengths may be anywhere from a few nanometers to tens of microns, but aggregates and bundles can be significantly longer and wider.

CNT have very high surface areas as a consequence of their structure. The surface area will also depend on the dimensions of the tubes, and the degree of bundling, but can be measured using standard adsorption iso-therm instruments (e.g., BET isotherm). Theoretical values for discrete SWCNT ($\sim$1300 m^2/g) and MWCNT ($\sim$100–800 m^2/g) have been estimated (12). In practice, bundling will reduce the surface area of SWCNT to $\sim$300 m^2/g, or less (13).

There are three major methods of CNT synthesis, viz., arc-discharge, laser ablation, and chemical vapor deposition (CVD) (14). The underlying principle involves producing fragments of carbon that are then reconstituted to form the tube, usually with the aid of a metallic catalyst, at quite high temp-eratures ($\sim$500–1200°C). It is possible to produce CNT without metal catal-ysts, although the yields are exceedingly low and SWCNT will be very rare.

By a mile, the most common method of synthesis is CVD. In addition to heat ($\sim$600 + °C), there are three key ingredients:

1. Carbon source (carbon precursor), e.g., methane, methanol, acetylene, benzene, or carbon monoxide.
2. Catalyst support: this could be a flat surface (e.g., SiO$_2$) for vertically aligned growth, a powder of finely divided particles (e.g., MgO, zeolite, aluminates, or silicates), or no support in the case where the metal catalyst is formed as an aerosol (e.g., in the high-pressure carbon monoxide conversion HiPco process) (15).

3. Metal catalyst: this is usually transition metals, commonly Fe, Co, Ni, and Mo, and sometimes a mix or alloy, of these. The form of the metal going in depends on the synthesis method and the type of support:
    a. for surfaces, a thin surface layer of metal (e.g., Ni);
    b. for powders, metal salts (e.g., iron nitrate) or preformed NP;
    c. for aerosol, an organometallic (e.g., iron pentacarbonyl) (16).

In addition to the above, additives may also be included. These additives might include an inert carrier gas (e.g., argon gas), a reducing agent (e.g., hydrogen gas), or a growth promoter (e.g., low concentrations of water vapor).

The basic mechanism for growth relies on the formation of metal NP, usually aided by the high temperatures (8,17). Carbon is formed by dissociation of the carbon source, preferentially at the catalyst, to produce fragments that can recombine to generate the CNT. The size of the nascent nanotube can be directly related to the size of the metal particle, which thus acts as a template (18). The support is also believed to play a role, not only by dispersing the catalyst, but by stabilizing the NP and assisting with decomposition of the carbon source. Exact details of the growth mechanism are still under debate, and will likely differ between methods.

What are the net results of the CVD recipe and basic mechanism? This might be quite a minefield of potential parameters for a toxicologist to deal with. Not only will there be variability between samples prepared with different (sometimes proprietary) ingredients, there will be some variability within and between batches prepared by the same method! The products will contain a number of non-CNT impurities: these are summarized in Figure 3. Scanning electron microscopy (SEM) or transmission electron microscopy (TEM) can indicate the presence of certain residuals, and also give an idea about dimensions. However, both methods are time intensive, and can look at only a small amount of the sample material: therefore, caution should be used when making conclusions. The overall carbon content can be measured by thermogravimetric analysis (TGA), which is used to detect loss of materials due to burning (as carbon does). TGA may even distinguish between CNT and other types of carbon, which will burn at different temperatures. Support materials typically do not burn at temperatures used in TGA, whereas the metal catalyst may be seen to oxidize (gaining, rather than losing mass). There are three main classes of residual impurity, which we will discuss in more detail.

Residual Support

For some methods of CNT synthesis there may be no support to remove, e.g., aerosol methods, or the support may be included as part of the required product, e.g., the surface of an electronic wafer. Otherwise the support will

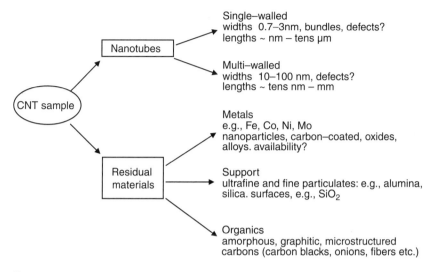

Figure 3 Summary of the possible components in a carbon nanotube sample. *Abbreviation*: CNT, carbon nanotube.

form a large percentage of the produced CNT, and there will normally be some attempt to remove it. The form of the support is typically as a finely divided powder: possibly a so-called nanopowder. The large surface area of the support is exploited to promote the synthesis. The chemical makeup of the support is usually some type of silicate or oxide: it must survive the harsh reaction conditions required for CVD, and should not hinder the CVD process. Removal of the support can be made difficult if carbon is deposited directly onto the support causing it to become encased and protected to some extent.

Residual Metal

The most common catalytic metal used is Fe, although a wide range of transition metals have been shown to catalyze CNT growth. Small percentages of other metals, e.g., Mo, can be added to promote fine division of the NP during initial heating: this will tend to promote SWCNT growth. The amount of residual iron can vary between a few percent to tens of percent by mass of the CNT, and most of this is in the form of NP, although larger aggregates can form. Postproduction processing can remove some—*but typically not all*—of the residual metal. There can be no easy rules about the availability, or inertness, of the metal remaining in the sample even after postproduction processing. This is because processing may make available some previously inaccessible metal, e.g., by creating defects in CNT.

After growth, metal NP can often be seen under TEM as being encapsulated somewhere inside a tube that has grown (19). Metal NP can also be seen as spherical encapsulates in carbon ("failed" CNT) (20): this carbon may be graphitic or amorphous soot. Since most samples are subsequently exposed to air, any exposed metal NP will oxidize. The speed, and extent to which oxidation occurs will depend on the environment of the exposed metal. In some cases a metal oxide shell can protect a metal core. Also, it can not be assumed that any carbon encapsulated metal NP are not in fact metal oxides: this will depend on exposure to air via defects in the carbon coatings, and whether the atmosphere during synthesis was a reducing environment (e.g., containing H_2). Transition metals have an ability to dissolve carbon in small amounts, as in bulk carbon steel, and these alloys may also be present. Selective area X-ray diffraction might be used to determine what forms of metal are present: like electron microscopy, however, this is a very selective analytical method. Inductively coupled plasma-optical emission spectroscopy (ICP-OES) can be used to accurately quantify metal content, both of the CNT, and of solutions made to test *in vitro* for metal availability. Such tests, however, may still not reveal what form of metal is present.

Residual Organics

Residual organics could mean almost any carbon-containing species, aside from the CNT. The sizes and shapes of these can vary from molecular (residual organic molecules, e.g., benzene) to bulk carbon. The bulk carbon can be present in a spectrum of forms. Amorphous carbon has no long-range order, and can be classified as diamond-like or graphite-like depending on the density of C atoms and how they are bonding to each other. Microstructured carbon is a generic classification that includes carbon blacks and carbon fibers, and could include any structures that can be made out of layers of graphite, e.g., carbon "onions" or "horns" (20). Postproduction processing generally relies on residual organics being more easily broken up, dispersed, and removed.

POSTPRODUCTION PROCESSING

Purification

In practice, purification can involve both chemical and high-energy physical methods. The general premise is to exploit the resistance of CNT to the harsh processing conditions, so that impurities are more easily broken into pieces, dispersed, converted (e.g., oxidized), and removed (e.g., by filtration and washing, or centrifugation). Such treatments might include high temperature treatment with oxidizing agents or acids, sometimes for long periods.

The CNT are not completely infallible, and many will be damaged or oxidized in a survival of the fittest. The most vulnerable points under attack are the more highly curved SWCNT, defects, and end caps. The processing will create defects (e.g., missing C atoms) and other functional groups (e.g., –COOH carboxylic groups (Fig. 2) on CNT at these vulnerable points. Creation of a defect causes a nonnative chemical site and therefore potential vulnerability, possibly enough to split an existing tube at that point: tube shortening may indeed be a desired result (21). Processing may erode the protection of residual materials that were previously protected, e.g., metals or support particles. These residual materials may not be immediately exposed during processing, but become more liable to exposure during later handling.

Ultimately, the survival of the fittest will leave a different material from the prepared sample. The survivors may in some cases be more vulnerable or chemically active, or conversely they may be more inert having survived a harsh process. Some further processing may be carried out to mitigate against damage caused, this can take the form of a long, slow annealing at high temperature under an inert gas, where the CNT graphite can retile to repair itself. This will produce the highest grade of CNT product, and it seems unlikely that a manufacturer would go to such lengths where a less perfect product would suffice. Even after all efforts to purify CNT, commercial samples are not usually more than 95% nominal purity. Much of the remainder will be residual metal, mostly encapsulated in the tubes themselves, with residual non-CNT carbon.

Functionalization

One of the attractive features of CNT has been as material building blocks that may be opened-up to the vast array of modern chemical synthetic methods available. Functionalization (or, derivatization) of CNT is used to attach chemical groups to modify their properties and handling. Discussion of the possible routes achieved so far could fill an entire review article: therefore, we will limit this to giving a brief overview relevant to toxicology. The reader is directed to two recent reviews that cover the topic in more detail (22,23).

Functionalization falls into two categories: physical (noncovalent) and chemical (covalent, or ionic). *Physical functionalization* includes use of surfactants, e.g., to exfoliate and disperse tubes. This is distinct from *chemical functionalization* in that no direct chemical bonds are made between the surfactant and CNT, only weak physical (noncovalent) forces are involved (e.g., van der Waals forces).

Surfactants greatly increase the usability of CNT, because they are not generally inclined to disperse in water or other solvents. Pristine CNT can only be dispersed in small quantities in polarizable solvents such as dichlorobenzene (0.095 mg/cm) or chloroform (0.031 mg/cm) (24). A wide range of surfactants have been used, including common surfactants such as sodium dodecyl sulfate (SDS, 0.1 mg/cm), or—arguably the best—sodium dodecylbenzenesulfonate (SDBS, 10 mg/cm) (25). Such surfactants have an inherent toxicity, which may complicate toxicological studies of CNT. Other surfactants include polymers such as poly(ethyleneglycol) (26), or biopolymers such as single-stranded DNA (27), which are believed to wrap around the tube.

Dispersal in surfactant is usually assisted by ultrasonication, or other vigorous action. Sonication can temporarily increase the dispersability of tubes in surfactant: although the tubes will tend to reaggregate and settle-out over time. Moreover, it is known that intense sonication can tend to damage tubes (28).

Besides attachments to the outside of tubes, it is possible to fill the insides of tubes with various species: including metals (29), C_{60} (SWCNT "peapods") (30), and a number of proteins (31). It has been shown that the filling materials are largely protected by the nanotube shell, but are effectively immobilized. A study of β-lactamase I catalyzed hydrolysis of penicillin showed that it retained catalytic activity, suggesting that no significant conformational distortion had occurred (31).

The study of the interactions between CNT and biomolecules has become especially popular recently, with interest in the use of CNT for biological sensors and drug delivery (23). Proteins are found to noncovalently bind very strongly to CNT, with their flexibility allowing them to wrap and fold over the CNT surface. The optical and electrical properties of SWCNT are very sensitive to adsorbates, and there is interest in combining adsorbate recognition with CNT to make nanoscale biosensors (32). CNT show a notable ability to traverse cell membranes. There has been intense debate over the mechanism for uptake, with two likely mechanisms being surface adsorption-mediated endocytosis (33,34) and direct diffusion (35,36).

The array of chemical groups successfully bonded to CNT is impressive: from halogens to (grafted) polymers (22). In general, the scale of chemical functionalization is mostly limited to research and development quantities. Some companies produce and sell functionalized tubes, e.g., with fluorine (CNT-F) groups, or partially oxidized with carboxylic (CNT-COOH) groups (Fig. 2). It seems increasingly likely, however, that practical applications of CNT will involve chemical functionalization. Both the type and degree of functionalization will likely affect the potential toxic properties of CNT (37).

There are some functional groups that will be of use to the toxicologist. SWCNT have been functionalized with fluorescent indicators, e.g., fluorescein, enabling the tracing of CNT entry into cells (38). Alternatively, it may be useful to label CNT with heavy metals, e.g., as contrast agents for electron microscopy (39). Carboxyl functionalized SWCNT have been labeled with radioactive ^{125}I nuclei, allowing researchers to follow the distribution of CNT with the bodies of mice (40).

SUMMARY AND OUTLOOK

CNT represent a fashionable icon of nanotechnology, whose popularity has grown out of massive investment and not just a little hype. In this short review, we hope to have given a flavor of the complicated variety of material that could be found in a supplier's catalog nominally labeled as CNT. A sample of CNT may contain many things besides the ideal SWCNT. There are many—possibly too many—parameters to be considered by the toxicologist. It is perhaps not surprising, therefore, that some of the first toxicological studies are at variance with each other over the potential risk of CNT to health and the environment. Many of the materials studied will have been obtained commercially, with limited data on their unique chemical and physical characteristics. The reproducibility of synthesis of CNT can be low, as synthesis parameters change, and manufacturers further develop their processes. It may help to define and narrow the source of different effects of these materials, perhaps targeting carbon materials other than CNT. Careful sample analysis and characterization will also be critical. The development of toxicological tests on CNT, and the analysis of the outcomes, would be significantly enhanced by collaborations with researchers who are expert in dealing with nanotubes or similar materials. Only with joint efforts from toxicologists and material scientists/chemists, may hold the key.

REFERENCES

1. ISI Web of Knowledge [database online]. Thomson Scientific; 2007. Available at: http://isiwebofknowledge.com/.
2. Scientifica: Nanotubes Production (http://www.scientifica.com), 2005.
3. Donaldson K, Aitken R, Tran L, Stone V, Duffin R, Forrest G, Alexander A. Carbon nanotubes: a review of their properties in relation to pulmonary toxicology and workplace safety. Toxicol Sci 2006; 92:5–22.
4. Dai H. Carbon nanotubes: synthesis, integration, and properties. Acc Chem Res 2002; 35:1035–44.
5. Pfeiffer R, Kuzmany H, Kramberger C, Schaman C, Pichler T, Kataura H, Achiba Y, Kurti J, Zolyomi V. Unusual high degree of unperturbed environment in the interior of single-wall carbon nanotubes. Phys Rev Lett 2003; 90:225501 (225501–4).
6. Zhang MF, Yudasaka M, Koshio A, Iijima S. Thermogravimetric analysis of single-wall carbon nanotubes ultrasonicated in monochlorobenzene. Chem Phys Lett 2002; 364:420–6.

7. Lin T, Pajpai V, Ji T, Dai LM. Chemistry of carbon nanotubes. Aust J Chem 2003; 56:635–51.

8. Ajayan PM, Ebbesen TW. Nanometre-size tubes of carbon. Rep Prog Phys 1997; 60:1025–62.

9. Radovic LR, Bockrath B. On the chemical nature of graphene edges: origin of stability and potential for magnetism in carbon materials. J Am Chem Soc 2005; 127:5917–27.

10. Jorio A, Saito R, Hafner JH, Leiber CM, Hunter M, McClure T, Dresselhaus G, Dresselhaus MS. Structural (n, m) determination of isolated single-wall carbon nanotubes by resonant Raman scattering. Phys Rev Lett 2001; 86:1118–21.

11. Hou PX, Xu ST, Ying Z, Yang QH, Liu C, Cheng HM. Hydrogen adsorption/ desorption behavior of multi-walled carbon nanotubes with different diameters. Carbon 2003; 41:2471–6.

12. Peigney A, Laurent C, Flahaut E, Basca RR, Rousset A. Specific surface area of carbon nanotubes and bundles of carbon nanotubes. Carbon 2001; 39:507–14.

13. Ye Y, Ahn CC, Witham C, Fultz B, Liu J, Rinzler AG, Colbert D, Smith KA, Smalley RE. Hydrogen adsorption and cohesive energy of single-walled carbon nanotubes. Appl Phys Lett 1999; 74:2307–9.

14. Popov VN. Carbon nanotubes: properties and application. Mater Sci Eng R 2004; 43:61–102.

15. Nikolaev P, Bronikowski MJ, Bradley RK, Rohmund F, Colbert DT, Smith KA, Smalley RE. Gas-phase catalytic growth of single-walled carbon nanotubes from carbon monoxide. Chem Phys Lett 1999; 313:91–7.

16. Rao CNR, Govindaraj A. Carbon nanotubes from organometallic precursors. Acc Chem Res 2002; 35:998–1007.

17. Cassell AM, Raymakers JA, Kong J, Dai H. Large-scale CVD synthesis of single-walled carbon nanotubes. J Phys Chem B 1999; 103:6484–92.

18. Cheung CL, Kurtz A, Park H, Lieber CM. Diameter-controlled synthesis of carbon nanotubes. J Phys Chem B 2002; 106:2429–33.

19. Zhang Y, Li Y, Kim W, Wang D, Dai H. Imaging as-grown single-walled carbon nanotubes originated from isolated catalytic nanoparticles. Appl Phys A 2002; 74:325–8.

20. Subramoney S. Novel nanocarbons—structure, properties, and potential applications. Adv Mater 1998; 10:1157–71.

21. Liu J, Rinzler AG, Dai H, Hafner JH, Bradley RK, Boul PJ, Lu A, Iverson T, Shelimov K, Huffman CB, Rodriguez-Macias F, Shon Y-S, Lee TR, Colbert DT, Smalley RE. Fullerene pipes. Science 1998; 280:1253–6.

22. Tasis D, Tagmatarchis N, Bianco A, Prato M. Chemistry of carbon nanotubes. Chem Rev 2006; 106:1105–36.

23. Klump C, Kostarelos K, Prato M, Bianco A. Functionalized carbon nanotubes as emerging nanovectors for the delivery of therapeutics. Biochim Biophys Acta 2006; 1758:404–12.

24. Bahr JL, Mickelson ET, Bronikowski MJ, Smalley RE, Tour JM. A Dissolution of small diameter single-wall carbon nanotubes in organic solvents? Chem Comm 2001:193–4.

25. Islam MF, Rojas E, Bergey DM, Johnson AT, Yodh AG. High weight fraction surfactant solubilization of single-wall carbon nanotubes in water. Nano Lett 2003; 3:269–73.

26. Jin Z, Sun X, Xu G, Goh SH, Ji W. Nonlinear optical properties of some polymer/multi-walled carbon nanotube composites. Chem Phys Lett 2000; 318:505–10.

27. Zheng M, Jagota A, Strano MS, Santos AP, Barone P, Chou SG, Diner BA, Dresselhaus MS, McLean RS, Onoa GB, Samsonidze GG, Semke ED, Usrey M, Walls DJ. Structure-based carbon nanotube sorting by sequence-dependent DNA assembly. Science 2003; 302:1545–8.

28. Shelimov KB, Esenaliev RO, Rinzler AG, Huffman CB, Smalley RE. Purification of single-wall carbon nanotubes by ultrasonically assisted filtration. Chem Phys Lett 1998; 282:429–34.

29. Sloan J, Hammer J, Zwiefka-Sibley M, Green MLH. The opening and filling of single walled carbon nanotubes (SWTs). Chem Comm1998:347–8.

30. Monthioux M. Filling single-walled carbon nanotubes. Carbon 2002; 40: 1809–23.

31. Davis JJ, Green MLH, Hill HAO, Leung YC, Sadler PJ, Sloan J, Xavier AV, Tsang SC. The immobilisation of proteins in carbon nanotubes. Inorg Chim Acta 1998; 272:261–6.

32. Katz E, Willner I. Biomolecule-functionalized carbon nanotubes: applications in nanobioelectronics. Chemphyschem 2004; 5:1085–104.

33. Kam NWS, Jessop TC, Wender PA, Dai HJ. Nanotube molecular transporters: internalization of carbon nanotube–protein conjugates into mammalian cells. J Am Chem Soc 2004; 126:6850–1.

34. Kam NWS, Dai HJ. Carbon nanotubes as intracellular protein transporters: generality and biological functionality. J Am Chem Soc 2005; 127:6021–6.

35. Pantarotto D, Singh R, McCarthy D, Erhardt M, Briand JP, Prato M, Kostarelos K, Bianco A. Functionalized carbon nanotubes for plasmid DNA gene delivery. Angew Chem Int Ed 2004; 43:5242–6.

36. Cai D, Mataraza JM, Qin ZH, Huang ZP, Huang JY, Chiles TC, Carnahan D, Kempa K, Ren ZF. Highly efficient molecular delivery into mammalian cells using carbon nanotube spearing. Nat Meth 2005; 2:449–54.

37. Sayes CM, Liang F, Hudson JL, Mendez J, Guo W, Beach JM, Moore VC, Doyle CD, West JL, Billups WE, Ausman KD, Colvin VL. Functionalization density dependence of single-walled carbon nanotubes cytotoxicity in vitro. Toxicol Lett 2006; 161:135–42.

38. Pantarotto D, Briand JP, Prato M, Bianco A. Translocation of bioactive peptides across cell membranes by carbon nanotubes. Chem Comm2004:16–7.

39. Smith BW, Luzzi DE, Achiba Y. Tumbling atoms and evidence for charge transfer in La-2@C-80@SWNT. Chem Phys Lett 2000; 331:137–42.

40. Wang HF, Wang J, Deng XY, Sun HF, Shi ZJ, Gu ZN, Liu YF, Zhao YL. Biodistribution of carbon single-wall carbon nanotubes in mice. J Nanosci Nanotech 2004; 4:1019–24.

3

Effect-Oriented Physicochemical Characterization of Nanomaterials

Stefano Zuin

Venice Research Consortium and Department of Environmental Science, University Cà Foscari, Venice, Italy

Giulio Pojana and Antonio Marcomini

Venice Research Consortium and Department of Environmental Science, University Cà Foscari, Venice, Italy

BACKGROUND

It is well established (from which the general interest arises!) that nanomaterials (NM) display properties and behavior that can be very different compared to the corresponding bulk materials of the same chemical composition. Size, shape, and surface state are properties accounting for most of their differences (1,2). The physical and chemical characterization of NM are important steps in toxicological and ecotoxicological studies in order to correctly evaluate and assess their potential exposure routes, toxicity, and related risk.

Although little data are currently available on the ecotoxicological and toxicological effects associated with NM (3), their physicochemical properties are expected to influence their biological response (4). Recent toxicity studies on engineered nanoparticles (NP) such as carbon nanotubes (CNT), fullerenes, metal oxides (e.g., titanium dioxide, iron oxide), silica and quantum dots (QD), have highlighted the need to carefully and thoroughly characterize NM when investigating their potential biological effects (5–12). Ideally, each toxicological assay should be accompanied by a detailed characterization of all the physicochemical properties of the investigated material that could have biological relevance.

NM exhibit peculiar characterization challenges because of their diversity, in comparison to traditional materials and chemicals. Both physical (e.g., particle size and morphology, water solubility) and chemical (e.g., chemical composition and structure, type of coating) properties are important, but other parameters, such as surface/volume ratio, phase transfer, chemical stability, tendency to aggregation, may be important as well. No individual characterization technique can provide adequate information to completely support the potential risk assessment for a given NM. In addition, information about supplied and as-produced batches are very important to understand the product composition variability, the technical performance and most appropriate application procedures and the optimal storage condition. Even the synthesis route is a key aspect, since a given NM can be produced by different processes yielding formally the same composition, but with quite different exhibited properties: CNT, for example, can be produced by a variety of synthesis methods that can also generate (in percentages as high as 50% or more) amorphous and graphitic nano-particulate by-products, metallic catalyst residues both in complex association with nanotube cavities or as particles encapsulated by carbonaceous shells, and, consequently, with different toxicological properties (13).

The most noticeable example is probably that of fullerenes. Recent studies have shown that significant differences exist between the conventional, hydrophobic, and not water-soluble fullerene (C_{60}) and the stable, "aqueous" nC_{60} suspension prepared by solvent dispersion and stirring procedures. The latter, which is not soluble in organic solvents but readily soluble in water, is thought to contain residual solvent molecules inside the fullerene aggregates, so strongly modifying their physical aggregation state and, in all probability, influencing their biological behavior (14). In the case of metal and metal oxide NP synthesized in a liquid phase, size and shape are often controlled by addition of organic stabilizers such as thiols, phosphanes, phosphines, amines, carboxylates, polymers, and/or surfactants (15), which are in some cases actually chemically bonded to the particle and not simply sorbed to its surface. Such molecules may affect the cellular internalization of NP in living organisms and their diffusion through tissues, as well as their biological behavior (16).

The various synthetic routes developed for NM may be very important in influencing their biological activity, but are often overlooked by researchers interested in this field, especially biologists and toxicologists, as demonstrated by the currently reported scientific literature. It is indeed necessary to measure or derive not only the NM characteristics but also to assess and document the NM involved synthetic methods and its related properties (e.g., dispersion media, dispersion procedure, solution pH, stabilization procedures) in order to understand the associations between NM features and observed biological responses. Although the interpretation of conventionally applied biological markers of toxicity are well developed, a series of issues related to the characterization and detection of NM in toxicity studies still need to be addressed.

This chapter aims to identify and describe the major characterization parameters that should be investigated before, during and after a toxicity test is performed, and evaluate whether currently available analytical techniques, methods, and procedures are capable of detecting and quantifying NM during in vivo/in vitro studies in order to generate scientifically meaningful dose–response relationships. The essential physicochemical properties of NM are considered from a toxicological perspective, as well as their properties that can better describe the behavior as mediators of the toxicity. In this context, the needed characterization of NM has been divided into three topics:

- Characterization of NM "as-produced" or provided by the manufacturer before being tested.
- Characterization of NM during the dosing formulation (administrated NM).
- Characterization of NM after administration.

These topics provide a comprehensive review of more adequate characterization techniques, methods, and procedures.

PHYSICOCHEMICAL PROPERTIES OF NANOMATERIALS AS MEDIATORS OF TOXICITY

The interaction of NM with biological systems is affected by several factors. A tentatively comprehensive list of physicochemical properties of NM that can influence the toxicity is described here below. All these parameters should be characterized and determined during in vivo/in vitro experimentation as a preliminary activity included in the adopted experimental protocol.

Size

Size in NM matters. It plays a key role in determining the final properties of NM. The size can modify the physicochemical properties of the material as well as create the opportunity for increased uptake and interaction with biological tissues. Particle size is, actually, the most investigated factor (17). The biological activity of NM is already known to increase as the particle size decreases: nanometer-sized particles are being discovered to be more biologically active (more toxic) than the same material of larger (even in the microrange) size (4,18), since they can reach places not accessible to larger particles, as when they are inhaled (19). Unfortunately, in the literature the size is often taken from the nominal size declared by the supplier, or determined only in the supplied/synthesized material. Moreover, the size refers very often to the individual particle, not to the potential aggregates that can be formed during handling, storage, and synthesis.

Surface Area

In addition to the size, also the surface area is an important feature from a toxicological perspective. Reduction in size to the nanoscale level causes a steady increase of the surface/volume ratio, and therefore a greater percentage of atoms to be displayed on the surface rather than in the inner bulk lattice. The increase in surface area boosts exponentially the number of potentially active groups per mass unit, thus enhancing the overall material reactivity. One simple example is gold, which is known to be very stable to oxidation, while at sizes below a few nm it can burn spontaneously (20). Moreover, smaller particles mean a much larger number per mass unit, with an increased potential for biological interaction (21). As an example, during inhalation experiments on rats with TiO_2 and $BaSO_4$, the first was shown to induce a greater lung inflammation than the second, but the effects were actually similar when related to the overall surface area exhibited (22).

Shape

NM can exhibit various shape and structures, such as spheres, needles, tubes, rods, platelets, etc. The shape can have two main effects: one, in solution and under aerosol form, is the variation of the hydrodynamic radius between spherical particles and oblong ones (larger for the latter) with the same mass, which triggers a variation in their mobility and diffusion in both gas and liquid phases. The second effect is that the shape influences the deposition and adsorption kinetics in biological media, since the blocking mechanisms of ion channels in cell walls appear to be dependent on the shape of tested NP (23,24). Some results from reported in vitro toxicity studies pointed out that CNT stimulate platelet aggregation, while fullerene do not (25). Indeed, the particular shape of cylindric, rolled-up graphene layers in CNT may influence their biological activity, since single-walled carbon nanotubes (SWNT) seem to be more toxic than multiwalled carbon nanotubes (MWNT) with the same length (26). The long, thin geometry and practical water insolubility of CNT may have the potential to cause effects similar to those arising from inhalation of asbestos fibres, even if the chemical composition is completely different (27). Currently, no detailed investigations have been carried out on inorganic NP of similar chemical composition but different shape, and shape/composition relationships remain largely unexplored.

Chemical Composition

The chemical composition, in terms of elemental composition and chemical structure, is an intrinsic property of all materials and it is consequently an important parameter for the comprehension of NM biological behavior.

NM can have very different chemical compositions, from completely inorganic, e.g., metals (iron, nickel, zinc, titanium, gold, silver, palladium, iridium, and platinum), and metal oxides (titanium oxide, zinc oxide, silica, iron oxide, etc.), to entirely organic (fullerenes, CNT, nanopolymers, biomolecules). Some NM can exhibit a hybrid, "core-shell" structure, as the semiconductor nanocrystal QD: they consist of a metalloid crystalline "core" and an inorganic shell that shields and stabilizes the QD core for specific applications, such as biomedical imaging and electronic applications. QD may be biocompatible, but the physical (thermal) and chemical (photochemical, oxidative) degradation of the coating can reveal the inner core (often composed by elements such as Cd, Zn, Te, Se, In, As), which may exhibit toxic effects as NP or upon dissolution of the core itself into elemental constituents (28). Even the chemical purity is an important chemical parameter to be taken into consideration, since some NM (i.e., CNT, metal NP) can contain metal impurities, such as Fe, Ni, Co, which could affect the biological response by masking the NP behavior with their intrinsic toxicity (29,30). As example, manganese doping on micronized sunscreen titania particles, has been shown to reduce free radical generation rates and to enhance the photostability to ultraviolet A (UVA) radiation, in comparison with undoped titania (31). The cytotoxicity caused by SWNT, MWNT, and fullerenes on alveolar macrophages has been recently investigated (32). In some experiments, the purity of the selected CNT seemed to be the main factor responsible for the exhibited differences in cytotoxic effects (33).

Lattice Structure

Many materials with the same chemical composition can have different lattice structures, and exhibit different physical and chemical properties, as it is well known for quartz, made of silicon and oxygen atoms with the same ratio Si:O 1:2 that can be arranged into different lattice structures depending on the synthetic route and temperature conditions involved. Several structural investigations on inorganic NM indicate that also the crystal lattice type may have an important role on the overall structure of NP, because of the very high portion of surface atoms with respect to the bulk lattice. The size reduction may create discontinuous crystal planes that increase the number of structural defects, as well as disrupt the electronic configuration of the material, with possible toxicological consequences (22,34). As example, the rutile and anatase phases of TiO_2 are known to be stable and metastable, respectively, but when the particle size is reduced below 20 nm their stability is reversed (35). This is a critical aspect, since rutile and anatase react very differently as oxidation catalyst when exposed to light (36).

Surface Chemistry

NP exhibit an high tendency to aggregate. This is a typical behavior of ultrafine particles, because of largely increased specific surface/volume ratios that enhance their interparticle attraction by London and van der Waals forces, as well as electrostatic interactions (37). Engineered NP, especially those for biomedical applications, are often "stabilized" with specific coatings also to avoid the formation of aggregates. Surface-functionalized NP are usually coated with organic molecules containing hydrophilic (in some cases biocompatible) terminal functional groups such as $-SH$, $-CN$, $-OH$, $-COOH$, $-NH_2$, etc., bonded to the surface atoms through covalent bonds (38). These surface groups can transform insoluble and/or unstable NP into highly soluble (in the desired solvent, usually water) depending on the specific application. The cytotoxic response of CNT in cultured cells has been revealed to depend on surface functionalization (39,40). Surface modifications of quartz affect the cytotoxicity, inflammogenicity and fibrogenicity of silica (41), and DNA damage in lung epithelial cells (42,43). Therefore, the coating and chemical nature of a NM surface should be known before starting an experiment (44). Suppliers sometimes report limited information (often for patent reasons) about the coating, if any, in the specification sheet, and the researchers should be aware of its presence and physicochemical behavior.

Surface Charge

NP, when dispersed in liquid media, may carry an electric charge on their surface. This charge can depend upon the particle nature and the surrounding medium (45). Their size and surface charge are major factors affecting the NM dispersion characteristics. Also, size and charge can influence the adsorption of ions, contaminants, and biomolecules, and the way cells react when exposed to them (46). Surface charge is also known to influence the biological response to NM, including phagocytosis, genotoxicity, and inflammation (47). Not only the coating type but also the surface charge resulting from the density and spatial arrangement of the coating itself on the surface particles is a factor that can affect the administration pathway, as diffusion within the organs, cellular uptake mechanisms, and cytotoxicity (48). Particle surface charge has been shown to alter blood–brain barrier integrity in rats after exposure to emulsifying wax, which NP are prepared from warm oil-in-water microemulsion precursors in the presence of surfactants (49). The decrease of surface charge have been shown to reduce their toxicity of amine-terminated poly(amidoamine) dendrimers for drug delivery applications (50–52).

Aggregation State

As discussed above, NP can form aggregates in both solution and powder form, as well as in the gas phase, depending on the size, chemical composition, surface charge, and chemical composition. The aggregation can depend also from storage and handling conditions, and it can occur even in freshly prepared NM. It can be also a function of the synthesis procedure: CNT can be present as complex aggregates of ropes and bundles even just after their synthesis by gas-phase reaction (53,54). The aggregation affects the stability of NM suspensions that are usually prepared for toxicological experiments. Even if the toxicological consequences of aggregation are currently largely unknown, some evidences indicate that the type and the aggregation degree of NP may influence the inflammation and oxidative stress after administration (55–57). Also, the extent of aggregation should be taken into account during the characterization of NM.

CHARACTERIZATION OF AS-PRODUCED OR SUPPLIED NANOMATERIALS

The characterization of NM freshly prepared or provided by the manufacturer is usually the main approach applied during toxicity test planning in order to obtain useful physicochemical information for the explanation of the exhibited biological behavior. A very broad range of analytical methods and procedures can be used to perform a detailed characterization, including microscopic, spectroscopic, chromatographic, and nuclear techniques. The selection of the most adequate techniques is not simple, since it depends mainly on the type of NM to be tested, on the test to be performed and on the data quality required. Current toxicological research does not take into enough consideration the characterization of investigated NM. As a matter of fact, only a very few of the currently available techniques are employed, and in some cases researchers discuss their results and deductions simply relying on data provided by the supplier in the technical specification sheet, which are usually limited to average size and purity. In some cases the declared characterization is insufficient since improper techniques, deriving from bulk or macrosize analysis, are employed. It has to be stressed out that the combination of more than one technique is fundamental to adequately characterize a selected NM and avoid the misinterpreting of the obtained toxicological results. Due to the current lack of standardized characterization procedures for NM, it is strongly suggested to carry out an independent characterization of each tested NM. The researcher should also keep in mind that most NM exhibit an high product variability, since the usually small production amount involved and the reaction types. As a consequence, the characterization should be performed on a larger than planned amount of material, in order to create a small "bank" of NM useful for confirmatory or later experiments (provided that the selected NM are stable enough to be stored for the entire experimental activity period, otherwise the characterization should be repeated with a new batch for more safety). Table 1 shows the more widely applied characterization techniques. They have been classified on the basis of their applicability to acquire physicochemical information of as-produced or supplied NM, as dosed NM during experiments, and finally after their administration in biological (in vivo, in vitro) matrices.

Determination of Size, Shape, and Aggregation State

Size and shape of NM are usually measured by electron microscopy, which include many qualitative and semiquantitative techniques widely used to investigate the morphology (size and shape) and also the aggregation state of NP (58–62). Scanning electron microscopy (SEM) spatial resolution is theoretically below 5 nm, with magnification up to × 100,000, even if the resolution and image depth of field are actually determined by the beam current and the final spot size. In contrast, Transmission Electron Microscopy (TEM) resolution is in the 0.5–3 nanometers, and it is the most useful and appropriate technique for the direct investigation of NM (63). In particular, TEM resolution is nominally below 1 nm for high-resolution transmission electron microscopy (HRTEM) (64). SEM and TEM observations must be performed in a vacuum environment, and can be applied only to solid samples. Very recently, accessories for the investigation of liquid dispersions with SEM have been commercially available. Moreover, SEM provides information only for conductive materials. Nonconductive materials can be observed as well, but the sample needs to be coated with a several-nanometer layer of conductive material, such as gold; this process may potentially modify the sample. The sample preparation is usually a long, laborious, and critical step that can affect the ultimate resolution and the ability to get the required information on a given sample. Size distribution may be obtained by TEM simply counting (performed through a software feature) the number of particles as a function of size, but it is made only on a small portion of the sample, with no high statistical reliability (65,66). The TEM technique can provide additional crystallographic information, such as the surface atoms arrangement, defects at atomic scale: if the energy dispersive spectrometry (EDS) option is applied, detailed information on the chemical composition of the sample surface can be obtained. Figure 1 is a TEM image of a commercial CNT sample showing the high complexity of such organic NM.

Other microscopy techniques are also available for the determination of size and shape, as well as the aggregation state, such as scanning probe microscopy (SPM). SPM includes both atomic force microscopy (AFM) and

Table 1   Analytical Techniques Applicable for the Characterization of Nanomaterials

	SEM	TEM	SPM (AFM, STM)	ATOF-MS	DIC, CLSM, FLM	DMA, CPC	SMPS, DLPI	EPI, DC	DLS	ζ-pot
Size distribution	● □ ■ ◆	● □ ■ ◆	● ■ ◆						● □ ■	
Surface area				□		□	□			
Shape	● □ ■ ◆	● □ ■ ◆	● □ ■ ◆		◆			□		
Chemical composition				□	◆					
Purity				□						
Surface chemistry										
Surface charge									●	● ■
Aggregation state	● □ ■ ◆	● □ ■ ◆	● ■ ◆		◆					
Crystal structure	● □ ■ ◆ ● □	● □ ■ ◆ ● □								
Porosity										

(Continued)

Table 1 Analytical Techniques Applicable for the Characterization of Nanomaterials *(Continued)*

	XRD	AES	TGA, DSC	XPS	FTIR	RS	NMR	UV-Vis	FlFFF	BET	ICP-MS, AS	HPLC, GPC	ESR
Size distribution	••								•• ■ ◆			• ■ ◆	
Surface area										••			
Shape													
Chemical composition		••	•	•	•	•	••	• ■	• ■ ◆		•• □ ■ ◆	• ◆	• ■ ◆
Purity			•		•	•							
Surface chemistry		•	•	••	•	•	••	••	•• ■ ◆			• ◆	• ◆
Surface charge													
Aggregation state							••		• ■ ◆				
Crystal structure	•• □		•		•	•	•						• ◆
Porosity										••			

Note: For the acronym descriptions, please refer to the list of abbreviations at end of chapter.

Legend: ••, Highly applicable for as-produced or as-supplied NM; •, applicable in some cases: may provide some information for as-produced or as supplied NM; ■, applicable for administered NM as suspension in biological fluid; □, applicable for administered NM in aerosol form; ◆, applicable for NM characterization after administration in biological matrices.

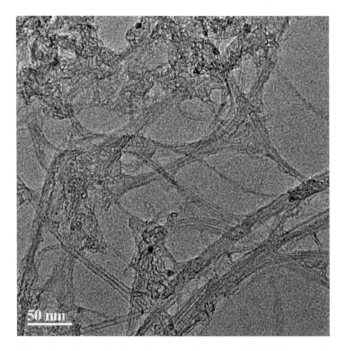

Figure 1 Transmission electron microscopy (TEM) image of a commercial carbon nanotube (CNT) sample. Note the high complexity of this specific nanomaterial, including individual tubes (both linear and bended), as well as nanotube muddles and elemental carbon impurities.

scanning tunneling microscopy (STM), which are all based, with some minor modifications, on a scanning probe (called the tip), which is moved above a grate where particles have been firmly deposited, and feels the height variation due to the presence of particles similarly to a pickup on a turntable for vinyl records (67). By applying these techniques, individual NP and aggregates can be easily recorded along the three dimensions, while SEM and TEM can measure only two dimensions. Similarly to SEM and TEM, AFM data can provide quantitative information about the size distribution with a software-based image processing, even if limited to a small sample surface (usually $10 \times 10 \, \mu m$). An advantage over TEM is that both liquids and solids can be analyzed and the images can be measured in all environments (68,69). STM images give directly the three-dimensional morphology of complex samples such as CNT and can resolve simultaneously both their atomic structure and the electronic density (70,71). As for TEM and SEM, the deposition process is mainly responsible for the overall result, and many fluctuations can occur in the obtained size distribution.

In some specific cases, as for QD, a simple fluorescence spectrum determination combined with quantomechanic equations, can give reliable size distribution data, which are commonly supplied by producers of these NM (72).

Photon correlation spectroscopy (PCS), in its subtechniques dynamic light scattering (DLS) and quasielastic light scattering (QELS), can measure the particle size of NM in liquid dispersions, with the great advantage of being a nondestructive technique (73–77). The obtained dimension is actually the "hydrodynamic radius," since it describes the radius of a spherical particle moving as an individual unit in a fluid, surrounded by the solvation layer. It is derived from the intensity of scattered light, usually coherent light generated by a multiangle laser unit, and it can provide distributions in terms of number (i.e., number of particles and agglomerates), volume (i.e., volume of particles and agglomerates), and intensity distribution (of the light scattered by examined particles) as function of size. A correct laser diffraction measurement requires the knowledge of the solution viscosity and refractive index, which for some samples could be difficult to obtain. In addition, the overall sensitivity is highly dependent on the investigated size range (78). The accuracy and precision are very good provided that the exhibited size distribution is very narrow, due to the physical approach applied. If the size distribution is broad, or aggregates are present, the autocorrelation function applied to derive the intensity fluctuation of the scattered light will be dominated by their signals, so the interpretation of obtained data requires high care. It assumes spherical particles, so the shape effects on the size distribution are unknown (46,78). Other different scattering techniques (including DLS), or a combination of other techniques, such as small angle X-ray scattering (SAXS), wide angle X-ray diffraction (WAXD), and small angle neutron scanning (SANS) may be also used. The theory governing the scattering process (by light in DLS and SLS, X-ray in SAXS and WAXD, and neutrons in SANS) is the same, while the difference stays in the mechanism of interaction between the incident radiation and the sample, and the structural (i.e., size, shape, and internal structure as well as interparticle interactions) information that can be obtained (79).

Field flow fractionation (FFF) is a very powerful technique (with both analytical and preparative capabilities), although its potential is currently underestimated. Although not recent (it was developed in the 1960s), this chromatographic technique can in principle separate particles from < 1 nm to several μm size with no regard to their chemical composition according to different mobility induced by a force (electric, thermal, gravitational, or flow, depending on the instrumental configuration) orthogonal to a main laminar flow where the particle is injected in (80). This nondestructive technique, when coupled with PCS detectors, can easily overtake their drawbacks and increase significantly the quality of the size distribution data, especially for very complex mixtures, permitting also the collection of the injected sample for further chemical and physical characterization of the separated fractions (81–83).

For some specific NP, such as gold, ultraviolet-visible spectroscopy (UV-Vis) spectra can also give very accurate information on the size distribution and their aggregation (84).

Surface Area and Porosity

A porosity measurement can supply information on the specific surface area of investigated NM and on the pore presence, distribution, average size and shape, indicating possible biochemical interactions with proteins and enzymes during administration. Specific surface area (total surface per mass unit) and porosity of NM can be easily obtained using the Brunauer–Emmett–Teller (BET) method. The determination is based on the measurement of the adsorption isotherm of an inert gas (usually N_2) into a dry, solid material (85). Although the BET is a standard measurement for solid NP characterization, such as nano-sized catalysts (86,87), the obtained results depend on the employed instrumentation and on the operator ability. In some cases, depending on the preanalysis procedures employed (vacuum, samples drying, temperature gradients), some degradation and/or contamination of the material can occur. Moreover, the technique cannot be applied to liquid suspensions. Porosity can be also measured by using mercury, although special techniques and higher vacuum conditions are needed for analysis (46,88). The typical purification of commercial CNT, based on strong oxidation followed by acid treatment, has been already shown to modify their porosity and specific surface area (89).

Chemical Stability and Surface Charge in Solution

NM characteristics such as aggregation, dispersion, surface charge, may be altered if the sample is prepared in solution for in vivo (e.g., intradermal injection, intratracheal instillation) or in vitro (e.g., cell uptake) tests, or even if the sample is aerosolized during an inhalation study. The stability of NP dispersions has been definitely little investigated. In fact, it is well established that NP dispersions, both in water or in organic solvents, tend to aggregate with time. The aggregation state and the kinetic of this phenomenon depend on many factors, such as NP type, concentration, coating, solvent, temperature, pH, salt concentration, ionic strength, presence of surfactant and/or dispersants, etc. Many of the commercially available NP dispersions (the typical solvent being water) are actually composed of both individual NP and their aggregates, in variable percentages. Some NP dispersions can be stable for months, others only for minutes, and often suppliers do not provide time-life values, as well as proper storage conditions and handling precautions. All these features need to be preliminarily investigated in order to avoid to get misleading toxicological results. The determination of the dispersion stability is fundamental prior to any biological experiment, especially if solid NP have to be dispersed in a medium prior to dosing. DLS with zeta potential (ζ-pot) option is usually applied for this purpose, by measuring the charge carried by the suspended NP. The zeta potential is a function of the particle surface charge and of any adsorbed solvent or stabilizer layer at the interface, and it depends also on the nature and composition of the surrounding medium where the particles are suspended in (90). If the dispersion exhibits a sufficient negative (i.e., < -30 mV) or positive (i.e., $> +30$ mV) zeta potential, particles repel enough each other, giving a stable dispersion. Vice versa, if the zeta potential values are within this range, there are not sufficient interparticle repulsive forces to prevent aggregation with time. Small changes of pH, concentration of ions and ligands can lead to dramatic changes in the zeta potential, and as a consequence, the aggregation tendency of dispersed particles. It is strongly advisable to measure the zeta potential as function of pH, and also calculate the isoelectric point (IEP), the pH value at which the zeta potential is equal to zero (91–93). A correct evaluation of the time stability of dispersed NP would require the development of standardized experimental protocols, which are currently lacking.

Chemical Composition, Purity, and Crystal Structure

The chemical composition of NM requires the concurrent application of several spectroscopic techniques such as inductively coupled plasma (ICP), X-ray diffraction (XRD), nuclear magnetic resonance (NMR), UV-Vis and fluorescence, which are widely used to measure the atomic structure and composition of pure NM. According to the carbon content, organic and inorganic NM should be distinguished.

The ICP is a well-suited technique for a detailed chemical composition analysis, since it benefits of its destructive ability to simultaneously produce individual ions of theoretically each atomic element, which can be combined with the selectivity and sensitivity of optical emission spectrophotometry (OES) and mass spectrometry (MS), so permitting to qualitative identify and quantify the main components, as well as trace impurities, in all NM. The fundamental prerequisite is a complete mineralization of the sample prior to analysis, which can be a critical and laborious step for very stable NM, both of organic and inorganic nature. It cannot provide information about the chemical structure of the investigated material, and it offers a relatively low sensitivity with regard to some lighter elements, such as H, O, N, C, S. Elemental analysis is in principle more appropriate for organic NM, but the high carbon content and the relatively high thermal stability of some NP, such as fullerenes and CNT, could be over the instrumental oxidation capabilities. A very recently commercially available technique, the aerosol time of flight–mass spectrometry (ATOF-MS), allows to get a detailed chemical analysis of NP under aerosol form, also subdividing the analyzed particles into size, with results similar to those attainable by FFF coupled with TOF-MS (94).

In comparison to inorganic NM, much less investigation has been performed on the presence of potentially bioavailable organic chemicals in NM. High performance liquid chromatography coupled with fluorescence detection (HPLC-FL) has been applied to the determination of polycyclic aromatic hydrocarbons (PAHs) in carbon-based NP such as carbon black (CB) (95,96).

XRD is a powerful technique to investigate the surface atomic structure (e.g., crystal structure, lattice defects, charge distribution) of NM. It has been already applied to QD (97) and metal Fe, Ni, and Co NP (98,99). The chiral distribution in Ag and Pt NP, as well as the sample purity (residual catalyst, functional groups) in MWNT, can be examined by XRD (62,100).

The electron paramagnetic resonance (EPR) and electron spin resonance (ESR) are versatile, nondestructive, analytical qualitative and quantitative techniques that can provide very valuable structural information of investigated material, such as defects in crystals and magnetic properties, but it is mainly applied for the determination of paramagnetic elements and free radicals. They have been applied to the characterization of metallic NM such as Au, Pd, Ni, and Fe (101,102), ZnO (103), and TiO$_2$ (104).

Fourier transform infrared spectroscopy (FTIR) and Raman spectroscopy (RS) are two simple qualitative techniques that can give qualitative information about organic structures by means of the analysis their bond vibrational energies. FTIR is widely used for the characterization of fullerene and CNT (105,106), CdS nanocrystal (107), metal and metal oxide NP such as gold and zinc oxide (108,109). The Raman scattering (RS) can also provide a fast and nondestructive method to investigate the phase changes (amorphous or crystalline), the size variations, and the lattice stress. For example, dimension and periodicity of nanocrystal QD may be obtained (110), as well as information on structural organization and interfacial characteristics of CNT (111,112).

NMR is another sophisticated, nondestructive technique used to investigate the surface and bulk chemical features of chemicals, eliciting the electronic structure and the surrounding electronic environment of contained elements, so allowing the accurate identification of individual atom position in a given chemical structure, with the only limitation that some elements exhibit too low or no signal. It can be used with both organic and inorganic NM, either in solid state or solvent dispersion, and its applicability in this field is steadily increasing (113–116).

In some cases, the Auger electron spectroscopy (AES) can also be used to examine elemental compositions of surface, providing compositional information for NM such as CNT (70) and Si and TiO$_2$ NP (117,118).

Conventional UV-Vis and fluorescence measurements can also provide valuable information, as about the optical property of core-shell NP (119). Absorption spectra are used to investigate the size quantization effects as well as to estimate the electron band gap of QD, as well as their surface functionalization (120).

Surface Chemistry and Contamination

X-ray photon spectroscopy (XPS) is a nondestructive technique well suited for the investigation of surface elemental composition of NM. It is currently the most widely used surface-analysis technique, and it supplies detailed, qualitative only, information about chemical elements on the surface and their chemical environment, such as coating type and coverage extent, binding states, oxidation states, etc. (121). XPS requires vacuum conditions to maintain the surface free from contamination, so it cannot be directly applied to liquid samples. It is usually applied to the surface characterization of metallic NP, such as aluminum, nickel, and gold NP, as well as CdS (122–125), CNT (126), and core-shell structures (127,128).

Differential scanning calorimetry (DSC) technique can give qualitative and quantitative information about physical and chemical changes that involve endothermic and exothermic processes, while thermogravimetric analysis (TGA) can provide information regarding the presence of volatile contaminants or labile components in the NM measuring changes in weight of a sample with increasing temperature (129–131). The coating degree of functional groups such as carbonyl, phenols, lactones, and carboxyl can be quantitatively measured also by simple procedures such as Boehm's titration (132), while the content of dextran (DEX) at the poly (ε-caprolactone) (PCL) NP surface was measured by a enzymatic degradation of NP with endodextranase (133). In some cases, the ESR technique can be successfully applied to the characterization of magnetic NP surface, such as Fe_3O_4 (134).

The surface contamination of provided NM is another parameter rarely investigated during their characterization. The presence of CO_2 impurities in ZnO NP was studied by infrared (IR) absorption spectroscopy (135). More advanced surface chemistry characterization should be welcome in order to correctly ascertain the coverage degree by coating reactions and to measure the thickness of mono/multilayer coating, because these features are rarely reported by suppliers.

CHARACTERIZATION OF ADMINISTERED NANOMATERIALS

The characterization of administered NM during toxicity studies is essential to ascertain the interaction pathways and the physicochemical properties modification that occur in the NM during the experiment (4). In order to correctly determine the dose of NM that might cause physiological response in vivo/in vitro assays, it is moreover necessary, in addition to discerning their physicochemical properties, to set the correct exposure conditions and correctly quantify the administered NM. The ways NM are placed in contact with biological systems (e.g., dermal penetration, intradermal injection, intratracheal instillation, inhalation of aerosol, cells uptake pathways, etc.) require special consideration, because there are several issues associated with the selected exposure conditions. NP aggregate naturally in aqueous medium (136) and some are even theoretically insoluble (e.g., fullerene) (137,138). Some procedures proposed to avoid aggregation of dispersed NP such as pH alteration or addition of surfactants may change the surface chemistry of the investigated materials during their administration and affect their interaction with cells, and, consequently, their biological effects (139,140). Moreover, often experimental conditions reported in the literature do not mimic realistic exposure conditions.

As described in the previous paragraph, physiological response to NM depends on their physicochemical properties, but it can depend also on the adopted administration conditions. Selected biological culture media and dispersion procedures, such as stirring and sonication, as well as the addition of stabilizers, salts, might potentially influence the biological effects of NM. The characterization at this stage is very important to understand the relationship between NM physicochemical features and the exposure, uptake, effect response, in order to establish a correct exposure–dose relationship. Unfortunately, very few reports include a detailed characterization at this stage. The most suitable characterization techniques and procedures depend strongly on the adopted experimental design, exposure route (e.g., in vitro such as cells uptake, or in vivo, such as inhalation, instillation, dermal uptake) and conditions in which cell culture (in vitro assay) systems or animals (in vivo assay) are exposed to NP. It is firstly essential to assess the behavior of the investigated NM in the medium (water, air, cell culture) of destination. Several in vivo inhalation toxicity studies are conducted by intratracheal instillation (6,8), or by aerosol generation (10,141). In the first case, particles need to be suspended in a suitable exposure medium prior to application, and then need to be characterized as liquid suspensions, while in the second case NP are dispersed by a jet airstream through a mixing chamber, and thus a generated aerosol, not a water dispersion, needs to be characterized.

Nanomaterial Characterization in Liquid Media

Currently, no standardized methods for the dispersion of NM during *in vitro* and in vivo toxicological studies have been proposed, because of the high variety of investigated NM and adopted testing protocols. In addition to a detailed characterization of the supplied NM, a well-designed experiment should include also their characterization during the dispersion procedure to obtain at least, size distribution, actual concentration, surface charge, and suspension stability of the administered NM. All tested NM should be subjected to standardized storage and application procedures and explicit handling instructions should be reported. Unfortunately, NM are currently administered according to very qualitative criteria. Many literature reports include a simple suspension of the selected NP in a suitable biological medium (e.g., cell culture medium, sterile saline solution), or even in water. The obtained suspension is often sonicated or stirred prior to incubation with cell or to administration to animals, in order to avoid aggregation (142,143). Many different sonication and stirring conditions have been proposed, often without explanation, although it should be known that the resulting dispersion can vary depending on the adopted experimental conditions: stirring time and speed can modify the aggregation state of NM, while too high sonication power, such as that attainable by probe sonicators, can even partially modify the NM structure and conformation, as highlighted for CNT (136). Only in few cases, the aggregation state of NP, as well as their stability over time when suspended, have been checked in toxicity studies. Often, the description of the adopted dispersion procedure is even not described in detail, or not reported at all, so experiments cannot be easily reproduced by others. The lack of standardized procedures is probably the main reason of so many debates about the reported toxicological results. Fullerene, as example, is sometimes dissolved in toluene (144,145), tetrahydrofuran (THF) (76) or other organic solvents, and then transferred into water by extracting the organic phase with water, in order to obtain a "water-soluble C_{60}," as already reported. It has been suggested that this "aqueous" C_{60} is toxic to cultured cells (39,146,147), while more recent studies reported that C_{60} prepared with a different method appears vice versa to be not toxic (148–151). It derives that the preparation method requires attention and has to be documented, because C_{60} dispersion seems to undergo modifications during the preparation of water-soluble aggregates that are responsible for the exhibited cytotoxic effects (152,153). Similarly, in vitro cytotoxicity testing of SWCNT typically involves their preliminary dispersion within a cell culture medium, followed by their subsequent addition to a cell line of interest. However, the degree of interaction between the SWCNT and the medium in which they are dispersed and the influence of such interactions on cell viability remains currently unexplored (154).

Various sonication procedures have been found to change the NP chemistry and they have been also applied for synthesis purposes (155). The sonication procedure, including time, frequency, and energy of the applied ultrasound conditions, as well as type of sonication and probe, and time interval between dispersion and administration, should be investigated, optimized and validated before starting an experiment, and then detailed in the analytical report. The same conditions should be adopted along a quite large set of experiments, in order to produce reproducible results. Also the selection of vehicle and media, pH solution, addition of surfactants and/or other stabilizers should be investigated in terms of potential side effects and described.

There are many available techniques for detecting and accurately characterizing the size, the aggregation state, and the stability of NP in liquid media. The most commonly used method is, as described previously, DLS, or a combination of SAXS, WAXD, and SANS. Also, electron microscopy (TEM, SEM) may provide valuable information on size, shape, and aggregation state, provided the solvent evaporation step does not induce structural modifications.

Methods for NP characterization in solution include flow FFF (FlFFF) coupled online with multiangle light scattering (MALS) and UV-Vis spectrophotometry to measure respectively the size and concentration of NP (156). ICP can also be used for concentration determination of TiO_2 and Au NP in solutions (157,158).

Nanomaterial Characterization in Aerosol

Several toxicological studies are based on a deliberate in vivo inhalation of aerosol containing NP (159–162). Depending on the experiment, aerosolization is obtained by nebulization of NP liquid suspensions or powders (163–165). Inhaled NP may deposit in each of the three regions of the human respiratory tract (nasopharyngeal, tracheobronchial, and alveolar regions) on the basis of their size, while their aggregation may change the preferential deposition site (19). In the same way, size distribution, morphology, density, and composition of the generated aerosolized particles, can influence the location of deposition during inhalation toxicological studies, which in turn control the potential rate and route of entry into the circulatory system (166). The characterization of these generated aerosols is therefore a key aspect. It can include parameters such as concentration measurements (e.g., particle number per unit volume), size distribution, surface area, morphology, and composition.

The condensation particle counter (CPC) technique is often used to determine the particle number concentration (167,168). This technique is based on the principle of growing the particles in a saturated vapor atmosphere so that they become large enough to be detected by optical counters, and can reveal particles in the 3 to 1000 nm size range (169). The scanning mobility particle sizers (SMPS) and electrical low pressure impactors (ELPI) can also be applied (170). A nanometer aerosol differential mobility analyzer (DMA) is placed before the CPC in order to analyze the size distribution of particles, covering currently an approx. size range from 3 to 50 nm (171). However, since the passage of the aerosol flow in the DMA is relatively slow, a significant loss of smaller ($<$ 5 nm) particles by Brownian diffusive deposition can occur (172). Recently, a low pressure DMA (LPDMA) has been developed for the in situ measurement of nanosized aerosol particles under subatmospheric (i.e., 65–760 Torr) pressure (173,174). However, mass measurements methods for aerosol are not sufficiently sensitive to NP, because of losses and decreasing counting efficiency with decreasing particle size (175).

DLS may be used to measure the diffusion particle size weighted by light scattering intensity, with a measuring size range between 50 and 1000 nm (167). As for suspended particles in liquid, DLS can measure the scattered light by generated aerosol, but the sampling equipment and instruments are different between those cited above. The major limitation of these techniques is that they cannot discriminate agglomerates of NP from individual, larger particles (176).

A recently developed technique, the time of flight mobility (TOFM) spectrometer, is able to determine the elemental distribution of aerosolized NP. Depending on sampling inlet configuration, size separation method, vaporization method, and type of mass spectrometer coupled to it, is it possible to obtain a size-resolved chemical composition of NP in gas suspension. The TOFM is currently limited by its sampling capabilities and its requirement for a relatively high concentration (167,177,178). A simultaneous system has been developed to measure the size-dependent concentration and chemical composition of particles smaller than 40 nm using an ICP-MS combined with a DMA (179).

The availability of NP standards is a key aspect for the measurement of aerosol. There is an urgent need for appropriate particle size standards for instrument calibration. There is only one calibration standard in the nanometer size range, the NIST SRMr 1963, a water suspension of polystyrene nanospheres with a mean size of 100.7 nm (180). Standards are needed for verifying and improving the accuracy and precision of the obtained measure. In addition, other problems still need to be solved, such as adequate sampling protocols to ensure reproducibility and accuracy in aerosol size analysis, and portable instruments.

Relatively few techniques are available to monitor exposures with respect to aerosol surface area (181,182). Available techniques to measure aerosol surface area are the epiphaniometer (EPI), diffusion charging (DC), and scanning mobility particle sizer (SMPS) (183–186). However, instruments capable of measuring the total NP surface area fractions are currently not commercially available (175).

Particles may be also collected on surface (e.g., filters, baffles) and later analyzed in order to obtain their size, shape, structure, aggregation state, and in some case compositional information by specific analysis of the collected fractions, by applying the same techniques mentioned above. Sample collection can also be performed by an electrostatic precipitator (ESP) (170). In the ESP, the charged particles are transported by the electric field of the instrument, and, finally, deposited on the sampling surface (169). A homogeneous deposition of NP on a sampling surface can be obtained by adjusting the flow conditions and the electric field. Assuming that NP are collected and homogenously distributed on the surface, they can be analyzed in different ways to determine their size, shape, and aggregation state by SEM, TEM and scanning transmission electron microscopy (STEM) (187,188).

NANOMATERIAL CHARACTERIZATION AFTER THE ADMINISTRATION EXPERIMENT

The characterization of NM in biological media after their administration is probably the most demanding task in nanotoxicology research. Such characterization is fundamental for correctly evaluating the interaction with biological tissues and explaining the observed biological effects and the involved mechanisms. In principle, almost all the techniques described above can be applied to NM after administration, but the concentration levels are usually very low, and the complex biological matrices renders this task most demanding for both qualitative (presence, distribution) and quantitative (actual concentration in specific tissues or cell components) information requirements. Currently, the determination of internal doses of NM after toxicological experiments, as well their final fate, are actually limited by methodological capabilities (4). Some analytical methods are already available to detect and quantify specific NM in biological media, while procedures to evaluate modifications in NM physical and chemical properties due to interactions with the biological matrix are not commonly applied (46,189). Moreover, studies on the identification of fate of administered NM in blood circulation and as well as their accumulation, renal excretions and organ distribution, and the determination of clearance half-life, have been little investigated (190).

Qualitative Characterization of Nanomaterials in Biological Matrices

The NP internalization (uptake) in cell, may be monitored by common cell and molecular biology methods, such as fluorescence microscopy (FLM), TEM, SEM, differential interference contrast microscopy (DIC), and confocal laser scanning microscopy (CLSM) (142,191–197). By these microscopy techniques, the presence and distribution of individual particles and their aggregates with components at the cellular level can be observed, but it is impossible to ascertain if the aggregation took place before or after particle uptake by the cells (46). Whatever the situation, sample preparation may be very time consuming and complex, since it includes different steps such as fixation, dehydration, staining, sectioning, stabilization, etc. Cryogenic SEM and TEM, as well as scanning transmission ion microscopy (STIM), are microscopy techniques specifically modified to be applied to unfixed, unstained vitrified biological samples as diagnostic tools in structural cell biology. The percutaneous penetration of TiO_2 of cross-sections of pig skin has been recently investigated by STIM (198), while cryo-TEM has been used to detect the dermal penetration of TiO_2 contained in sunscreen formulation into the underlying living tissue by a cryosectioning of biological material (199,200). While conventional SEM and TEM analysis require a chemical fixation of the investigated sample, which may induce structural modifications, a quick freezing permit to observe the biological samples in their native state. One of the important factors of the cryo-TEM or cryo-SEM success is the sample thickness that can be analyzed: the vitreous sample must be sectioned with a cryomicrotome to a thickness suitable for high-quality cryoimaging, and this is often a laborious task to obtain (201).

Fluorescence detection has been also shown to be applicable to NM. Nanometer-sized luminescent materials, such as QD (202,203), silver NP (204), gold dye-doped silica NP (205,206), are used as luminescence probes for their detection in biological media. Compared with conventional organic dyes, such as fluorescein, cyanine, amino dyes, and carboxylic acids, luminescent NP exhibit higher photostability and stronger luminescence. The luminescence is often affected by scattering phenomena, such as Tyndall, Rayleigh, and Raman scattering (207). In some cases fluorescent groups can be bonded to the NM as markers, but it is an open issue whether these added fluorophores can alter NM surface chemistry and their biochemical activity and fate in organisms, or be released by the particles during the experiment (13).

CLSM can be applied to a wide range of investigations in the biological and medical sciences for imaging thin (up to 100 µm) optical sections in living and fixed cells and tissues. Current instruments are equipped with a laser source and filters that allow very precise regulation of wavelength and excitation intensity. When coupled with dedicated photomultipliers these microscopes are capable of examining fluorescence emission ranging generally from 400 to 750 nm. A CLSM image of cells after administration of fluorescent polystyrene nanobeads is shown in Figure 2.

Also, AFM is an emerging diagnostic tool for biological studies, and it has been successfully applied to investigate the interaction between the NP, such as QD, and cell systems (208,209).

Radioactivity measurements can be applied to ascertain the adsorption and distribution of specific radiolabeled (such as those containing ^{14}C) NM administered in vivo, with the great advantage of accurately identifying and

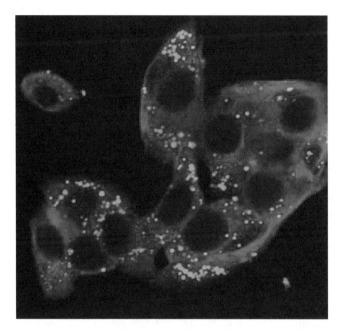

Figure 2 Confocal laser scanning microscopy (CLSM) image of HepG2 cell after administration of 20 nm fluorescent carboxylate-modified microsphere polystyrene beads. *Source*: Courtesy of Prof. V. Stone, Napier University, Edinburgh, U.K.

quantifying presence and distribution even in living organisms ("whole body measurements"), so permitting to follow their administration into the biological system (210–213). The main limitations are the applicability to only some specific NM types (mainly carbon based), the specific, and often very expensive, synthetic route involved, and the safety precautions to be followed. Radioactive elements can be included in the surface coating of the investigated NM. Special care should be spent to check the chemical stability of the coating when dispersed in the biological matrix to avoid misleading results due to coating release and diffusion into other tissues.

Characterization of Inorganic NM in Biological Matrices

Elemental analysis has been already successfully applied to both qualitative and quantitative determination of inorganic NM in biological media because of its high selectivity and sensibility (in the ppt to ppq range), by analyzing their distinctive elements (generally the heavier ones), such as titanium for TiO_2, Cd for CdSe QD, etc. Atomic absorption spectroscopy (AAS) or ICP (with OES and MS detectors) can be used, depending on the element, on its concentration level and on the matrix to be investigated (214–216). It cannot be applied to organic NM or to lighter elements, such as O, N, S, or to biological oligoelements such as Fe or Zn, being naturally contained in living materials. In this case, elemental analysis can be applied if the investigated NM are specifically enriched with not naturally occurring isotopes or elements, which can be used as "tracers" for their identification and quantification. The potential release of such elements by the NP core must be investigated in advance. In addition to the same procedure adopted for their determination in pure NM, a digestion step of the biological sample is additionally required prior to analysis. The digestion procedure is the most critical aspect and it needs to be specifically developed and validated for both the selected NM and the investigated matrix. An accurate separation of specific tissues can permit to get a more detailed distribution pathway of the adsorbed particles. It should be noted that this procedure can not distinguish the adsorbed NM from the dissolved forms due to biochemical degradation of the administered material: in this case a preliminary size-based separation of the extracted components, for instance by gel permeation chromatography (GPC) or FFF, is suggested. Some analytical methods are already available for selected elements and matrices. ICP determination after pressurized acid digestion of the tissue samples has been used to quantify the systemic distribution of inhaled silver NP in rats (214), of intravenous injected cobalt-ferrite NP in mice (215), and to measure oxides (Fe_2O_3, Y_2O_3, and ZnO) NP uptake by cells (216). Magnetite NP internalization into mouse macrophage and human breast cancer cells was visualized using both fluorescence and confocal microscopy, and quantified by ICP-MS (217).

Characterization of Organic Nanomaterials in Biological Matrices

The determination of organic NM in biological media is probably the most demanding analytical task in nanotoxicology. Their chemical structure is often very similar to those of many other synthetic organic molecules (e.g., polystyrene beads and polystyrene), while the size is much larger, or similar to those of biomolecules already existing in the examined medium. It follows that conventional techniques developed for organics can be only partially applied to their determination. In some cases, such as for nano-CB and CNT, the high variability in their chemical structure and size distribution renders very difficult the correct identification and quantification of these NM in such complex environments at the administrated concentration level applied, even if the most sensitive detectors, such as MS, are used. Moreover, current purification procedures, developed for small (i.e., < 2000 Da) molecules, cannot be easily applied. In principle, separation techniques such as GPC, FlFFF, HPLC, and capillary electrophoresis (CE) can be applied, but the separation/detection method need to be specifically developed for each investigated NM and biological matrix. Among these, FlFFF seems the most promising technique, although very few applications have been proposed so far (218). As above underlined, the extraction and purification procedures are the most critical steps, because of the chemical similarity between administered NM and the surrounding environment. Currently, a very limited number of methods have been proposed: fullerenes have been successfully determined in biological media, by means of solvent extraction followed by HPLC coupled with UV and MS detection (219,220), while FlFFF has been proposed for the determination of CNT (221). The quantitative uptake by endothelial cells of biodegradable poly-*DL*-lactide-co-glycolide (PLGA) containing 6-coumarin as a fluorescent marker has been measured by centrifugation of biological sample and subsequent analysis by HPLC coupled with fluorescence detection (207).

LIST OF ABBREVIATIONS

AAS   atomic absorption spectroscopy
AES   Auger electron spectroscopy
AFM   atomic force microscopy
ATOF-MS   aerosol time of flight–mass spectrometry
BET   Brunauer–Emmett–Teller adsorption measurement method
CB   carbon black
CE   capillary electrophoresis
CLSM   confocal laser scanning microscopy
CNT   carbon nanotubes
CPC   condensation particle counter
DC   diffusion charging
DIC   differential interference contrast microscopy
DLS   dynamic light scattering
DMA   differential mobility analyzer
DSC   differential scanning calorimetry
EDS   energy dispersive X-ray spectroscopy
ELPI   electrical low pressure impactors
EPI   epiphaniometer
EPR   electron paramagnetic resonance
ESP   electrostatic precipitator
ESR   electron spin resonance
FL   fluorescence
FFF   field flow fractionation
FlFFF   flow field flow fractionation
FLM   fluorescence microscopy
FTIR   Fourier transform infrared spectroscopy
GC   gas chromatography
GPC   gel permeation chromatography
HPLC   high performance liquid chromatography

HRTEM   high resolution transmission electron microscopy
ICP-OES   inductively coupled plasma–optical emission spectroscopy
ICP-MS   inductively coupled plasma-mass spectroscopy
MALS   multiangle light scattering
MWNT   multiwalled carbon nanotubes
NM   nanomaterial(s)
NMR   nuclear magnetic resonance
NP   nanoparticle(s)
PCS   photon correlation spectroscopy
QD   quantum dots
QELS   quasielastic light scattering
RS   Raman spectroscopy
SANS   small angle neutron scanning
SAXS   small-angle X-ray scattering
SEM   scanning electron microscopy
SLS   static light scattering
SMPS   scanning mobility particle sizer
SPM   scanning probe microscopy
STEM   scanning transmission electron microscopy
STIM   scanning transmission ion microscopy
STM   scanning tunneling microscopy
SWNT   single-walled carbon nanotubes
TEM   transmission electron microscopy
TGA   thermogravimetric analysis
UVA   Ultraviolet A radiation
UV-Vis   ultraviolet–visible spectroscopy
WAXD   wide-angle X-ray diffraction
XPS   X-ray photoelectron spectroscopy
XRD   X-ray diffraction
ζ-pot   zeta potential analysis

REFERENCES

1. Alivisatos AP. Perspectives on the physical chemistry of semiconductor nanocrystals. J Phys Chem 1996; 100:13226–39.
2. Wautelet M, Dauchot JP, Hecq M. Size effects on the phase diagrams of nanoparticles of various shapes. Mater Sci Eng 2003; C23:187–90.
3. Dreher KL. Health and environmental impact of nanotechnology: toxicological assessment of manufactured nanoparticles. Toxicol Sci 2004; 77:3–5.
4. Oberdörster G, Maynard A, Donaldson K, et al. Principles for characterizing the potential human health effects from exposure to nanomaterials: elements of a screening strategy. Review. Part Fibre Toxicol 2005; 2:1–35.
5. Shvedova AA, Castranova V, Kisin ER, et al. Exposure to carbon nanotube material: assessment of nanotube cytotoxicity using human keratinocyte cells. J Toxicol Environ Health A 2003; 66:1909–26.

6. Warheit DB, Laurence BR, Reed KL, et al. Comparative pulmonary toxicity assessment of single-wall carbon nanotubes in rats. Toxicol Sci 2004; 77:117–25.

7. Sayes C, Fortner J, Guo W, et al. The differential cytotoxicity of water-soluble fullerenes. Nano Lett 2004; 4:1881–7.

8. Lam C, James JT, McCluskey RM, et al. Pulmonary toxicity of single-wall carbon nanotubes in mice 7 and 90 days after tracheal installation. Toxicol Sci 2004; 77:26–34.

9. Long TC, Saleh N, Tilton R, et al. Titanium dioxide (P25) Produces reactive oxygen species in immortalized brain microglia (BV2): implications for nanoparticle neurotoxicity. Environ Sci Technol 2006; 40:4346–52.

10. Bermudez E, Mangum JB, Wong BA, et al. Pulmonary responses of mice, rats, and hamsters to subchronic inhalation of ultrafine titanium dioxide particles. Toxicol Sci 2004; 77:347–57.

11. Brunner TJ, Wick P, Manser P, et al. In vitro cytotoxicity of oxide nanoparticles: comparison to asbestos, silica, and the effect of particle solubility. Environ Sci Technol 2006; 40:4374–81.

12. Austin M, Chan WCW, Bhatia SN. Probing the cytotoxicity of semiconductor quantum dots. Nano Lett 2004; 4:11–8.

13. Hurt RA, Monthioux M, Kane A. Toxicology of carbon nanomaterials: status, trends, and perspectives on the special issue. Carbon 2006; 44:1028–33.

14. Brant J, Lecoanet H, Hotze M, et al. Comparison of electrokinetic properties of colloidal fullerenes (n-C_{60}) formed using two procedures. Environ Sci Technol 2005; 39:6343–51.

15. Masala O, Seshadri R. Synthesis routes for large volumes of nanoparticles. Annu Rev Mater Res 2004; 34:41–81.

16. Brayner R, Ferrari-Iliou R, Brivois N, et al. Toxicological impact studies based on *Escherichia coli* bacteria in ultrafine ZnO nanoparticles colloidal medium. Nano Lett 2006; 6:866–70.

17. Nel A, Xia T, Madler L, et al. Toxic potential of materials at the nanolevel. Rev Sci 2006; 311:622–7.

18. Donaldson K, Stone V, Tran CL, et al. Nanotoxicology. Occup Environ Med 2004; 61:727–8.

19. Oberdorster G, Oberdorster E, Oberdorster J. Nanotoxicology: an emerging discipline evolving from studies of ultrafine particles. Environ Health Perspect 2005; 113:823–39.

20. Donaldson K, Tran CL. Inflammation caused by particles and fibres. Inhal Toxicol 2002; 14:5–27.

21. Warheit DB. Nanoparticles: health impacts? Mater Today 2004; 7:32–5.

22. Tran CL, Buchanan RT, Cullen RT, et al. Inhalation of poorly soluble particles. II. Influence of particle surface area on inflammation and clearance. Inhal Toxicol 2000; 12:1113–26.

23. Scientific Committee on Emerging and Newly Identified Health Risks (SCENIHR). Opinion on the appropriateness of existing methodologies to assess the potential risks associated with engineered and adventitious products of nanotechnologies. Adopted by the SCENIHR during the 7th plenary meeting of 28–29 September 2005. European Commission. Health & Consumer Protection Directorate-General. Directorate C – Public Health and Risk Assessment. C7 – Risk Assessment. SCENIHR/002/05.

24. Park KH, Chhowalla M, Iqbal Z, et al. Single-walled carbon nanotubes are a new class of ion channel blockers. J Biol Chem 2003; 278:50212–26.
25. Radomski A, Jurasz P, Alonso-Escolano D, et al. Nanoparticle-induced platelet aggregation and vascular thrombosis. Br J of Pharmacol 2005; 146:882–93.
26. Jia G, Wang H, Yan L, et al. Cytotoxicity of carbon nanomaterials: single-wall nanotube, multi-wall nanotube, and fullerene. Environ Sci Technol 2005; 39: 1378–83.
27. Seaton A, Donaldson K. Nanoscience, nanotoxicology, and the need to think small. Lancet 2005; 365:923–4.
28. Hardman R.A. Toxicologic review of quantum dots: toxicity depends on physicochemical and environmental factors. Environ Health Perspect 2006; 114:165–72.
29. Maynard AD, Baron PA, Foley M, et al. Exposure to carbon nanotube material during the handling of unrefined single walled carbon nanotube material. J Toxicol Environ Health A 2004; 67:87–107.
30. Pulskamp K, Diabaté S, Krug HF. Carbon nanotubes show no sign of acute toxicity but induce intracellular reactive oxygen species in dependence on contaminants. Toxicol Lett 2007; 168:58–74.
31. Wakefield G, Lipscomb S, Holland E, et al. The effects of manganese doping on UVA absorption and free radical generation of micronised titanium dioxide and its consequences for the photostability of UVA absorbing organic sunscreen components. Photochem Photobiol Sci 2004; 3:648–52.
32. Jia G, Wang H, Yan L, et al. Cytotoxicity of carbon nanomaterials: single-wall nanotube, multi-wall nanotube, and fullerene. Environ Sci Technol 2005; 39: 1378–83.
33. Bianco A, Wu W, Pastorin G, et al. Carbon nanotube-based vectors for delivering immunotherapeutics and drugs. In: Kumar Challa SSR, ed. Nanomaterials for Medical Diagnosis and Therapy. Nanotechnologies for the Life Sciences. Vol. 10. Weinheim: Wiley-VCH, 2007:85–142.
34. Jefferson DA. The surface activity of ultrafine particles. Phil Trans R Soc Lond A 2000; 358:2683–92.
35. Barnard AS, Curtiss LA. Prediction of TiO_2 nanoparticle phase and shape transitions controlled by surface chemistry. Nano Lett 2005; 5:1261–6.
36. Barnard AS. Nanohazards: knowledge is our first defence. Nat Mater 2006; 5: 245–8.
37. Werth JH, Linsenbühler M, Dammer SM, et al. Agglomeration of charged nanopowders in suspension. Powder Technol 2003; 133:106–12.
38. Dutta J, Hofmann H. Self-organization of colloidal nanoparticles. In: Nalwa HS, ed. Encyclopedia of Nanoscience and Nanotechnology. Vol. 10. California: American Scientific Publisher, 2004:617–40.
39. Sayes CM, Fortner JD, Guo W, et al. The differential cytotoxicity of water-soluble fullerenes. Nano Lett 2004; 4:1881–7.
40. Sayes CM, Liang F, Hudson JL, et al. Functionalization density dependence of single-walled carbon nanotubes cytotoxicity in vitro. Toxicol Lett 2006; 161:135–42.
41. Borm PJA, Robbins D, Haubold S, et al. The potential risks of nanomaterials: a review carried out for ECETOC. Particle Fibre Toxicol 2006; 3:11.

42. Knaapen AK, Albrecht C, Becker A, et al. DNA damage in lung epithelial cells isolated from rats exposed to quartz: role of surface reactivity and neutrophilic inflammation. Carcinogenesis 2002; 23:1111–20.

43. Schins RPF, Duffin R, Höhr D, et al. Surface modification of quartz inhibits toxicity, particle uptake, and oxidative DNA damage in human lung epithelial cells. Chem Res Toxicol 2002; 15:1166–73.

44. Yina H, Toob HP, Chowa GM. The effects of particle size and surface coating on the cytotoxicity of nickel ferrite. Biomaterials 2005; 26:5818–26.

45. Eastman J. Colloid stability. In: Cosgrove T, ed. Colloid Science: Principles, Methods and Applications. Oxford: Blackwell Publishing, 2005:36–49.

46. Powers KW, Brown SC, Krishna VB, et al. Research strategies for safety evaluation of nanomaterials. Part VI. Characterization of nanoscale particles for toxicological evaluation. Toxicol Sci 2006; 90:296–303.

47. Schins RP, Duffin R, Hohr D, et al. Surface modification of quartz inhibits toxicity, particle uptake, and oxidative DNA damage in human lung epithelial cells. Chem Res Toxicol 2002; 15:1166–73.

48. Hoet PHM, Brüske-Hohlfeld I, Salata OV. Nanoparticles—known and unknown health risks. Rev J Nanobiotechnol 2004; 2:12.

49. Lockman PR, Koziara JM, Mumper RJ, et al. Nanoparticle surface charges alter blood–brain barrier integrity and permeability. J Drug Target 2004; 12: 635–41.

50. Malik N, Wiwattanapatapee R, Klopsch R, et al. Dendrimers: relationship between structure and biocompatibility in vitro, and preliminary studies on the biodistribution of ^{125}I-labeled polyamidoamine dendrimers in vivo. J Control Release 2000; 65:133–48.

51. Nigavekar SS, Sung LY, Llanes M, et al. [3]H dendrimer nanoparticle organ/ tumor distribution. Pharm Res 2004; 21:476–83.

52. Quintana A, Raczka E, Piehler L, et al. Design and function of a dendrimer-based therapeutic nanodevice targeted to tumor cells through the folate receptor. Pharm Res 2002; 19:1310–6.

53. Cheng HM, Li F, Su G, et al. Large-scale and low-cost synthesis of single-walled carbon nanotubes by the catalytic pyrolysis of hydrocarbon. Appl Phys Lett 1998; 72:3282–4.

54. Rinzler AG, Liu J, Dai H, et al. Large-scale purification of single-wall carbon nanotubes: process, product, and characterization. Appl Phys A 1998; 67:29–37.

55. Duffin R, Clouter A, Brown DM, et al. The importance of surface area and specific reactivity in the acute pulmonary inflammatory response to particles. Ann Occup Hyg 2002; 46:242–5.

56. Wilson MR, Lightbody JH, Donaldson K, et al. Interactions between ultrafine particles and transition metals in vivo and in vitro. Toxicol Appl Pharmacol 2002; 184:172–9.

57. Wick P, Manser P, Limbach LK, et al. The degree and kind of agglomeration affect carbon nanotube cytotoxicity. Toxicol Lett 2007; 168:121–31.

58. Soto KF, Carrasco A, Powell TG, et al. Comparative in vitro cytotoxicity assessment of some manufactured nanoparticulate materials characterized by transmission electron microscopy. J Nanoparticle Res 2005; 7:145–9.

59. Chen Q, Saltiel C, Manickavasagam S, et al. Aggregation behavior of single-walled carbon nanotubes in dilute aqueous suspension. J Colloid Interf Sci 2004; 280:91–7.

60. Sun YP, Li X, Cao J, et al. Characterization of zero-valent iron nanoparticles. Adv Colloid Interf Sci 2006; 120:47–56.

61. Wang ZL, Poncharal P, de Heer WA. Measuring physical and mechanical properties of individual carbon nanotubes by in situ TEM. J Phys Chem Solids 2000; 61:1025–30.

62. Belin T, Epron F. Characterization methods of carbon nanotubes: a review. Mater Sci Eng B 2005; 119:105–18.

63. Andrievsky GV, Klochkov VK, Karyakina EL, et al. Studies of aqueous colloidal solutions of fullerene C60 by electron microscopy. Chem Phys Lett 1999; 300:392–6.

64. Ramallo-López JM, Giovanetti L, Craievich AF, et al. XAFS, SAXS and HREM characterization of Pd nanoparticles capped with *n*-alkyl thiol molecules. Phys B: Condensed Mater 2007; 389:150–4.

65. Yee C, Scotti M, Ulman A. One-phase synthesis of thiol-functionalized platinum nanoparticles. Langmuir 1999; 15:4314–6.

66. Tilaki RM, Irajizad A, Mahdavi SM. The effect of liquid environment on size and aggregation of gold nanoparticles prepared by pulsed laser ablation. J Nanoparticle Res 2002, online 23 September 2006. http://www.springerlink. com/content/a0w0435560741242/?p = 1fd3b36fcfe74d58a0c6cb5c76abc6e3 &pi=0.

67. Gu Y, Xie H, Gao J, et al. AFM characterization of dendrimer-stabilized platinum nanoparticles. Langmuir 2005; 21:3122–31.

68. Islam MF, Rojas E, Bergey DM, et al. High weight fraction surfactant solubilization of single-wall carbon nanotubes in water. Nano Lett 2003; 3: 269–73.

69. Paredes JI, Burghard M. Dispersions of individual single-walled carbon nanotubes of high length. Langmuir 2004; 20:5149–52.

70. Terrones M, Jorio A, Endo M, et al. New direction in nanotube science. Mater Today 2004; 7:30–45.

71. Wang ZL, Poncharal P, de Heer WA. Measuring physical and mechanical properties of individual carbon nanotubes by in situ TEM. J Phys Chem Solids 2000; 61:1025–30.

72. Parak WJ, Manna L, Simmel FC, et al. Quantum Dots. In: Schmid G, ed. Nanoparticles: From Theory to Application. Weinheim: Wiley-VCH, 2004: 4–49.

73. Lee JY, Kim JS, An KH, et al. Electrophoretic and dynamic light scattering in evaluating dispersion and size distribution of single-walled carbon nanotubes. J Nanosci Nanotechnol 2005; 5:1045–9.

74. Sano M, Kamino A, Okamura J, et al. Self-organization of PEO-graft-single-walled carbon nanotubes in solutions and Langmuir-Blodgett films. Langmuir 2001; 17:5125–8.

75. Bowen P. Particle size distribution measurement from millimeters to nanometers and from rods to platelets. J Disper Sci Technol 2002; 23:631–62.

76. Deguchi S, Alargova RG, Tsujii K. Stable dispersions of fullerenes, C60 and C70, in water. Preparation and characterization. Langmuir 2001; 17:6013–7.
77. Jillavenkatesa A, Kelly JF. Nanopowder characterization: challenges and future directions. J Nanoparticle Res 2002; 4:463–8.
78. Pecora R. Dynamic light scattering measurement of nanometer particles in liquids. J Nanoparticle Res 2000; 2:123–31.
79. Chu B, Liu T. Characterization of nanoparticles by scattering techniques. J Nanoparticle Res 2000; 2:29–41.
80. Giddings JC. The field-flow fractionation family: underlying principles. In: Schimpf M, Caldwell K, Giddings JC, eds. Field-Flow Fractionation Handbook. New York: Wiley-Interscience, 2000:3–30.
81. Cho J, Park YJ, Sun H, et al. Measurements of effective sizes and diffusivities of nano-colloids and micro-particles. Coll Surf A: Physicochem Eng Asp 2006; 274:43–7.
82. Tagmatarchis N, Zattoni A, Reschiglian P, et al. Separation and purification of functionalized water-soluble multi-walled carbon nanotubes by flow field-flow fractionation. Carbon 2005; 43:1984–9.
83. Jungmann N, Schmidt M, Maskos M. Characterization of polyorganosiloxane nanoparticles in aqueous dispersion by asymmetrical flow field-flow fractionation. Macromolecules 2001; 34:8347–53.
84. Amendola V, Rizzi GA, Polizzi S, et al. Synthesis of gold nanoparticles by laser ablation in toluene: quenching and recovery of the surface plasmon absorption. J Phys Chem B 2005; 109:23125–8.
85. Allen T. Surface area determination by gas adsorption. In: Allen T, ed. Particle Size Measurement. Surface Area and Pore Size Determination. 5th ed. Vol. II. London: Chapman & Hall, 1997:39–103.
86. Signoretto M, Breda A, Somma F, et al. Mesoporous sulphated zirconia by liquid-crystal templating method. Micropor Mesopor Mater 2006; 91:23–32.
87. Menegazzo F, Fantinel T, Signoretto M, et al. Metal dispersion and distribution in Pd-based PTA catalysts. Chem Commun 2007; 8:876–9.
88. Signoretto M, Oliva L, Pinna F, et al. Synthesis of sulfated-zirconia aerogel: effect of the chemical modification of precursor on catalyst porosity. J Non-Crystalline Solids 2001; 290:145–52.
89. Yang CM, Kaneko K, Yudasaka M, et al. Effect of purification on pore structure of HiPCO single-walled carbon nanotube aggregates. Nano Lett 2002; 2:385–8.
90. Staiger M, Bowen P, Ketterer J, et al. Particle size distribution measurement and assessment of agglomeration of commercial nanosized ceramic particles. J Disper Sci Technol 2002; 23:619–30.
91. Pochard I, Boisvert JP, Persello J, et al. Surface charge, effective charge and dispersion/aggregation properties of nanoparticles. Polym Int 2003; 52:619–24.
92. Zhao L, Gao L. Stability of multi-walled carbon nanotubes dispersion with copolymer in ethanol. Coll Surf A: Physicochem Eng Asp 2003; 224:127–34.
93. Basch A, Horn R, Besenhard JO. Substrate induced coagulation (SIC) of nano-disperse carbon black in non-aqueous media: the dispersibility and

stability of carbon black in *N*-methyl-2-pyrrolidinone. Coll Surf A: Physicochem Eng Asp 2005; 253:155–61.

94. DeCarlo PF, Kimmel JR, Trimborn A, et al. Field-deployable, high-resolution, time-of-flight aerosol mass spectrometer. Anal Chem 2006; 78: 8281–9.

95. Borm PJA, Cakmak G, Jermann E, et al. Formation of PAH–DNA adducts after in vivo and vitro exposure of rats and lung cells to different commercial carbon blacks. Toxicol Appl Pharmacol 2005; 205:157–67.

96. Jacobsen NR, Saber AT, Møller P, et al. Increased mutant frequency by carbon black, but not quartz, in the lacZ and cII transgenes of Muta™Mouse lung epithelial cells. Environ Mol Mutagen 2007. In Press.

97. He R, Gu H. Synthesis and characterization of mondispersed CdSe nanocrystals at lower temperature. Coll Surf A: Physicochem Eng Asp 2006; 272:111–6.

98. Peng S, Wang C, Xie J, et al. Synthesis and stabilization of monodisperse Fe nanoparticles. J Am Chem Soc 2006; 128:10676–7.

99. Ahmed OS, Dutta DK. Generation of metal nanoparticles on montmorillonite K 10 and their characterization. Langmuir 2003; 19:5540–1.

100. Zhu W, Miser D, Chan W, et al. Characterization of multiwalled carbon nanotubes prepared by carbon arc cathode deposit. Mater Chem Phys 2003; 82:638–47.

101. Hori H, Teranishi T, Taki M, et al. Magnetic properties of nano-particles of Au, Pd and Pd/Ni alloys. J Magn Magn Mater 2001; 226:1910–1.

102. Hseih CT, Huang WL, Lue JT. The change from paramagnetic resonance to ferromagnetic resonance for iron nanoparticles made by the sol–gel method. J Phys Chem Solids 2002; 63:733–41.

103. Jayakumar OD, Gopalakrishnan IK, Kadam RM, et al. Magnetization and structural studies of Mn doped ZnO nanoparticles: Prepared by reverse micelle method. J Cryst Growth 2007; 300:358–63.

104. Konovalova TA, Lawrence J, Kispert LD. Generation of superoxide anion and most likely singlet oxygen in irradiated TiO_2 nanoparticles modified by carotenoids. J Photochem Photobiol A: Chem 2004; 162:1–8.

105. Liang Y, Zhang H, Yi B, et al. Preparation and characterization of multi-walled carbon nanotubes supported PtRu catalysts for proton exchange membrane fuel cells. Carbon 2005; 43:3144–52.

106. Jiang G, Wang L, Chen C, et al. Study on attachment of highly branched molecules onto multiwalled carbon nanotubes. Mater Lett 2005; 59:2085–9.

107. Li Z, Du Y, Zhang Z, et al. Preparation and characterization of CdS quantum dots chitosan biocomposite. React Funct Polym 2003; 55:35–43.

108. Jiang G, Wang L, Chen W. Studies on the preparation and characterization of gold nanoparticles protected by dendrons. Mater Lett 2007; 61:278–83.

109. Ghule K, Ghule AV, Chen BJ, et al. Preparation and characterization of ZnO nanoparticles coated paper and its antibacterial activity study. Green Chem 2006; 8:1034–41.

110. Yang Z, Shi Y, Liu J, et al. Optical properties of Ge/Si quantum dot superlattices. Mater Lett 2004; 58:3765–8.

111. Delhaes P, Couzi M, Trinquecoste M, et al. A comparison between Raman spectroscopy and surface characterizations of multiwall carbon nanotubes. Carbon 2006; 44:3005–13.

112. Gruneis A, Rummeli MH, Kramberger C, et al. High quality double wall carbon nanotubes with a defined diameter distribution by chemical vapor deposition from alcohol. Carbon 2006; 44:3177–82.

113. Ladizhansky V, Hodes G, Vega S. Surface properties of precipitated CdS nanoparticles studied by NMR. J Phys Chem B 1998; 102:8505–9.

114. Garcia-Fuentes M, Torres D, Martin-Pastor M, et al. Application of NMR spectroscopy to the characterization of PEG-stabilized lipid nanoparticles. Langmuir 2004; 20:8839–45.

115. Zelakiewicz BS, De Dios AC, Tong YY. ^{13}C NMR spectroscopy of ^{13}C$_1$-labeled octanethiol-protected Au nanoparticles: shifts, relaxations, and particle-size effect. J Am Chem Soc 2003; 125:18–9.

116. Mayer C. NMR Studies of nanoparticles. Ann Rep NMR Spectrosc 2005; 55: 207–59.

117. Vdovenkova T, Strikha V, Tsyganova A. Silicon nanoparticles characterization by Auger electron spectroscopy. Surf Sci 2000; 454–56:952–6.

118. Kumar PM, Badrinarayanan S, Sastry M. Nanocrystalline TiO$_2$ studied by optical, FTIR and X-ray photoelectron spectroscopy: correlation to presence of surface states. Thin Solid Films 2000; 358:122–30.

119. Zhang L, Xia D, Shen Q. Synthesis and characterization of Ag@TiO$_2$ core-shell nanoparticles and TiO$_2$ nanobubbles. J Nanoparticle Res 2006; 8:23–8.

120. Rong MZ, Zhang MQ, Liang HC. Surface derivatization of nano-CdS clusters and its effect on the performance of CdS quantum dots in solvents and polymeric matrices. Appl Surf Sci 2004; 228:176–90.

121. Lojkowski W, Daniszewska A, Chmielecka M, et al. Nanometrology. In: Lojkowski W, Turan R, Proykova A, Daniszewska A, eds. Nanoforum. European Nanotechnology Gateway, July 2006. Available for download from www.nanoforum.org. Nanoforum consortium.

122. Zhang Y, Fu D, Liu J. Synthesis and characterization of CdS nanoparticles with strong electrolyte behaviour. J Nanoparticle Res 2000; 2:299–303.

123. Chena H, Wanga Y, Wanga Y, et al. One-step preparation and characterization of PDDA-protected gold nanoparticles. Polymer 2006; 47:763–6.

124. Phung X, Groza J, Stach EA, et al. Surface characterization of metal nanoparticles. Mat Sci Eng A 2003; 359:261–8.

125. Zhang HL, Evans SD, Henderson JR, et al. Spectroscopic characterization of gold nanoparticles passivated by mercaptopyridine and mercaptopyrimidine derivatives. Phys Chem B 2003; 107:6087–95.

126. Gabriel G, Sauthier G, Fraxedas J, et al. Preparation and characterisation of single-walled carbon nanotubes functionalised with amines. Carbon 2006; 44: 1891–7.

127. Hota G, Idage SB, Khilar KC. Characterization of nano-sized CdS–Ag$_2$S core-shell nanoparticles using XPS technique. Coll Surf A: Physicochem Eng Asp 2007; 293:5–12.

128. Bentzen EL, Tomlinson ID, Mason J, et al. Surface modification to reduce nonspecific binding of quantum dots in live cell assays. Bioconjug Chem 2005; 16:1488–94.

129. Sahoo Y, Pizem H, Fried T, et al. Alkyl phosphonate/phosphate coating on magnetite nanoparticles: a comparison with fatty acids. Langmuir 2001; 17: 7907–11.

130. Williams DN, Gold KA, Holoman TRP, et al. Surface modification of magnetic nanoparticles using gum arabic. J Nanoparticle Res 2006; 8: 749–53.

131. Inaba R, Fukahori T, Hamamoto M, et al. Synthesis of nanosized TiO_2 particles in reverse micelle systems and their photocatalytic activity for degradation of toluene in gas phase. J Mol Catal A: Chem 2006; 260: 247–54.

132. Toles CA, Marshall WE, Johns MM. Surface functional groups on acid-activated nutshell carbons. Carbon 1999; 37:1207–14.

133. Lemarchand C, Gref R, Lesieur S, et al. Physico-chemical characterization of polysaccharide-coated nanoparticles. J Control Release 2005; 108:97–111.

134. Köseoglu Y. Effect of surfactant coating on magnetic properties of Fe_3O_4 nanoparticles: ESR study. J Magn Magn Mater 2006; 300:327–33.

135. Hlaing Oo WM, McCluskey MD, Lalonde AD, et al. Infrared spectroscopy of ZnO nanoparticles containing CO_2 impurities. Appl Phys Lett 2005; 86: 073111.

136. Paredes JI, Burghard M. Dispersions of individual single-walled carbon nanotubes of high length. Langmuir 2004; 20:5149–52.

137. Beck MT. Solubility and molecular state of C60 and C70 in solvents and solvent mixtures. Pure Appl Chem 1998; 70:1881–7.

138. Ruoff RS, Tse DS, Malhotra R, et al. Solubility of C60 in a variety of solvents. J Phys Chem 1993; 97:3379–83.

139. Monteiro-Riviere NA, Inman AO, Wang YY, et al. Surfactant effects on carbon nanotube interactions with human keratinocytes. Nanomed: Nanotechnol, Biol Med 2005; 1:293–9.

140. Araujo L, Lobenberg R, Kreuter J. Influence of the surfactant concentration on the body distribution of nanoparticles. J Drug Target 1999; 6:373–85.

141. Oberdörster G, Sharp Z, Atudorei V, et al. Extrapulmonary translocation of ultrafine carbon particles following whole-body inhalation exposure of rats. J Toxicol Environ Health A 2002; 65:1531–43.

142. Rothen-Rutishauser BN, Schurch S, Aenni B, et al. Interaction of fine particles and nanoparticles with red blood cells visualized with advanced microscopic techniques. Environ Sci Technol 2006; 40:4353–9.

143. Brunner TJ, Wick P, Manser P, et al. In vitro cytotoxicity of oxide nanoparticles: comparison to asbestos, silica, and the effect of particle solubility. Environ Sci Technol 2006; 40:4374–81.

144. Andrievsky GV, Klochkov VK, Bordyuh AB, et al. Comparative analysis of two aqueous-colloidal solutions of C-60 fullerene with help of FTIR reflectance and UV-Vis spectroscopy. Chem Phys Lett 2002; 364:8–17.

145. Scharff P, Risch K, Carta-Abelmann L, et al. Structure of C-60 fullerene in water: spectroscopic data. Carbon 2004; 42:1203–6.

146. Oberdorster E. Manufactured nanomaterials (fullerenes, C60) induce oxidative stress in the brain of juvenile largemouth bass. Environ Health Perspect 2004; 112:1058–62.

147. Sayes CM, Gobin AM, Ausman KD, et al. Nano-C60 cytotoxicity is due to lipid peroxidation. Biomaterials 2005; 26:7587–95.

148. Gharbi N, Pressac M, Hadchouel M, et al. [60] Fullerene is a powerful antioxidant in vivo with no acute or subacute toxicity. Nano Lett 2005; 5: 2578–85.

149. Mori T, Takada H, Ito S, et al. Preclinical studies on safety of fullerene upon acute oral administration and evaluation for no mutagenesis. Toxicology 2006; 225:48–54.

150. Moussa F, Chretien P, Dubois P, et al. The influence of C-60 powders on cultured human leukocytes. Fullerene Sci Technol 1995; 3:333–42.

151. Moussa F, Chretien P, Pressac M, et al. Preliminary study of the influence of cubic C-60 on cultured human monocytes: lack of interleukin-1 beta secretion. Fullerene Sci Technol 1997; 5:503–10.

152. Levi N, Hantgan RR, Lively MO, et al. C60-fullerenes: detection of intracellular photoluminescence and lack of cytotoxic effects. J Nanobiotechnol 2006; 4:14.

153. Andrievsky G, Klochkov V, Derevyanchenko L. Is the C60 fullerene molecule toxic? Fullerenes Nanotubes and Carbon Nanostructures 2005; 13:363–76.

154. Casey A, Davoren M, Herzog E, et al. Probing the interaction of single walled carbon nanotubes within cell culture medium as a precursor to toxicity testing. Carbon 2007; 45:34–40.

155. Suslick KS, Fang MM, Hyeon T, et al. Applications of sonochemistry to materials synthesis. In:Crum LA, Mason TJ, Reisse J, Suslick KS, eds. Sonochemistry and Sonoluminescence. Netherlands: Kluwer Publishers, 1999: 291–320.

156. Fraunhofer W, Winter G, Coester C. Asymmetrical flow field-flow fractionation and multiangle light scattering for analysis of gelatin nanoparticle drug carrier systems. Anal Chem 2004; 76:1909–20.

157. Schmidt J, Vogelsberger W. Dissolution kinetics of titanium dioxide nanoparticles: the observation of an unusual kinetic size effect. J Phys Chem B 2006; 110:3955–63.

158. Demers LM, Mirkin CA, Mucic RC, et al. A fluorescence-based method for determining the surface coverage and hybridization efficiency of thiol-capped oligonucleotides bound to gold thin films and nanoparticles. Anal Chem 2000; 72:5535–41.

159. Oberdorster G, Sharp Z, Atudorei V, et al. Extrapulmonary translocation of ultrafine carbon particles following whole body inhalation exposure of rats. J Toxicol Environ Health A 2002; 65:1531–43.

160. Kreyling, WG, Semmler M, Erbe F, et al. Translocation of ultrafine insoluble iridium particles from lung epithelium to extrapulmonary organs is size dependent but very low. J Toxicol Environ Health A 2002; 65:1513–30.

161. Kapp N, Kreyling W, Schulz H, et al. Electron energy loss spectroscopy for analysis of inhaled ultrafine particles in rat lungs. Microsc Res Technol 2004; 63:298–305.

162. Bermudez E., Mangum JB, Asgharian B, et al. Long-term pulmonary responses of three laboratory rodent species to subchronic inhalation of pigmentary titanium dioxide particles. Toxicol Sci 2002; 70:86–97.

163. Grassian VH, O'Shaughnessy PT, Adamcakova-Dodd A, et al. Inhalation exposure study of titanium dioxide nanoparticles with a primary particle size of 2 to 5 nm. Environ Health Perspect, 2007; 115:397–402. In Press. Available via http://dx.doi.org/Online 4 December 2006.

164. Shama JOH, Zhang Y, Finlay WH, et al. Formulation and characterization of spray-dried powders containing nanoparticles for aerosol delivery to the lung. Int J Pharm 2004; 269:457–67.

165. Oberdörster G, Sharp Z, Atudorei V, et al. Translocation of inhaled ultrafine particles to the brain. Inhal Toxicol 2004; 16:437–45.

166. Kreyling WG, Semmler-Behnke M, Moller W. Health implications of nanoparticles. J Nanoparticle Res 2006; 8:543–62.

167. Pui DYH, Brock JR, Chen DR, et al. Instrumentation and measurement issues for nanometer particles: workshop summary. J Nanoparticle Res 2000; 2:103–12.

168. Dick WD, McMurry PH, Weber RJ, et al. White-light detection for nanoparticle sizing with the TSI ultrafine condensation particle counter. J Nanoparticle Res 2000; 2:85–90.

169. Fissan H. Ultrafine particles—measurement techniques. BIA-workshop ultrafine aerosols at workplace, Sankt Augustin, Germany, August 21–22, 2002. BG Institute for Occupational Safety and Health—BIA, BIA-Report 7/2003e.

170. Luther W. Industrial application of nanomaterials—chances and risks. Technology analysis. Published by: Future Technologies Division of VDI technologiezentrum GmbH Düsseldorf, Germany, 2004.

171. Chen DR, Pui DYH, Hummes D, et al. Design and evaluation of a nanometer aerosol differential mobility analyzer (Nano-DMA). J Aerosol Sci 1998; 29:497–509.

172. Kousaka Y, Okuyama K, Adachi M. Determination of particle size distribution of ultra-fine aerosols using a differential mobility analyzer. Aerosol Sci Technol 1985; 4:209–25.

173. Seto T, Nakamoto T, Okuyama K, et al. Size distribution measurement of nanometer-sized aerosol particles using DMA under low pressure conditions. J Aerosol Sci 1997; 28:193–206.

174. Kuga Y, Okauchi K, Takeda D, et al. Classification performance of a low pressure differential mobility analyzer for nanometer-sized particles. J Nanoparticle Res 2001; 3:175–83.

175. Fissan H, Neumann S, Trampe A, et al. Rationale and principle of an instrument measuring lung deposited nanoparticle surface area. J Nanoparticle Res 2007; 9:53–9.

176. HSE Health & Safety Executive. Nanoparticles: an occupational hygiene review. Prepared by the Institute of Occupational Medicine for the Health and Safety Executive, 2004.

177. Park K, Rai A, Zacharia MR. Characterizing the coating and size-resolved oxidative stability of carbon-coated aluminum nanoparticles by single-particle mass-spectrometry. J Nanoparticle Res 2006; 8:455–64.

178. Park K, Lee D, Rai A, et al. 2005. Size-resolved kinetic measurements of aluminium nanoparticle oxidation with single particle mass spectrometry. J Phys Chem B 2005; 109:7290–9.

179. Okada Y, Yabumoto J, Takeuchi K. Aerosol spectrometer for size and composition analysis of nanoparticles. Aerosol Sci 2002; 33:961–5.

180. Mulholland GW, Bauer BJ. Nanometer calibration particles: what's available and what's needed? J Nanoparticle Res 2000; 2:5–15.

181. Shi JP, Harrison RM, Evans D. Comparison of ambient particle surface area measurement by epiphaniometer and SMPS/APS. Atmos Environ 2001; 35: 6193–200.

182. Maynard AD. Estimating aerosol surface area from number and mass concentration measurements. Ann Occup Hygiene 2003; 47:123–44.

183. Gäggeler HW, Baltensperger U, Emmenegger M, et al. The epiphaniometer, a new device for continuous aerosol monitoring. J Aerosol Sci 1989; 20:557–64.

184. Burtscher H. Physical characterization of particulate emissions from diesel engines: a review. J Aerosol Sci 2005; 36:896–932.

185. Jung HJ, Kittelson DB. Characterization of aerosol surface instruments in transition regime. Aerosol Sci Technol 2005; 39:902–11.

186. Ku BK, Maynard AD. Generation and investigation of airborne Ag nanoparticles with specific size and morphology by homogeneous nucleation, coagulation and sintering. J Aerosol Sci 2005; 36:1108–24.

187. Karlsson LS, Deppert K, Malm JO. Size determination of Au aerosol nanoparticles by off-line TEM/STEM observations. J Nanoparticle Res 2006; 8:971–80.

188. Pui DYH, Flagan RC, Kaufman SL, et al. Experimental methods and instrumentation. NSF Workshop Report on Emerging Issues in Nanoparticle Aerosol Science and Technology (NAST). Los Angeles, California, June 27–28, 2003.

189. Bhattacharya J, Choudhuri U, Siwach O, et al. Interaction of hemoglobin and copper nanoparticles: implications in hemoglobinopathy. Nanomed: Nanotechnol, Biol, Med 2006; 2:191–9.

190. Wallace WE, Keane MJ, Murray DK, et al. Phospholipid lung surfactant and nanoparticle surface toxicity: lessons from diesel soots and silicate dusts. J Nanoparticle Res 2007; 9:23–38.

191. Singh R, Panzarotto D, Lacerda L, et al. Tissue biodistribution and blood clearance rates of intravenously administered carbon nanotube radiotracers. PNAS 2006; 103:3357–362.

192. Patra CR, Bhattacharya R, Patra S, et al. Inorganic phosphate nanorods are a novel fluorescent label in cell biology. J Nanobiotechnol 2006; 4:11.

193. Davda J, Labhasetwar V. Characterization of nanoparticle uptake by endothelial cells. Int J Pharm 2002; 233:51–9.

194. Kirchner C, Liedl T, Kudera S, et al. Cytotoxicity of colloidal CdSe and CdSe/ZnS nanoparticles. Nano Lett 2005; 5:331–8.

195. Bielinska A, Eichman JD, Lee I, et al. Imaging {Au^0-PAMAM} gold-dendrimer nanocomposites in cells. J Nanoparticle Res 2002; 4:395–403.

196. Ballou B, Lagerholm BC, Ernst LA, et al. Noninvasive imaging of quantum dots in mice. Bioconjug Chem 2004; 15:79–86.

197. Akerman ME, Chan WCW, Laakkonen P, et al. Nanocrystal targeting in vivo. PNAS 2002; 99:12617–21.
198. Menzel T, Vogt RJ, Butz T. Investigations of percutaneous uptake of ultrafine TiO₂ particles at the high energy ion nanoprobe LIPSION. Nucl Instrum Meth Phys Res Sec B: Beam Interact Mater Atoms 2004; 219–20:82–6.
199. Pflücker F, Wendel V, Hohenberg H, et al. The human stratum corneum layer: an effective barrier against dermal uptake of different forms of topically applied micronised titanium dioxide. Skin Pharmacol Appl Skin Physiol 2001; 14:92–7.
200. Mavon A, Miquel C, Lejeune O, et al. In vitro percutaneous absorption and in vivo stratum corneum distribution of an organic and a mineral sunscreen. Skin Pharmacol Physiol 2007; 20:10–20.
201. Ladinsky MS, Pierson JM, McIntosh JR. Vitreous cryo-sectioning of cells facilitated by a micromanipulator. J Microsc 2006; 224:129–34.
202. Taylor JR, Fang MM, Nie S. Probing specific sequences on single DNA molecules with bioconjugated fluorescent nanoparticles. Anal Chem 2000; 72: 1979–86.
203. Mitchell GP, Mirkin CA, Letsinger RL. Programmed assembly of DNA functionalized quantum dots. J Am Chem Soc 1999; 121:8122–3.
204. Schultz S, Smith DR, Mock JJ, et al. Single-target molecule detection with nonbleaching multicolor optical immunolabels. PNAS 2000; 97:996–1001.
205. Santra S, Zhang P, Wang K, et al. Conjugation of biomolecules with luminophore-doped silica nanoparticles for photostable biomarkers. Anal Chem 2001; 73:4988–93.
206. Dubertret B, Calame M, Libchaber AJ. Single-mismatch detection using gold-quenched fluorescent oligonucleotides. Nat Biotechnol 2001; 19:365–70.
207. Ye Z, Tan M, Wang G, et al. Preparation, characterization, and time-resolved fluorometric application of silica-coated terbium(III) fluorescent nanoparticles. Anal Chem 2004; 76:513–8.
208. Pan YL, Cai JY, Qin L, et al. Atomic force microscopy-based cell nanostructure for ligand-conjugated quantum dot endocytosis. Acta Biochim Biophys Sin 2006; 38:646–52.
209. McNeil SC. Nanotechnology for the biologist. J Leukoc Biol 2005; 78:585–94.
210. Singh R, Panzarotto D, Lacerda L, et al. Tissue biodistribution and blood clearance rates of intravenously administered carbon nanotube radiotracers. PNAS 2006; 103:3357–62.
211. Jani P, Halbert GW, Langridge J, et al. Nanoparticle uptake by the rat gastrointestinal mucosa: quantitation and particle size dependency. J Pharm Pharmacol 1990; 42:821–6.
212. Gulson B, Wong H. Stable isotopic tracing-a way forward for nano-technology. Environ Health Perspect 2006; 114:1486–8.
213. Cagle DW, Kennel SJ, Mirzadeh S, et al. In vivo studies of fullerene-based materials using endohedral metallofullerene radiotracers. PNAS 1999; 96: 5182–7.
214. Takenaka S, Karg E, Roth C, et al. Pulmonary and systemic distribution of inhaled ultrafine silver particles in rats. Environ Health Perspect 2001; 109: 547–51.

215. Kückelhaus S, Tedesco AC, Oliveira DM, et al. Optical emission spectroscopy as a tool for the biodistribution investigation of cobalt-ferrite nanoparticles in mice. J Appl Phys 2005; 97 :10Q910.
216. Gojova A, Guo B, Kota RS, et al. Induction of inflammation in vascular endothelial cells by metal oxide nanoparticles: effect of particle composition. Environ Health Perspect, In press. Available via http://dx.doi.org/. Online 11 December 2006.
217. Zhang Y, Kohler N, Zhang M. Surface modification of superparamagnetic magnetite nanoparticles and their intracellular uptake. Biomaterials 2002; 23: 1553–61.
218. Andersson M, Fromell K, Gullberg E, et al. Characterization of surface-modified nanoparticles for in vivo biointeraction. A sedimentation field flow fractionation study. Anal Chem 2005; 77:5488–93.
219. Moussa F, Pressac M, Genin E, et al. Quantitative analysis of C-60 fullerene in blood and tissues by high-performance liquid chromatography with photo-diode-array and mass spectrometric detection. J Chromatogr B-Anal Technol Biomed Life Sci 1997; 696:153–9.
220. Xia XR, Monteiro-Riviere NA, Riviere JE. Trace analysis of fullerenes in biological samples by simplified liquid–liquid extraction and high-performance liquid chromatography. J Chromatogr A 2006; 1129:216–22.
221. Chen B, Selegue JP. Separation and characterization of single-walled and multiwalled carbon nanotubes by using flow field-flow fractionation. Anal Chem 2002; 74:4774–80.

4

Physicochemical Characteristics of Nanoparticles that Determine Potential Toxicity

Bice Fubini, Ivana Fenoglio, and Maura Tomatis

Interdepartmental Center "G. Scansetti" for Studies on Asbestos and Other Toxic Particulates and Dipartimento di Chimica IFM, University of Torino, Torino, Italy

INTRODUCTION

Nanoparticles (NPs) are not, as media report, a toxic entity per se, for example, just because of their size. Some NPs, because of their physicochemical features, including size, may constitute a serious hazard to human health. NPs are not only a product of the new nanotechnologies. NPs are present in the environment, and nanoscale phenomena permeate and often control natural processes. Humans have always experienced exposure to some nanosized particles in nature, which could thus be an important source of information on how to make harmless NPs. With the advent of the industrial revolution, "anthropogenic" sources of NPs appeared (e.g., internal combustion engines, power plants, etc.), which are now scattered worldwide. Whether the smallest particle fraction in polluted air is the most responsible one for adverse health effects is still a matter of debate, which could be solved by a systematic approach on what makes an NP toxic.

Because of their peculiar physical and chemical features, the study of NPs as potential toxic agents requires an interdisciplinary approach, involving multiple aspects ranging from physics and chemistry to biology and medicine. In the past, it was assumed that ultrafine particles would be easily exhaled, as opposed to those that are micron-sized, which would be retained in the lung. Conversely to this hypothesis, an enhanced toxicity to experimental animals and cell cultures, which has been reported in some cases when passing from micron- to nanosized particles of the same composition (e.g., titania, carbon particles, etc.), has raised a serious alarm in the past few years. Was this due to small size, to the high amount of surface exposed, or to a specific reactivity toward biomolecules and cells? In all cases the different behavior was linked to some physicochemical features, which need to be elucidated and clarified in order to identify any hazard from manufactured NP as well as to identify a safe method for the production of NP to be used in biomedicine. Nanosized particles in fact constitute a double-edged sword for human health: on the one hand, as previously outlined, NPs may turn out to be a serious hazard, while on the other they also hold great potential as drug delivery system, diagnostic tool, and therapeutic to well-defined targets in the body.

PHYSICOCHEMICAL DETERMINANTS IN PARTICLE TOXICOLOGY

The widely accepted physicochemical determinants in traditional particle toxicology are:

- the form of the particle (e.g., fibers more potent toxicant than isometric particles, spiky fractured crystals more potent than smooth roundish particles);
- the chemical composition and related surface reactivity (free radical-generating surface sites, poorly coordinated and easily removable metal ions, strong adsorption and modification of endogenous antioxidants or of proteins);
- the time of residence in a given body compartment generally defined as biopersistence (a property related both to chemical factors, such as solubility, adsorption potential, and to the cellular and tissue response to it).

At what extent and in which direction such properties are modified when particles are ground or prepared down to the nanolevel? The data so far available are not sufficient to give any general indication on this point. Contrasting results in toxicological tests on titania isometric particles and nanorods (1,2) or on quartz NPs (3) mainly suggest that many factors, beside nanosize, regulate toxicity, e.g., preparation route, crystallinity, origin of the dust, etc.

NANOPARTICLES VS. MICRON-SIZE PARTICLES: WHAT ARE THE RELEVANT PHYSICAL AND CHEMICAL DIFFERENCES RELATABLE TO TOXICITY?

The physicochemical features that make NPs different from their larger counterparts, may be summarized as follows:

1. Nanosize

2. Extremely large specific surface (surface exposed per unit mass)
3. High ratio of surface to bulk atoms with consequently higher surface reactivity
4. Specific reactivity arising at the nanolevel
5. Chemical structure linked to nanosize: absence of any larger counterpart
6. Strong interparticle forces

Nanosize

Mobility within the body and various penetration routes due to the small size of NP have been largely described in exhaustive reviews (4,5) and in other chapters of this book.

Two things should be pointed out when considering the molecular mechanisms of interaction of inhaled NPs: the comparable size of NP with cell membrane receptors, and the lower uptake of NP compared with larger particles by alveolar macrophages (6). Figure 1 depicts the expected scenario in the alveoli when NPs are inhaled: while most of the effects of larger particles are explained by a persistent inflammatory effect, a lower macrophage uptake of NPs involves reduced clearance (step 2) and reduced inflammatory response (step 3). However a longer residence of free NP in the alveolar space may imply a major direct challenge to target cells e.g., through

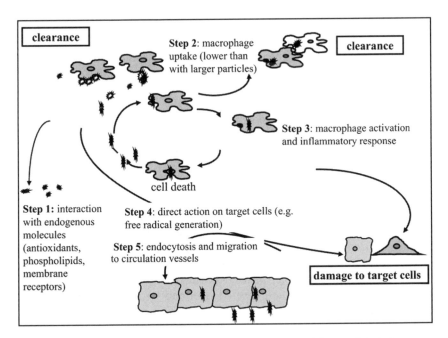

Figure 1 Expected scenario in the alveoli when nanoparticles are inhaled.

particle-generated free radical release (step 4), strong and prolonged interaction with endogenous molecules (antioxidants, phospholipids, membrane receptors) (step 1), and finally endocytosis and migration to circulation vessels (step 5).

Extremely Large Specific Surface

The much larger surface area exposed by any NP, with respect to the same mass of bigger particles, is a direct consequence of the small size of NPs, not a new property per se. This apparently obvious fact, however, highlights a crucial question, which was already put forward in "traditional" particle toxicology, i.e., which dose metric should be used when comparing the adverse effects of particles of different sizes and nature (7)? Expression of exposures (human data) and doses (animal and mechanistic data) could be given in different dose units but are commonly given per weight, which is the easiest one to measure, even if it is the least appropriate with poorly insoluble solid particles. When inhaled, particles usually act through their surface, which comes in contact with fluids and tissues, or as solid xenobiotics, whose biological activity is related to their form or number of particles. Thus, both surface area exposed and number of particles should be employed as dose units instead of weight (8–10).

Pulmonary toxicology studies in rats have reported that nanoscale particles, when administered to the lung of experimental animals, cause a greater inflammatory response when compared to micron-scale particles of identical composition at equivalent mass concentrations. In many of these studies, however, the experimental points did fit the same trend when doses were expressed per exposed surface instead than per weight (5). Thus it is questionable whether the nanosized particles are always intrinsically more toxic than their larger counterparts, or that the amount in weight which determines a given surface-dependent toxic effect, is much lower with nano than with micron-sized particles. Thus when comparing nano- versus micron-sized particles, the use of units of exposed surface is the most appropriate if there is evidence that the inflammatory response and mediators are surface dependent. In this context, the concept of overload—excess dusts in the lung, which causes cancer irrespective of the nature of the particles—should also be revisited, as carcinogenicity with NPs may originate in experimental animals as a consequence at weights below the overload values for micron-sized particles, but at surface areas exposed exceeding those corresponding to overload with micron-sized particles. In such cases, the overload registered with micron-sized particles should be converted into exposed surface area and the expected overload with corresponding NPs should be defined as the weight in NPs, which corresponds to the overload exposed surface area in the larger particle counterparts. Interestingly the International Agency for Research on Cancer, IARC, has recently classified

TiO_2 as 2B (possible animal carcinogen) mainly on the basis of positive results in experimental studies on TiO_2 NPs. Perhaps, once revisited on the basis of the newly defined overload, those studies would no longer indicate titania as a possible specific carcinogen.

Another consequence of the large exposed surface is the possibility that some of the products of a cellular reaction, and particularly those which are used to evaluate a biological activity might be simply adsorbed at the particle surface, thus inhibiting the correct evaluation of the test performed. Considerable amounts of the cytosolic enzyme lactate dehydrogenase (LDH), employed as a reflection of cytotoxicity, and the two most used cytokines to monitor inflammation, were adsorbed on carbon black NPs, suggesting that cytotoxicity and inflammatory responses to NPs could be underestimated because of such artifacts (11).

High Ratio of Surface to Bulk Atoms with Consequently Higher Surface Reactivity

Beside the extent of the surface area, which, as discussed above, is a quantitative measure, when approaching the smallest size, surface reactivity, even if measured per unit surface, is enhanced. Surface reactivity is usually linked to defective position of atoms or ions at the surface, with unsatisfied valencies or vacancies in the coordination sphere. Such sites, as illustrated in Figure 2, are often relatable to steps, kinks, and edges, or otherwise irregular atoms/ ions positions at the surface of the particles. Such sites are likely to be more abundant at the surface of small particles. Poorly coordinated transition metal ions or dangling bonds, caused by homolytic rupture of covalent bonds at the surface, are the catalytic sites where free radical generation, yielding formation of reactive oxygen species (ROS), takes place (12–14).

Specific Reactivity Arising at the Nanolevel

In the past few decades, the standard elementary school definition of the difference between atoms and molecules was: the molecule is the tiniest part of a substance, which keeps its properties unchanged. This, as is now clear to any chemist, is incorrect. How many molecules (or atoms or ions) do we need to obtain a piece of material, which bears the same properties of the bulk of it? Or conversely, until what point will a reduction in size not yield a marked variation in some physicochemical properties? Such variation may also reflect different biological activity of the NP with respect to the bulk. TiO_2 NPs and quantum dots (e.g., CdSe) belong to this category.

Titania has been employed in a large spectrum of products, including pharmaceutics and cosmetics. TiO_2 NPs are produced and largely employed in sunscreens, as they are powerful absorbent of UV radiations. Titania is a very white powder, but when the particle size becomes of the order of

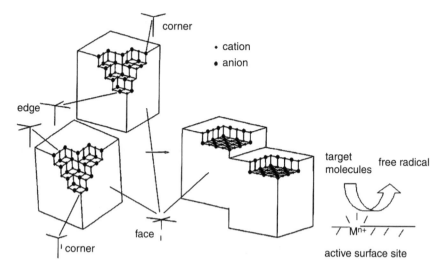

Figure 2 Enhanced surface reactivity: defective position of atoms or ions, with unsatisfied valencies or vacancies in the coordination sphere, at the surface.

magnitude of the visible wavelength it becomes transparent, thus much appropriate for its cosmetic usage. Unfortunately, in these circumstances the particles also exhibit a marked photocatalytic activity, which yields ROS release and which may damage the skin. In order to prepare safe powders to be used in sunscreen products, researchers have to look for conditions in which the transparency is maintained but the photocatalytic activity is inhibited. A major role is played by the crystal structure, rutile being much less photoactive than anatase (2), and by appropriate coating procedures.

CdSe nanocrystals are cytotoxic. When coated with a ZnS (CdSe/ZnS) the critical concentration, up to which no toxic effect is observed, is increased by a factor of 10 (15). Cytotoxicity also decreases when a ligand shell of mercaptopropionic acid coats the particles, even if such shell is not stable enough to prevent the release of Cd^{2+} ions from the particle surface, suggesting a role of surface phenomena. Moreover cytotoxicity correlated with the internalization of the particle and not only with the release of toxic Cd^{2+} ions. Thus, if such material is to be employed, research on the most appropriate coatings will be urgently required.

Chemical Structure Linked to Nanosize: Absence of Any Larger Counterpart

There are specific NP products that have no real larger equivalent, but exist in only a small number of nanoscale dimensions. This is the typical case for all the large known varieties of carbon nanotubes (singlewall, multiwall), all very biopersistent and made up of filaments a few microns long, with diameters of about 6 to 20 nm. Such compounds fall into the category of fibers because of their extremely high aspect ratio, and for this reasons they have been suspected to act on human health similar to asbestos (Fig. 3). Their chemical nature is complicated because they invariably contain a variety of residual impurities, mainly metals, organics, and support materials (16). The most commonly used metals for their growth are Fe, Co, Ni, and Mo. A large part of these impurities may be eliminated by chemical purification procedures, but traces often remain, and may be reactive. A few reviews have appeared reporting respiratory toxicity in experimental animals (17,18) and damage to cells in culture. The results are somewhat controversial, but there is a general consensus on the variability in the health effect caused by various kinds of CNTs, most likely related to the different preparation and purification routes. Those deprived of metals, particularly iron appear, similarly to asbestos, far less toxic (19). However, in contrast to asbestos, CNTs are hydrophobic, and in some cases do not generate free radicals, and rather act as quenchers (20). Thus their toxicity has to be ascribed to features different from those involved in asbestos toxicity.

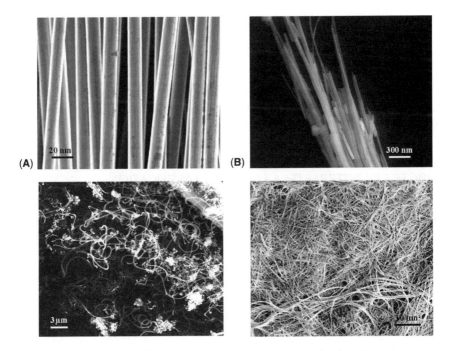

Figure 3 Scanning electron microscopy (SEM) images of (**A**) carbon nanotubes and (**B**) chrysotile asbestos fibers. *Source*: Courtesy of (**A**) Domenica Scarano and Federico Cesano and (**B**) Francesco Turci.

Strong Interparticle Forces

The smaller the particle, the stronger are the interparticle forces that attract NPs, with consequent aggregation and agglomeration. This is very important because aggregated particles behave in a different way from those that are isolated. When aggregation (van der Waals forces) evolves toward agglomeration (chemical bonds between the particles), what results is a nanostructured material, which can no longer be considered as NP. Surface charges, hydrophobicity, and adsorption of biomolecules from the media are the major determinants of such processes.

Interparticle forces act as strongly as intermolecular forces when particle size is very small. Is there a great difference between clustered carbon nanotubes and the graphite layers in graphite or chrysotile fibrils in a real fiber? Obviously such forces vary in different media, e.g., NPs, particularly when they are very hydrophobic, like CNTs, may be separated in air but clustered in water. Indeed this is great inconvenient when planning *in vitro* cellular tests or *in vivo* experiments, in which they should be administered to animal in a way close to the hypothesized exposure in humans. In some cases, clumping immediately killed the rats! Note that in water, individual NPs can seldom stay separated from those around them.

Hydrophobicity plays a major role in agglomeration in water via "hydrophobic interparticle forces," which means that one way to disperse some NPs, typically carbon nanotubes, is to oxidize them, in order to increase hydrophilicity due to formation of oxygen–carbon surface functionalities.

It is noteworthy that in the case of the above-mentioned CdSe and CdSe/ZnS surface modified nanodots their stability, with regard to aggregation, played an important role for cytotoxicity (15).

NANOPARTICLES: HIGHER OR LOWER TOXICITY THAN THEIR LARGER COUNTERPARTS? A POSSIBLE CLASSIFICATION

The alarm over the possible health effects caused by NPs began when several pulmonary toxicology studies in rats and mice revealed that many nanoscale particles, when administered to the lung of experimental animals, caused a large and persistent inflammatory response. NPs could be classified on the basis of such findings into three categories.

Greater Effect than Larger Particles per Unit Mass, but Same per Unit Surface

This mainly shows that the effect elicited is driven by the exposed surface area, thus bound to increase in intensity when particle size decreases and consequently the specific surface increases; e.g., intratracheal installation in rats and mice of 20 and 250 nm TiO_2 NPs induces a higher inflammatory response (measured as percentages of neutrophils) when compared per unit mass, while the effects were comparable when expressed at equal surface exposed.

Effect Similar to or Less than with Larger Particles

This indicates that other factors, besides exposed surface, play a role, which might play a greater role in larger particles than in those that are nanosized; e.g., the inflammatory effects of nanoscale TiO_2 rods as well as nano-TiO_2 dots (20 nm) were not significantly different from larger TiO_2 particles (300 nm) at equivalent weight doses (1). Thus, as inflammatory effects mainly depend on the exposed surface area, this suggests that features such as form (dots, rods) or the preparation route followed to obtain such forms involve a lowering and not an increase in toxicity. Crystalline silica NPs (quartz) have been prepared with the aim to detect whether nanosize would increase the toxicity of a highly toxic and inflammatory material, such as quartz. Unexpectedly, such material was less toxic than the commercial dust specimen usually employed as a reference (Min-U-Sil) even when simply compared at equal mass (3). We believe that in such case much has to be ascribed to the preparation route and not to the size of the examined particles. In order to prepare quartz in nanocrystalline form a hydrothermal preparation route was followed. This is the only known way for such preparation as grinding larger particle of quartz, in our experience, does create a small fraction in the nanosize range but the majority of the particles remain in the micron size range. The hydrothermal procedure, however, yields rather smooth particles with all valencies satisfied by the surrounding medium, i.e., fully hydrated. Such particles are quite different from the sharp ones generated by abrasion and grinding.

Higher Effect Even When Compared per Unit Surface

Only in such cases a true adverse surface reactivity appears specifically at the nanoscale; e.g., in Lison et al. (21) it was shown that the lung inflammatory response (LDH release), after intratracheal instillation in mice, of various MnO_2 dusts, with different size, increases when particle dimension decreases and regularly depends on the total surface area. But when the particles were ground, an enhanced cytotoxic activity was shown, indicating that new undefined reactive sites were produced at the particle surface by mechanical cleavage. The iron oxide hematite in nanosize released free radicals in different free radical generation models, while micron-sized particles of the same composition did not (22). This has to be ascribed to the much larger amount of surface iron atoms with free coordination positions at the surface. Accordingly, when tested on cell culture the nanosized samples showed a much higher toxicity (23).

THE REQUIREMENT FOR APPROPRIATE MODEL PARTICLES AND FOR THE ESTABLISHMENT OF A REPOSITORY OF PARTICLES FOR TESTING

One of the reasons of the relative insuccess in finding out the mechanisms of action at the molecular level of most pathogenic fibers and particles (even the most renown e.g., asbestos or silica) is, in our opinion, the lack of model solids in experimental studies. All real dusts have surface properties much linked to the history of the sample, the comminution routes, the presence of contaminants acquired during processing, etc. In order to know the role played by such factors a set of pure samples, only differing one from the other for a single property, should have been used. Instead, the employment of real dusts in virtually all experimental studies has brought up to what is called "The variability of quartz hazard" (24) in the case of the pathogenity of crystalline silica. A variability mainly linked to the variability in surface properties from one to the other sample (25). Similarly other toxic dusts e.g., asbestos, artificial mineral fibers, have also been tested without proper reference materials, e.g., a pure specimen of the mineral/material under study. This obviously reflects the whole history of particle toxicology in the past century. The awareness of the toxicity of some particles/fibers was mainly raised by large numbers of morbidity and death followed by epidemiological studies. The hypothesis on the mineral particle as causative agents was put forward and, only at the end, the interest was addressed to the possible mechanisms of action. With NP we need to follow the opposite way: i.e., identify adverse physicochemical properties before any toxic material has been largely produced and people is consequently exposed. This requires the accurate preparation of model solids to be employed in experimental studies along the following lines:

- Particles of different sizes, but prepared with the same procedure, thus with the same surface properties, in order to evaluate the effect of enhanced surface reactivity at the nanolevel. The test should be performed both in order to compare exposures to the same surface or to the same number of particles.
- Particles prepared via different routes, but with the same dimensions in order to evaluate the effect of different preparation procedures.
- Particles prepared in the different forms; e.g., rods, whiskers, etc., in which they are bound to be proposed for the market.
- Particles doped with the possible contaminants, which are likely to be adsorbed during usage.

REFERENCES

1. Warheit DB, Webb TR, Sayes CM, et al. Pulmonary instillation studies with nanoscale TiO_2 rods and dots in rats: toxicity is not dependent upon particle size and surface area. Toxicol Sci 2006; 91:227–36.

2. Sayes CM, Wahi R, Kurian PA, et al. Correlating nanoscale titania structure with toxicity: a cytotoxicity and inflammatory response study with human dermal fibroblasts and human lung epithelial cells. Toxicol Sci 2006; 92:174–85.

3. Warheit DB, Webb TR, Colvin VL, et al. Pulmonary bioassay studies with nanoscale and fine-quartz particles in rats: toxicity is not dependent upon particle size but on surface characteristics. Toxicol Sci 2007; 95:270–80.

4. Nel A, Xia T, Madler L, et al. Toxic potential of materials at the nanolevel. Science 2006; 311:622–7.

5. Oberdorster G, Oberdorster E, Oberdorster J. Nanotoxicology: an emerging discipline evolving from studies of ultrafine particles. Environ Health Perspect 2005; 113:823–39.

6. Oberdorster G, Ferin J, Gelein R, et al. Role of the alveolar macrophage in lung injury: studies with ultrafine particles. Environ Health Perspect 1992; 97: 193–9.

7. Fubini B. Use of physico-chemical and cell-free assays to evaluate the potential carcinogenicity of fibres. IARC Sci Publ 1996; 140:35–54.

8. Oberdorster G, Maynard A, Donaldson K, et al. Principles for characterizing the potential human health effects from exposure to nanomaterials: elements of a screening strategy. Part Fibre Toxicol 2005; 2:8.

9. Moss OR, Wong VA. When nanoparticles get in the way: impact of projected area on in vivo and in vitro macrophage function. Inhal Toxicol 2006; 18: 711–6.

10. Moss OR. Insights into the health effects of nanoparticles: why numbers matter. 2006; 26:1–7.

11. Monteiro-Riviere NA, Inman AO. Challenges for Assessing Carbon Nanomaterial Toxicity to the Skin. Carbon 2006; 44:1070–1078.

12. Fenoglio I, Prandi L, Tomatis M, et al. Free radical generation in the toxicity of inhaled mineral particles: the role of iron speciation at the surface of asbestos and silica. Redox Rep 2001; 6:235–41.

13. Fubini B, Fenoglio I, Elias Z, et al. Variability of biological responses to silicas: effect of origin, crystallinity, and state of surface on generation of reactive oxygen species and morphological transformation of mammalian cells. J Environ Pathol Toxicol Oncol 2001; 20 (Suppl. 1):95–108.

14. Fubini B, Hubbard A. Reactive oxygen species (ROS) and reactive nitrogen species (RNS) generation by silica in inflammation and fibrosis. Free Radic Biol Med 2003; 34:1507–16.

15. Kirchner C, Liedl T, Kudera S, et al. Cytotoxicity of colloidal CdSe and CdSe/ZnS nanoparticles. Nano Lett 2005; 5:331–8.

16. Donaldson K, Aitken R, Tran L, et al. Carbon nanotubes: a review of their properties in relation to pulmonary toxicology and workplace safety. Toxicol Sci 2006; 92:5–22.

17. Lam CW, James JT, McCluskey R, et al. A review of carbon nanotube toxicity and assessment of potential occupational and environmental health risks. Crit Rev Toxicol 2006; 36:189–217.

18. Muller J, Huaux F, Lison D, et al. Respiratory toxicity of carbon nanotubes: How worried should we be? Carbon 2006; 44:1048–56.

19. Kagan VE, Tyurina YY, Tyurin VA, et al. Direct and indirect effects of single walled carbon nanotubes on RAW 264.7 macrophages: role of iron. Toxicol Lett 2006; 165:88–100.

20. Fenoglio I, Tomatis M, Lison D, et al. Reactivity of carbon nanotubes: free radical generation or scavenging activity? Free Radic Biol Med 2006; 40: 1227–33.

21. Lison D, Lardot C, Huaux F, et al. Influence of particle surface area on the toxicity of insoluble manganese dioxide dusts. Arch Toxicol 1997; 71:725–9.

22. Fubini B, Fenoglio I, Martra G, et al. An overview on the toxicity of inhaled nanoparticles. In: Blitz JP, Gun'ko V, eds. Surface Chemistry in Biomedical and Environmental Science. NATO Science Series II: Mathematics, Physics and Chemistry. New York: Springer, 2006:241–52.

23. Ceschino R. Relazioni tra proprietà di superficie e potenziale patogeno di particolati tossici inalabili [PhD Thesis]. Italy: University of Turin, 2004.

24. Donaldson K, Borm PJ. The quartz hazard: a variable entity. Ann Occup Hyg 1998; 42:287–94.

25. Fubini B. Chemical aspects in the toxicity of mineral dusts and fibers. Mater Eng 1996; 7:249–75.

5

Exposure Assessment Considerations for Nanoparticles in the Workplace

Mark D. Hoover, Aleksandr B. Stefaniak, Gregory A. Day, and
Charles L. Geraci

*National Institute for Occupational Safety and Health, Morgantown, West Virginia
and Cincinnati, Ohio, U.S.A.*

INTRODUCTION

Engineered nanoparticles are increasingly being developed and used for myriad electronic, pharmaceutical, automotive, aerospace, and other product applications. During handling of nanoparticles throughout their lifecycle, the potential exists for inhalation, dermal, and possibly ingestion exposures of people to nanoparticles, as well as potential environmental impact. The exposures can involve a wide range of nanoparticle sizes, shapes, functionalities, concentrations and exposure frequencies and durations. Anticipating, recognizing, evaluating, and controlling those exposures is key to protecting the health of researchers, production workers, users, and members of the public. This chapter describes key issues for understanding, applying, and expanding the concepts of exposure assessment to make safe management of nanomaterials a reality. Focus is on measurement and exposure assessment in research and occupational settings, which provide early opportunities for prevention of potential illness and injury and for development and sharing of realistic experience and understanding of nanoparticle behavior. In conjunction with other chapters in this book, principles of exposure assessment can be combined with information on the characteristics, characterization methods, physicochemical properties, and biological behavior and associated toxicity of engineered nanoparticles to manage the development and use of nanotechnology in a safe manner.

EXPOSURE PATHWAYS AND THEIR SIGNIFICANCE

In an ideal world, a comprehensive exposure pathway model (Fig. 1) for transport of particles from a source such as a nanomaterial production or handling operation to air, to surfaces, and to workers or other individuals would be identified and understood. The pathway model would be accompanied by a comprehensive job-exposure matrix (Fig. 1) describing the temporal history of work jobs and associated exposure conditions for each potentially exposed individual. There would be an understanding of the particle size distribution of any potentially airborne nanoparticles or nanomaterial-containing particles and the likelihood that such particles might deposit in the various regions of the respiratory tract (Fig. 2). There would also be a scheme for selecting an appropriate level of control based on information about "determinants of exposure" such as the amount of material handled, its dustiness, flammability, reactivity, etc., and its potential toxicity due to particle size, mass, number, surface area, functionality, or other biologically relevant properties. To support decision making about measurement, exposure and control, there would be straightforward equations (see below) or comprehensive algorithms that would relate the conditions of work activities and worker exposure to estimated health effects from individual work tasks as well as throughout a nanoproduct life cycle and supply chain. There would also be an understanding of the inherent uncertainty or variability associated with key aspects of exposure situations (Figs. 2 and 3) and of how the various possible measures of exposure (e.g., average, cumulative, peak, or temporal patterns) relate to potential acute or chronic health effects such as irritation, sensitization, carcinogenicity, or toxicity to the skin or eyes, respiratory tract, central nervous system, or other target organs. *Prospectively*, the pathway model, job-exposure matrix, and relational equation approach would be used to design safe work facilities and practices. *Contemporaneously*, the modeling and exposure assessment approach would

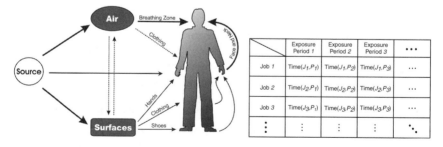

Figure 1 Comprehensive pathway model for use in task-specific assessment and control of exposures to nanoparticles and conceptual design of a comprehensive job-exposure matrix to document temporal work activities and exposure characteristics for each worker. *Source*: From Ref. 12.

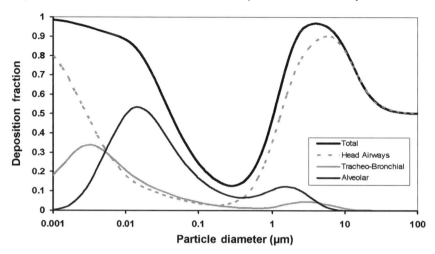

Figure 2 Illustration of particle size-dependent deposition of airborne particles in the human respiratory tract based on the ICRP 66 Human Respiratory Tract Model relationships for an adult, nose-breathing male during light exercise. *Abbreviation*: ICRP, International Commission on Radiological Protection. *Source*: From Ref. 1.

be used to monitor and verify that exposures are under control. *Retrospectively*, the approach could be used in health surveillance to reevaluate and understand any dose-response relationships between exposures to nanoparticles and unexpected health effects, if sufficient information about the material characteristics and behavior were available.

Relating Key Exposure Assessment Parameters

The following simple linear equation provides useful insights into key considerations for an effective exposure assessment:

$$\text{Risk of Health Effect} = (\text{MAR} * \text{DR} * \text{ARF} * \text{RF} * \text{CF} * \text{BR} * \text{T} * \text{DCF}) / \text{V}.$$

- MAR is the material-at-risk (nanograms, milligrams, grams, kilograms, or megagrams).
- DR is the damage ratio (what fraction of the material is disrupted or subject to dispersion during the work activity). This term takes into account the fact that not all of the material that may be present in a process is subject to disruption. A consistent approach must be used to associate a DR with a corresponding MAR. For example, material in storage would not have the same DR factor for mechanical disruption and dispersion as material being processed in a manufacturing step.
- ARF is the Airborne Release Fraction (or rate for a continuous release). This term takes into account the fact that only a small fraction of the disrupted material may be actually dispersed into the air by the process or event of interest, and that the airborne release fraction will depend on the physical

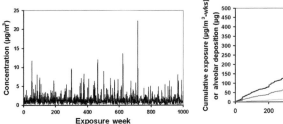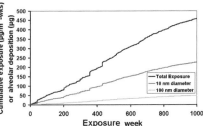

Figure 3 Illustration of the temporal variability (*left*) and cumulative exposure profile (μg/m³-weeks) (*right*) that may be encountered during assessment of occupational exposures to airborne nanoparticles. Population of values is lognormally distributed with a median geometric standard deviation for total exposure variability of 2.4, as observed by Kromhout et al. for a wide range of exposures to chemical agents. The individual values were obtained using the Crystal Ball Monte Carlo simulation tool. The median concentration value of 1 μg/m³ and the sampling frequency of once per week were arbitrarily selected for the illustration. Estimates of the cumulative amounts of airborne material (μg) actually deposited in the alveolar region of the respiratory tract are shown for assumed particle diameters of 10 nm and 100 nm, based on the alveolar lung deposition efficiency values of 0.49 and 0.11, respectively, presented 3 for the ICRP 66 Human Respiratory Tract Model. *Sources*: From Refs. 1, 22, and 23.

form of the material (perhaps 0.00002 for a vitrified source material in a closed metal container, 0.0001 for a solid, 0.001 for a liquid, and 0.01 for a powder). If a variation of this equation is being used for assessment of dermal exposure, the release fraction would be associated with those particles that could present themselves for skin exposure.

■ RF is the Respirable Fraction (particles smaller than 10 μm aerodynamic diameter, if concern is only for particles that may deposit in the alveolar region of the respiratory tract). There may be opportunities to reduce the magnitude of the ARF and RF values by controlling environmental factors such as humidity, temperature, conditions of material aging or storage, and methods of equipment or facility operation and housekeeping. Figure 3 uses the particle-size dependent relationships of the International Commission on Radiological Protection (ICRP) Human Respiratory Tract Model (1) to illustrate how regional deposition in the respiratory tract varies with particle size. For health concerns related to exposure to nanoparticles, deposition in all regions of the respiratory tract may be of concern. Other chapters in this book can be consulted regarding the concerns for direct actions of nanoparticles in the human body or the effects following translocation from the point of exposure to other organs. In a variation of this equation for assessing dermal exposure, considerations might be given to particles that have diameter smaller than 1 μm, which is a size that the studies of Tinkle et al. (2) have demonstrated are, in conjunction with motion, as at the wrist, capable of penetrating the stratum corneum of human skin and reaching the epidermis and, occasionally, the dermis. Different considerations might be given to larger diameter particles that may only have potential to enter damaged skin.

■ CF is the control factor (0.05 for a control system that captures 95% of the airborne particles). This factor would preferentially be used to characterize the engineered control practices put in place to reduce potential exposures to a safe level, and where ever possible to levels that are as low as practicable.

■ BR is the Breathing Rate (0.025 m^3/min for the ICRP standard reference man (3) involved in light work activity). Note that some work activities may involve greater levels of exertion than the standard assumption of light exercise, and other activities may require less.

■ T is the time duration of exposure (minutes or other time units consistent with anticipating or documenting the exposure). Time periods can be used that are consistent with the job-exposure matrix, or when statutory or administrative occupational exposure limits are available, the time periods can be consistent with determining compliance with those limits (8 hour time-weighted averages or 15 minute short-term exposure limits).

■ DCF is the dose conversion factor (e.g., injury or illness per unit of delivered dose of nanoparticles to the body or affected organ of the exposed individual). This parameter is likely to be the most problematic factor in the equation. Note that in the case of radiation exposure assessment and control, the unifying DCF approach of "latent cancer fatalities per unit of radioactivity inhaled" and the associated extensive understanding of the relationships between the physicochemical properties and biological behavior of inhaled radioactive materials has provided a harmonized basis for the development and implementation of material-specific radiation protection programs. In the myriad potential health outcomes that may need to be addressed for exposures to nanoparticles, it will be necessary to seek unifying bases for relating the probability of potential health effects to the various potential measures of exposure. It is likely that an entire scheme of DCF relationships and values will be needed to address the full range of general and organ-specific health outcomes that may result from biological exposures to nanoparticles. Thus, multiple applications or summations of the equation may be needed to address the range of health effects that might be associated with exposures to a given material. This is particularly true in light of the fact that the effects may vary by intensity and duration of exposure, physical form of the toxicant, environmental conditions and other considerations. As noted in the other chapters of this book, work is still underway to adequately understand the dose-response relationships between exposures to nanoparticles and health effects.

■ V is the effective volume in which the nanoparticles are dispersed (m^3 or other volume units, and with appropriate considerations for the rate of air exchange or exhaust).

Note that the equation described above is based on historical decision analysis techniques and methods for estimating potential associated health effects to humans from accidental releases of radioactive materials (4,5). Because DCF values (latent cancer fatalities per unit of radioactivity inhaled) for materials of known radiation type, biological solubility, and aerodynamic particle size have been provided in guidance by authoritative bodies such as the ICRP, the equation can provide an actual numerical value. As noted below, the equation can also be used to build an understanding of the relative magnitudes and importance of the variability and uncertainties associated with each of the parameters. In situations where not all parameters are known, the equation can still function as a useful heuristic device to guide occupational health and environmental protection strategies, especially in conjunction with a checklist and ranking system for relative values of the equation parameters.

Although more complicated equations and models can be used, the use of this relatively straightforward equation in the present discussion illustrates that managing potential health risks in nanotechnology can take advantage of proven approaches and good practices from traditional industrial hygiene experience. For example, application of a variation of this equation in the U.S. Department of Energy Safety Notice on Decision Analysis Techniques (4) was to estimate the inhalation dose to a worker from a fire involving plutonium-contaminated rags in a glovebox enclosure. Concerns exist for pyrophoricity of nanoparticles and for potential dispersion of nanoparticles during fires. Similarly, application of the calculation approach in the U.S. Department of Energy handbook on *Airborne Release Fractions/Rates and Respirable Fractions for Nonreactor Nuclear Facilities* (5) documents a wide range of experimental results from spilling, pouring, ignition, and other disruption and handling activities involving uranium, plutonium and other nuclear materials.

Ramachandran (6) has summarized a number of exposure modeling approaches based on their level of sophistication regarding details of the determinants of exposure and the degree and uniformity of mixing phenomena between the source and the exposed individuals. He notes that, although a number of studies over the last several decades (e.g., see references 7; 8; 9; 10) have identified and modeled important determinants of exposure such as throughput rate in a production facility, local exhaust ventilation, etc., the field of exposure modeling is still relatively new. Nicas and Jayjock (11) have described the value of mathematical modeling for exposure assessment when the availability of actual exposure data is limited.

A Source-receptor Model for Assessing Exposures to Nanoparticles

Figure 1 illustrates a multiple pathways model to describe the manners in which workers and others may be exposed to nanoparticles. Day et al. (12) recently applied this model to assess workplace exposures to beryllium. The model incorporates the comprehensive source-receptor relationships developed by Schneider et al. (13) to describe the multiple compartments (air, surfaces, clothing, skin) and the mass transport processes (emission, deposition, resuspension/evaporation, transfer, removal, redistribution, decontamination, penetration/permeation) that contribute to exposures of the skin. Sources (research and development or production processes in nanotechnology) can result in transfer of nanoparticles directly to skin, clothing, or other objects, and can generate airborne nanomaterial-containing particles, some of which may be removed by ventilation systems, some of which may settle onto surfaces, and a smaller fraction that may be inhaled. Contaminated surfaces can include equipment, tools, floors and stairs, clothing, and areas of exposed skin. Some settled nanoparticles may become resuspended, and subsequently may settle onto other surfaces, may be inhaled, or may be removed by ventilation systems. Settled particles may also be transferred to clothing or hands through direct contact with contaminated surfaces.

According to Fenske (14), surface sampling can be considered a first approximation of personal dermal exposure, and the dynamics of surface-to-skin transfer is a complex process involving factors including contact pressure and motion, work practices, and hygienic behavior. Day et al. (12) observed strong relationships between the levels of beryllium on cotton gloves and on necks and faces. The potential for skin exposure can be assessed through a variety of techniques, including the use of interception (cotton gloves) and removal techniques (surface wipes and skin wipes) (15,16). Maynard et al. (17) used a cotton glove interception technique to assess dermal contact with carbon nanotubes during handling and pouring operations. The major assumption underlying all interception techniques is that the collection medium captures and retains chemicals in a relative manner to that of the skin.

Brouwer et al. (18) investigated the transfer of particles from contaminated surfaces to uncontaminated hands and to cotton gloves through a set of controlled laboratory experiments. Their results indicated that the mass of particles transferred from contaminated surfaces to cotton gloves was approximately 70-fold higher than was transferred to uncovered hands. Thus, the analytical results from cotton glove samples may considerably overestimate exposure. In contrast, the major assumption underlying all removal techniques is that the majority of the contamination residing on a surface is captured by the collection medium. In a dermal contamination and assessment study involving lead-containing dust, Que Hee et al. (19) observed experimentally that serial wipe sampling is insufficient to remove all lead-containing dust from the hands of study subjects. Thus, results from surface and skin wipe samples may underestimate total mass exposure, and may best be considered an index of exposure and be used as an assessment guide to improve the effectiveness of nanoparticle migration control.

In regard to skin sampling, interception and removal techniques consider only the level of contaminant deposited on the skin surface over a given period of time. According to Cherrie and Robertson (20), a biologically relevant measure of dermal exposure includes consideration not only for the level of contamination and duration of exposure, but also the area of exposed skin. When a permeability coefficient is available for the contaminant of interest, then it may be possible to estimate total mass uptake through the skin. Given the lack of a permeability coefficient or a validated biological monitoring technique for nanoparticle-containing particles, the results of cotton glove and skin wipe samples may provide an estimate of relative skin exposure, but not uptake, among workers assigned to various processes in a facility. Additional discussion of issues and concerns for dermal exposure and effects of nanoparticles can be found in Chapter 19.

DOCUMENTING THE OCCURRENCE AND NATURE OF EXPOSURES

It is desirable to document and record the details of the material characteristics and transfer rates to the exposed individual in a job-exposure matrix (Fig. 1). In practice, it is seldom possible to measure all exposure characteristics for all workers at all times. Whenever possible, it is desirable to reduce the costs and time requirements for exposure sampling and characterization and improve the statistical value of results by identifying groups of individuals who may be similarly exposed. A similar exposure group (SEG) is defined as a group of workers likely to have the same general exposure profile because of the tasks they perform, the similarity of the way tasks are performed, and the materials and processes with which they work (21). Table 1 illustrates a manner in which SEGs might be established to classify workers at a nanotechnology research or production facility. In the Table 1 example, the administrative group, production group, and production support group have different potential pathways for nanoparticle exposure and different exposure protection practices to mitigate those potential exposures. Note that many groups may need to be established in some facilities. In anticipating potential exposures or evaluating actual exposures it should be recognized that there can be significant differences between exposures over time for an individual worker (within worker variation) and significant differences between exposures over time for workers who are ostensibly exposed under "the same" work conditions (between worker variation). Between-worker variations can result from individual differences in how workers carry out specific work tasks. Within-worker variation can result from inherent day-to-day differences in factors such as the material at risk, damage ratio, airborne release fraction, etc.

In a comprehensive evaluation of within- and between-worker components of occupational exposure to chemical agents, Kromhout et al. (22) found that the median geometric standard deviation for total exposure variability was 2.4. As illustrated in Figure 3 using a statistical simulation model (23), that level of variability translates into temporal exposure concentration differences of

Table 1   Illustration of Similar Exposure Groups (SEGs) to Classify Workers at a Nanotechnology Research or Production Facility

Similar exposure groups (SEGs)	Potential nanoparticle exposure pathways	Exposure protection work practices
Administrative	1. Skin contact with nanoparticles carried from the facility into office areas 2. Inhalation of nanoparticles resuspended from contaminated surfaces in office areas 3. Inhalation of nanoparticles released from the facility	1. No use of gloves, respiratory protection, or other personal protective clothing or equipment while in office areas 2. Possible use of personal protective equipment while in production areas
Production (with task-specific SEG designations)	1. Skin contact with nanoparticles during production 2. Inhalation of nanoparticles released from processes 3. Inhalation of nanoparticles resuspended from contaminated surfaces	1. Incidental exposure protection from gloves or special clothing that may be worn in some circumstances to protect against cuts, abrasions, chemicals, and thermal injuries 2. Task-specific use of respiratory protection and other personal protective clothing or equipment for nanotechnology processes
Production support, including janitorial and maintenance staff (may also require task-specific SEG designations)	1. Skin contact with nanoparticles during time spent in the facility 2. Inhalation of released or resuspended nanoparticles during time spent in the facility	1. No use of gloves, respiratory protection, or other personal protective clothing or equipment while in office areas 2. Possible use of personal protective equipment while conducting certain operations in production areas

more than a factor of 10. The cumulative exposure profile (Fig. 3) resulting from such a concentration distribution will increase monotonically with time, and the amount actually deposited in a region of interest in the respiratory tract (e.g., the alveolar region, in this example) will depend on the actual particle size deposition efficiency (Fig. 2) of the inhaled material. Because the health consequences of inhalation exposures depend on both the mechanism of biological interaction and the extent to which deposited material is retained in the lung, the biological solubility and lung-retention properties of the inhaled particles should also be evaluated. If the particles of interest are rapidly cleared from the lung, then the temporal profile of particle lung burden will have a shape that mirrors the original exposure profile as shown in Figure 3. If the particles of interest are retained with little clearance, then the temporal profile of particle lung burden will have a shape that mirrors the cumulative exposure profile as shown in Figure 3. For particles of intermediate clearance (e.g., weeks instead of hours or years), then the temporal profile of particle lung burden will have the shape illustrated in Figure 4. Thus, sufficient measurements of both concentration and relevant particle properties such as size must be made using statistical approaches such as those described in Bullock and Ignacio (21) to support a meaningful assessment of the exposure profile and its potential health consequences.

The work of Kromhout and Vermeulen (24) can be consulted for additional information about assessing temporal, personal, and spatial variations for dermal exposures. Nieuwenhuijsen (26) can be consulted for a wide range of aspects for exposure assessment in occupational and environmental epidemiology, including the use of questionnaires, source dispersion modeling, geographical information systems, collection and modeling of personal exposure data, use of exposure surrogates such as self-reports and expert evaluations, use of physiologically based pharmacokinetic modeling, biological monitoring for indicators of exposure, and sources and consequences of exposure measurement errors, including how errors can be avoided by proper

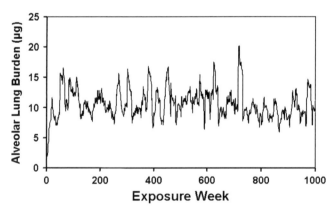

Figure 4 Temporal variability of particle lung burden for the exposure profile illustrated in Figure 3, assuming a particle diameter of 10 nm and a relatively insoluble particle clearance halftime of 350 days. The shape of this profile can be compared to the original exposure profile which would apply if the particles of interest were rapidly cleared from the lung and the cumulative exposure profile which would apply if the particles were retained with little clearance.

study design. Checkoway, Pearce, and Kriebel (26) provide a useful text on research methods in occupational epidemiology, including a dedicated chapter on exposure and dose modeling. Smith (27) addresses issues in exposure and dose assessment for epidemiology and risk assessment, especially related to the lack of clear specification of exposure and dose. These questions for traditional occupational exposure assessment and epidemiology for chemical exposures are directly relevant to exposure assessment for engineered nanoparticles.

CONCLUSION

Many of the exposure assessment issues presented in this chapter indicate that most nanomaterial can be approached as a logical subset of traditional exposure assessment for chemical hazards in the workplace and environment. In a manner similar to concerns for special formulations of chemicals, the challenge for providing effective exposure assessment and protection of human and environmental health rests in recognition of when the unique size, surface, and compositional properties of nanomaterials may alter their ability to interact with biological systems. The question of what aspects of exposure should be assessed will continue to challenge heath protection professionals. A goal of the nanotechnology community should be to develop a nanomaterial-specific compendium of information on materials at risk, damage ratios, airborne release fractions, respirable fractions, and biologically relevant particle characteristics for representative research, development, and manufacturing processes, handling and disposal situations, and potential accident scenarios. This will require a large number of site-specific studies. Not everything can be measured at all times, but intelligent approaches to exposure assessment can reduce risks from the outset and enable rapid learning of lessons with minimal risks to workers and members of the public.

DISCLAIMER

The findings and conclusions in this report are those of the authors and do not necessarily represent the views of the National Institute for Occupational Safety and Health.

REFERENCES

1. International Commission on Radiological Protection. Human Respiratory Tract Model for Radiological Protection, ICRP Publication 66. Ann ICRP 1994; 24(1–3).
2. Tinkle SS, Antonini JM, Rich BA, Roberts JR, Salmen R, DePree K, Adkins EJ. Skin as a route of exposure and sensitization in chronic beryllium disease. Environ Health Perspect 2003, 11:1202–1208.

3. International Commission on Radiological Protection. Reference Man: Anatomical, Physiological and Metabolical Characteristics, ICRP Publication 23. Amsterdam, The Netherlands: Elsevier, 1975.

4. U.S. Department of Energy, Airborne Release Fractions/Rates and Respirable Fractions for Nonreactor Nuclear Facilities, U.S. Department of Energy Handbook DOE-HDBK-3010-94, Washington, DC: U.S. Department of Energy, December 1994.

5. U.S. Department of Energy, Decision Analysis Techniques, Safety Notice Issue No. 95-01, Office of Nuclear and Facility Safety, Office of Operating Experience Analysis and Feedback, Washington, DC: U.S. Department of Energy, August 1995.

6. Ramachandran G, ed. Occupational Exposure Assessment for Air Contaminants. Boca Raton, FL: CRC Press, 2005.

7. Keil CB, ed. Mathematical models for estimating occupational exposures to chemicals. Fairfax, VA: AIHA Press, 2000.

8. Burstyn I, Teschke K. Studying the determinants of exposure: a review of methods. Am Ind Hyg Assoc J 1999; 60:57–72.

9. Nicas M. Estimating exposure intensity in an imperfectly mixed room. Am Ind Hyg Assoc J 1996; 57:542–550.

10. Cherrie JW, Schneider T. Validation of a new method for structured subjective assessment of past concentrations. Ann Occup Hyg 1999; 43:235–245.

11. Nicas M, Jayjock M. Uncertainty in exposure estimates made by modeling versus monitoring. Am Ind Hyg Assoc J 2002; 63:275–283.

12. Day GA, Dufresne A, Stefaniak AB, Schuler CR, Stanton ML, Miller WE, Kent MS, Deubner DC, Kreiss K, Hoover MD. Exposure pathway assessment at a copper-beryllium alloy facility. Ann Occup Hyg 2007; 51:67–80.

13. Schneider T, Vermeulen R, Brouwer DH, Cherrie JW, Kromhout H, Fogh CL. Conceptual model for assessment of dermal exposure. Occup Environ Med 1999; 56:765–773.

14. Fenske RA. Dermal exposure assessment techniques. Ann Occup Hyg 1993; 37:687–706.

15. CEN, European Committee for Standardization. Workplace Exposure—Strategy of the Evaluation of Dermal Exposure. TC137/WG 6 (prCEN/TR 15278), Berlin: European Committee for Standardization, 2005.

16. CEN, European Committee for Standardization. Workplace Exposure—Measurement of Dermal Exposure—Principles and Methods. TC137/WG 6 (prCEN/TR 15279), Berlin: European Committee for Standardization, 2005.

17. Maynard AD, Baron PA, Foley M, Shvedova AA, Kisin ER, Castranova V. Exposure to carbon nanotube material: aerosol release during the handling of unrefined single walled carbon nanotube material. J Toxicol Environ Health 2004; 67:87–107.

18. Brouwer DH, Kroese R, van Hemmen JJ. Transfer of contaminants from surface to hands: experimental assessment of linearity of the exposure process, adherence to the skin, and area exposed during fixed pressure and repeated contact with surfaces contaminated with a powder. Appl Occup Environ Hyg 1999; 14:231–239.

19. Que Hee SS, Peace B, Clark CS, Boyle JR, Bornschein RL, Hammond PB. Evolution of efficient methods to sample lead sources, such as house dust and hand dust, in the homes of children. Environ Res 1989; 38:77–95.
20. Cherrie JW, Robertson A. Biologically relevant assessment of dermal exposure. Ann Occup Hyg 1995; 39:387–392.
21. Bullock WH, Ignacio JS, eds. A Strategy for Assessing and Managing Occupational Exposures, 3rd ed. Fairfax, VA: American Industrial Hygiene Association Press, 2006.
22. Kromhout H, Symanski E, Rappaport SM. A comprehensive evaluation of within- and between-worker components of occupational exposure to chemical agents. Ann Occup Hyg 1993; 37(3):253–270.
23. Decisioneering, Inc. Crystal Ball Version 5.2 User Manual: Forecasting and Risk Analysis for Spreadsheet Users. Denver, CO: Decisioneering, Inc., 2002.
24. Kromhout H, Vermeulen R. Temporal, personal and spatial variability in dermal exposure. Ann Occup Hyg 2001; 45:257–273.
25. Nieuwenhuijsen MJ, ed. Exposure Assessment in Occupational and Environmental Epidemiology. Oxford, England: Oxford University Press, 2003.
26. Checkoway H, Pearce N, Kriebel D, eds. Research Methods in Occupational Epidemiology. Oxford, England: Oxford University Press, 2004.
27. Smith TJ. Issues in Exposure and Dose Assessment for Epidemiology and Risk Assessment. Human and Ecological Risk Assessment 2002; 8(6): 1267–1293.

6

Biodistribution of Nanoparticles: Insights from Drug Delivery

Martin C. Garnett
School of Pharmacy, University of Nottingham, Nottingham, U.K.

INTRODUCTION

Medical scientists have long dreamt of drugs that would accumulate specifically in target tissues; either disease targets, or particular tissues in order to increase the specificity of their medicines. In the last 20 to 25 years, a number of groups have pursued this objective using a variety of materials formulated into "drug delivery systems" (1,2). Drug delivery systems is a catch-all term used to describe any formulation in which drugs are encapsulated or attached to various materials, which may modify the properties of the drug in terms of its localization in the body, its pharmacokinetics, or its uptake into particular cells or tissues. Drug delivery systems relevant to nanotoxicology may comprise macromolecules such as proteins, DNA, natural or synthetic polymers or constructs of nanoparticulate size such as micelles, polymeric micelles, polyelectrolyte complexes, liposomes, or nanoparticles prepared from polymers or lipids. These delivery systems have now been brought together under the heading *nanomedicines* (3). A significant amount of in vivo work has been done to determine how such systems behave and to understand why these constructs behave in a particular way to exploit delivery systems more effectively. This understanding is clearly the inverse of nanotoxicology where we wish to know where nanoparticles go to so we can assess their toxicity at that site.

In this chapter a number of aspects of drug delivery are examined, which may offer insights into where nanoparticles could conceivably get to in the body and whether this is a place where small or large amounts of material may accumulate. This chapter assumes as a starting point that material has already entered the body and accessed the bloodstream, and considers where it can get to from there. This chapter is divided into two areas. First, a consideration of physiology and anatomy that may help us to understand the possible routes by which materials are distributed or prevented from being distributed in the body. Second, a look at where materials have been successfully delivered to (or accumulated in) particular tissues or organs. The final part a discusses what this may mean for nanotoxicology.

BARRIERS TO NANOPARTICLE DISTRIBUTION

Small hydrophobic molecules can be carried around the body by the bloodstream, and can reach most tissues in the body fairly readily by processes of partitioning and diffusion, these processes largely being dependent on the physicochemical properties of the molecule. However, for larger molecules and particles, biodistribution is dependent more on the physiology and anatomy of the body, which presents a range of barriers and restricts the distribution in a number of different ways, dependent partly on the size of the particle. In view of this we should briefly consider the size and homogeneity of particles, which may be encountered as toxic threats.

Typically many of the particles which are being considered in industrial nanoparticles are found to be in the range of 5 to 50 nm in diameter when considered at the level of the individual particles. However, due to their properties many of these particles tend to aggregate and form particles with a much larger effective diameter. Particles found in airborne pollutants may have a route into the body via the lungs, due to the filtering effects of the airways, which have sizes from 2 to 4 μm downward. Because of this large possible range of sizes, this chapter will consider not just the very small nanometer sizes, which fall within the usual definition of nanotechnology, but the definition usually adopted in drug delivery where materials less than 1 μm in diameter are considered to be nanoparticles.

The first barrier to consider in the biodistribution of nanoparticles is a physiological one, that of clearance of particulate materials from the bloodstream.

Physiological Barriers: Opsonization and Clearance to the Liver

The body has evolved a series of complex processes to protect it against invading microorganisms, typically fungal spores, bacteria, and viruses, which are in the size range from about 50 nm up to a few micrometers. Particulates in the bloodstream are rapidly coated in a cocktail of serum proteins. In some cases this may be due to the recognition of common antigens by antibodies, but such specific binding events are unnecessary. In general particulate materials tend to have relatively hydrophobic surfaces, and an array of blood proteins will bind quite strongly to such surfaces in a random and nonspecific manner (4). It is very likely that among the bound proteins will be particular proteins such as antibodies and complement factors, which are then recognized by macrophages or other phagocytic cells in the body. These factors are known as opsonins and greatly facilitate the uptake of particulate material by phagocytic cells. Opsonins are not essential for phagocytosis to take place, as the phagocytic cells themselves can also interact with particle surfaces triggering uptake, however, these processes are significantly slower in the absence of opsonins (5,6).

Phagocytic cells are typically neutrophils or macrophages, of which the latter are most common. Macrophages are found in various guises in all tissues of the body, so they can take up particles from anywhere they may accumulate. However, the principal organs in which they are found are the spleen, liver, and lymph nodes. Because of the architecture of these tissues, spleen tends to be involved in the clearance of larger particles (>250 nm diameter), which become trapped, while liver is more involved in clearance of smaller particles. In the liver, structure is again important. The liver is designed as a filtration unit. It is built in hexagonal blocks called lobules in which blood enters from the outer corners of the units and flow along large vessels called sinusoids to the central vein that drains the lobule. Lying in wait along the sinusoids are the macrophages, known in the liver as Kupffer cells, to trap any particles passing by. The endothelial cells lining the sinusoids have holes called fenestrae, which are typically about 100 to 150 nm in diameter, which lead to the underlying liver parenchymal cells. The surface of the parenchymal cells is covered with microvilli and the parenchymal cell surface is thought to be responsible for uptake of smaller particulates by endocytic processes (7).

The blood flow to the liver is from two sources, the hepatic artery from the heart and the hepatic portal vein, from the gut. From these two sources about 25% of the blood flow around the body passes through the liver from each pump of the heart. This clearly makes for a very efficient filtration system. The liver is well known for its role in metabolism of small molecules and rendering them harmless, but this architecture is clearly designed to trap and metabolize a range of nanoparticulate materials as well.

Anatomical Barriers

Assuming that particles avoid uptake by the liver and spleen, they continue to circulate in the bloodstream, where can they get to? Blood vessels are lined by a layer of cells, the endothelium, which controls what materials can enter and leave the bloodstream and consequently what tissues the particles can get to.

Endothelium

In most tissues, the endothelium has a set of characteristics designed to prevent egress of materials. There are two possible routes by which materials could pass through the endothelium, either by passage through the gaps between the cells, the paracellular route, or by passage through the cells themselves. Most endothelium is continuous, that is, the cells are fixed together by tight junctions, a band around the top edges of the cells act like rivets pinning the membranes together. The tight junctions hold the membranes close together structurally and effectively prevent materials greater than 2 nm in diameter passing through the paracellular route. In general, larger molecules and particles do not readily pass through membranes, because they cannot partition in the same way as smaller molecules. However, there are mechanisms for materials to pass through the endothelium. Endothelial cells are very active at their membrane surfaces, being active in pinocytic uptake of materials. In this process, a miniature version of phagocytosis, materials are enveloped and incorporated into a spherical intracellular compartment. The size of the vesicles entrapping material is mainly in the region of 70 to 150 nm, although some larger vesicles are formed. In the endothelium, it appears that most of the material entrapped in this way has passed across the thin endothelial cells, and deposited on the other side of the cell in a process called transcytosis. The vesicle size would suggest that quite large particles should be able to participate in this process of transcytosis; however, there are other limitations. Under most epithelial and endothelial tissues is another feature, the basement membrane, part of the connective tissue. The basement membrane consists of fibrils of biological polymers composed of type IV collagen, laminin, entactin, nidogen, and heparan sulfate proteoglycans. These fibrils form a dense network attaching the endothelial cells to the underlying connective tissue (8). Examination of the basement membrane by transmission electron microscopy suggests that the interfibril network has a mesh size of about 13 to 15 nm, which would be expected to restrict passage of particles through this layer to this size range.

Fluid passes through the endothelial layer to form the lymph, which bathes all cells in the tissues. Analysis of lymph from various tissues should give us a good idea of what can pass through the endothelium. Analysis of proteins in lymph shows that as proteins get bigger, the relative proportions of those molecules in lymph gets smaller, and the largest protein molecules cannot pass through the endothelium in significant amounts.

Not all endothelium is the same in terms of its permeability properties. Brain endothelia have particularly effective tight junctions, which effectively eliminate the paracellular route of transport and also have minimal pinocytosis greatly reducing the transcellular route (9). However, in other conditions such as inflammation, the endothelium can become leaky allowing the accumulation of nanoparticulate material into inflamed tissues (10).

Cellular Uptake Processes

Once particles have reached the extracellular fluid we need to consider how they can get into cells. There are a number of mechanisms designed to facilitate uptake of macromolecules and small particles into cells for physiological reasons (11). One of the earliest to be described was pinocytosis, believed to be a nonspecific uptake mechanism related to cell nutrition. In this mechanism a cup-shaped invagination forms at the cell membrane, which encloses material in the extracellular fluid. From this mechanism either material bound to the membrane (adsorptive pinocytosis) or material contained in the fluid (fluid-phase pinocytosis) can be taken up. This was believed to be a nonspecific uptake mechanism. Two types of pinocytosis were described, a micropinocytosis involving vesicles up to about 150 nm in diameter, and macropinocytosis involving vesicles up to 300 nm in diameter. Uptake by pinocytosis results in formation of an endosome that eventually becomes converted to a lysosome. Lysosomes are an acidic compartment of about pH 4.5 to 5.0 containing a wide variety of degradative enzymes. Recently, a process known as membrane ruffling has been described, which results in particle uptake in a similar size to that of macropinocytosis and it has been suggested that these processes may be equivalent.

There are also endocytic processes by which molecules are taken up after specific recognition processes. The best described of these processes is clathrin dependent receptor-mediated uptake. In this process a receptor on the cell surface, is associated with coated pits (11). Interaction of a physiologically important molecule with the receptor triggers the formation of a vesicle which entraps the ligand and internalizes it into the cell to form an endosome. The vesicles generated in this process are a very strictly defined size of around 100 nm. Once the endosome has formed the receptor and ligand can be treated in a number of different ways depending on the receptor. These include recycling to the cell surface, being taken to the lysosomes for degradation, or in a few cases an alternative form of transcytosis for transport across the cell. Another form of endocytosis has also been described involving flask-shaped structures on membranes known as caveolae (12). These structures are about 70 nm in diameter, but their exact mechanisms of action are unclear. These structures have also been implicated in uptake of nanomaterials, and it is believed that they are responsible for the transcytosis seen across endothelia and some epithelia. These are also believed to mediate a form of receptor-mediated uptake into cells.

Recently, a further uptake process has been described in macrophages termed patocytosis, which applies to particles not larger than 500 nm (13). In this report, hydrophobic particles become trapped in membrane folds open to the extracellular space.

All the above mechanisms are natural physiological mechanisms designed to allow the cells to take up important physiological molecules and particles, and all end up in an intracellular vesicles surrounded by a membrane. In addition, there appear to be some other mechanisms that may depend on the physicochemical properties of particles. It has been reported that small hydrophobic particles can be taken up into macrophages and a range of other cell types including red blood corpuscles. In this mechanism the particles taken up were in the cytoplasm in direct contact with intracellular proteins and organelles (14). A similar uptake may also occur with positively charged particles. It is well known that positively charged polymers and particles interact with cell surfaces and can cause toxicity mediated by membrane effects. Work with positively charged dendrimers has shown the appearance of membrane defects 15 to 40 nm in diameter, which can allow egress of cellular proteins and ingress of small particles (15).

LOCALIZATION OF PARTICLES IN SPECIFIC TISSUES

Lung

Very large particles or particle masses of 5 to 7 μm in diameter or greater can become trapped in capillary beds, and these typically appear in the lung, but it seems unlikely that nanoparticles would accumulate in the body to a significant enough extent for aggregates of this size to occur (16).

Spleen and Liver

The role of the liver and spleen in the very efficient removal of particulates from the bloodstream was demonstrated in the early 1980s using model polystyrene nanoparticles. Hydrophobic 150 nm model polystyrene particles were removed from the bloodstream within about 5 min, and experiments using gamma scintigraphy and counting of radioactively labeled particles demonstrated that the majority of these particles accumulated in the liver (17). This behavior is typical of particulate materials injected into the bloodstream. It was found however, that coating of the particulates with poly(ethylene glycol) (PEG) containing surfactants such as poloxamers could greatly modify the behavior of nanoparticulates in vivo. The PEG polymer chains are very mobile and highly hydrated, forming a sterically stabilizing surface layer (18), which reduces serum protein binding and allowing a longer circulation time for particulates in the bloodstream (19). However, the biodistribution of the coated particles is greatly affected by particle size. Model poloxamer coated nanoparticles of 60 nm avoided the spleen completely, 150 nm particles showed some spleen uptake, but 250 nm particles were taken up significantly by the spleen, and this was due initially to mechanical trapping by the interendothelial cell slits (Table 1) (20).

Table 1 Effect of Nanoparticle Size on Spleen Uptake in the Rat after 24 h.
Labeled Polystyrene Particles Uncoated or Coated with Poloxamer 407.

Nanoparticle size (nm)	% of injected dose	
	Uncoated nanoparticles	Poloxamer 407 coated nanoparticles
60	0.3 ± 0.00	1.1 ± 0.2
150	2.6 ± 0.5	15 ± 6.3
250	6.3 ± 1.2	39.5 ± 1.7

Note: Values taken from the literature showing accumulation of nanoparticles in the brain with various surfactant coatings. *Source*: From Ref. 20.

Particles remaining in the circulation are usually eventually taken up by the liver. Nanoparticles and liposomes which are very small-coated particles of less than 60 to 70 nm in diameter can become taken up by the liver (7). In this case, uptake is by the liver parenchymal cells because smaller particles come into contact with these cells and are small enough to pass through the fenestrae in the endothelium.

Changing the amount or characteristics of the PEG surface layer can result in different biodistribution effects. A less dense PEG layer will usually result in a less effective protection against uptake of particles by the liver and therefore a shorter circulation half-life in the blood. Different surfactants have a different effect on biodistribution. In the following examples of localization to different tissues, these have been found by coating particles with a range of surfactants either with different anchoring moieties or with different PEG lengths. It is thought that these different localizations are the results of a preferential binding of particular serum components recognized by specific tissue endothelia.

Bone Marrow

The exact properties of the coating are very important in determining the final location and biodistribution of nanoparticles. Early studies with poloxamer 407 coated nanoparticles showed that long circulating nanoparticles could reach other destinations. Coated 60 or 100 nm polystyrene particles injected into rabbits showed a significant localization, around 50% of injected dose, to the bone marrow in rabbits (21). This illustrates the effects of different surfactant coatings on the localization of particles in rabbits.

Brain

Currently, there is a large body of evidence that nanoparticles coated with particular PEG-containing surfactants, can accumulate in the brain (22).

This effect was initially shown with poly(butylcyanoacrylate) nanoparticles coated with polysorbate 80 (23), but has also been seen with cyanoacrylate particles with different hydrophobicities with different types of PEG coatings (24) and poly(glycerol adipate) nanoparticles prepared in our laboratory (Table 2). The level of nanoparticle uptake is fairly low but histological examination clearly shows the presence of labeled particles within brain tissue. The mechanism of this uptake is reported to be due to the adsorption of apolipoprotein E (ApoE) onto the surface of the nanoparticles. ApoE is known to act as a ligand for the transcytosis of low-density lipoprotein across the blood–brain barrier (25). A number of other ligands are known to be involved in transcytosis of ligands across the blood–brain barrier, but whether these can also adsorb to nanoparticles is not known (Table 2).

Lipid-coated positively charged nanoparticles (26) have been reported to be taken up across the blood–brain barrier in vitro. Cationized proteins (27) are also known to get into the brain, but in this case this is a general effect seen in many endothelia, and consequently leads to a more general uptake across various epithelia, rather than specifically into the brain.

For all of these studies involving nanoparticles and the localization to different tissues, species effects are likely to be present. For example, bone marrow localization is seen in rabbits but not in rats due to differences in anatomy of rabbits. Recent data by Dr. P. Kallinteri from our laboratories comparing localization of the same particles in mice and rats also shows significant differences between these species (see Fig. 1). Differences between localization of nanoparticles in brain tissue of rats and mice have also been noted by Calvo et al. (24) (Fig. 1).

Table 2 Uptake of Coated Nanoparticles into the Brain

Nanoparticle and surfactant	% injected dose/g in brain at 1 h
PHDCA[a]	0.003
PHDCA + 1% poloxamer 908[a]	0.005
PHDCA + polysorbate 80[a]	0.002
PBCA + 1% polysorbate 80[b]	0.006
40%C$_{18}$PGA + 0.1% polysorbate 80[c]	0.029

Note: Values taken from the literature showing accumulation of nanoparticles in the brain with various surfactant coatings.
[a] Calvo et al. (24).
[b] Gulyaev et al. (23) (value for PBCA calculated from localization of doxorubicin adsorbed to particles).
[c] Garnett and Kallinteri unpublished data.
Abbreviations: PBCA, polybutylcyanoacrylate; 40%C$_{18}$PGA, poly(glycerol adipate) with 40% of pendant hydroxyl groups substituted with C$_{18}$ acyl groups; PHDCA, polycyanoacrylate-*co*-hexadecyl cyanoacrylate.

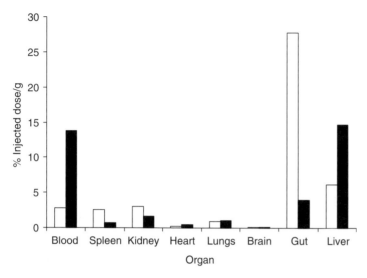

Figure 1 The biodistribution of 40% $C_{18}PGA$ particles coated with 0.1% polysorbate 80 3 hours after injection into mice open columns and rats filled columns. (40% $C_{18}PGA$, poly(glycerol adipate) with 40% of pendant hydroxyl groups substituted with C_{18} acyl groups.)

Lymph Nodes

Particles present in tissues can also have different localizations and fate, which is again dependent on particle size and coating. Larger particles 100 nm or greater cannot penetrate through tissue very well and so will tend to get taken up by resident macrophages in the tissue. However, particles of 60 nm with a sufficient PEG coating can penetrate through tissue and pass into the lymphatics. Particles with a thick coating will avoid uptake by the phagocytes in the lymph nodes and pass through to the circulation, but if the coating is not sufficiently good, the particles will accumulate in the lymph nodes (28).

Small superparamagnetic iron particles of around 30 nm coated with dextran are known to show some accumulation in lymph nodes, and this is believed to occur by extravasation through endothelia into tissues followed by drainage into lymph ducts and accumulation in lymph nodes (29). However, a recent report of starch-coated iron oxide particles suggested a different route. These were 60 to 90 nm particles, which had relatively short half-life in the circulation of 13 min. Both the size of the particles and the short half-life made it unlikely that the particles could extravasate into tissues and then accumulate in the lymph nodes. The localization of the particles within the lymph nodes was strongly suggestive that endothelial transcytosis into the lymph node was the pathway of uptake in this case (30).

RELEVANCE OF DRUG TARGETING STUDIES TO NANOTOXICOLOGY

Nanoparticles developed for diagnostic and therapeutic purposes are tested in a number of ways to determine their toxicology, but these studies are likely to be of limited help in determining the toxicology of nanoparticles in general. Drug delivery systems have been designed from the outset with the knowledge that they could accumulate and cause toxic effects. Consequently much effort is expended in ensuring that as far as possible, the materials from which they are constructed are nontoxic, biodegradable, and nonimmunogenic. Despite this, some toxic effects are seen with these materials with various cell types, including cationic polymers used in polyelectrolyte complexes for DNA delivery (31) and even poly(lactide-*co*-glycolide) particles (32), a polymer which has been approved for medical use. However, for nanoparticles that may be produced industrially or nanoparticulate pollutants, these are likely to contain materials, which are far less benign.

We can imagine from the pathways of biodistribution and uptake described, that ultimately most of these particles will end up in some tissue or cell. The possibilities for tissue localization are summarized in Figure 2. In addition to the known sites of localization, it is possible that further serum factors may be identified, which may lead to access to other tissue locations not yet documented.

Once accumulated in a tissue, the particles may or may not be taken up into cells. If taken up, the final subcellular localization could be in a lysosome or cytoplasm of the cell depending on the nanoparticle characteristics. If it is located in the cytoplasm, the presence of some bulk material

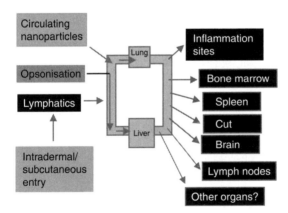

Figure 2 Summary diagrams showing the possible areas of localization of nanoparticles to various tissues from the blood circulation. Opsonization can result in uptake to the liver, but changes in size or surface characteristics can result in accumulation in a wide range of other tissues.

could cause direct harm or cell death by its interactions. If it is located in the lysosome we can look to the lysosomal storage diseases to see what harmful effects might result from accumulation of significant amounts of materials in this compartment (33). Even if nanoparticulate material is cleared by liver macrophages, the phagocytic process itself involves an oxidative step resulting in the generation of harmful oxygen radicals, the respiratory burst. Repeated insults and continuous production of these oxygen radicals is likely to be harmful.

Looking at the sort of tissues in which accumulation is likely will clearly depend on size, surface characteristics, and state of aggregation. In their normal unmodified state, it seems that the majority of materials finding their way into the circulation will end up in the liver or spleen. It is possible that some of the material may be taken up directly by the endothelium as this is in intimate contact with the blood. There is some possibility that airborne pollutants entering via the lung may acquire coatings of lung surfactants that may modify their behavior, but we are unaware of any current publications on the effect of natural surfactants on nanoparticle biodistribution.

For most industrial and pollutant nanoparticles, highly hydrophobic surfaces and aggregation is the norm. To make these industrial particles usable however, it is likely that many will eventually end up with some sort of sterically stabilizing surface coating to prevent or reduce aggregation and make them handleable. In these circumstances accumulation of particles at other sites is a possibility as we have seen from drug delivery systems.

Accumulation in bone marrow has been shown to occur at significant levels, but accumulation in brain is a much smaller percentage of total doses. We may therefore expect that any toxic effects are to be in the order of liver and spleen > bone marrow > brain, and that for brain damage to be significant, particles would have to have significant intrinsic toxicity. Effects on endothelium are more difficult to predict. The endothelium is a tissue, which is intimate contact with the blood so has the opportunity to take up nanoparticulates, and is also known to be a key mediator in many responses by the body. However, toxic effects are likely to be dependent on whether the endothelium is an endpoint where accumulation will occur, or whether, when uptake occurs it is mainly a staging post *en route* to somewhere else. We must also bear in mind the variability between species, and until more clinical studies are carried out with nanoparticles in different species it will be difficult to predict which animal model will be most relevant to the biodistribution of particles in humans.

REFERENCES

1. Stolnik S, Illum L, Davis SS. Long circulating microparticulate drug carriers. Adv Drug Del Rev 1995; 16:195–214.

2. Soppimath KS, Aminabhavi TM, Kulkarni AR, et al. Biodegradable polymeric nanoparticles as drug delivery devices. J Control Rel 2001; 70:1–20.
3. Moghimi SM, Hunter AC, Murray JC. Nanomedicine: current status and future prospects. FASEB J 2005; 19:311–30.
4. Young BR, Pitt WG, Cooper SL. Protein adsorption on polymeric biomaterials. I. Adsorptive isotherms. J Colloid Interface Sci 1988; 124:28–43.
5. Van Oss CJ. Phagocytosis: an overview. In: Di Sabato G, Everse J, eds. Immunological Techniques, vol. 132 Part J, Phagocytosis and Cell Mediated Cytotoxicity. San Diego, CA: Academic Press, 1986:3–15.
6. Absolom DR. Opsonins and dysopsonins: an overview. In: Di Sabato G, Everse J, eds. Immunological Techniques Part J, Phagocytosis and Cell Mediated Cytotoxicity. San Diego, CA: Academic Press, 1986:281–318.
7. Litzinger DC, Buiting AMJ, Van Rooijen N, et al. Effect of liposome size on the circulation time and intraorgan distribution of amphipathic poly(ethylene glycol)-containing liposomes. Biochem Biophys Acta 1994; 1190:99–107.
8. Inoue, S. Ultrastructure of basement membranes. Int Rev Cytol 1989; 117: 57–98.
9. Brightman MW. Morphology of blood–brain barrier interfaces. Exp Eye Res 1977; 25(Suppl.):1–25.
10. Schoefl G. Electron microscopic observations on the regeneration of blood vessels after injury. NY Acad Sci 1964; 116:789–902.
11. Van Deurs B, Peterson OW, Olsnes S, et al. The ways of endocytosis. Int Rev Cytol 1989; 117:131–77.
12. Schnitzer JE. Caveolae: from basic trafficking mechanisms to targeting transcytosis for tissue specific drug and gene delivery in vivo. Adv Drug Del Rev 2001; 49:265–80.
13. Kruth HS, Chang J, Ifrim I, et al. Characterisation of patocytosis: endocytosis into macrophage surface-connected compartments. Eur J Cell Biol 1999; 78: 91–9.
14. Geiser M, Rothe-Rutishauser B, Kapp N, Schürch S, Kreyling W, Schulz H, Semmler M, Im Hof V, Heyder J, Gehr P. Ultrafine particles cross cellular membranes by nonphagocytic mechanisms in lungs and in cultured cells. Environ Health Perspect 2005; 113:1555–60.
15. Hong S, Bielinska, AU, Mecke A, et al. Interaction of poly(amidoamine) dendrimers with supported lipid bilayers and cells: hole formation and the relation to transport. Bioconj Chem 2004; 15:774–82.
16. Illum L, Davis SS. Specific intravenous delivery of drugs to the lungs using ion-exchange microspheres. J Pharm Pharmacol 1982; 34(Suppl.):89P.
17. Davis SS, Illum L. Microspheres as drug carriers. In: Roerdink FHD, Kroon AM, eds. Drug Carrier Systems, vol. 9Horizons in Biochemistry and Biophysics. Chichester, UK: John Wiley & Sons, 1989:131–53.
18. Tadros FT. Polymer adsorption and dispersion stability. InTadros FT, ed. The Effect of Polymers on Dispersion Properties. London, UK: Academic Press, 1982, 1–18.
19. Stolnik S, Daudali B, Arien A, et al. The effect of surface coverage and conformation of poly(ethylene oxide) (PEO) chains of poloxamer 407 on the biological fate of model colloidal drug carriers. Biochim Biophys Acta 2001; 1514:261–79.

20. Moghimi SM, Porter CJH, Muir IS, et al. Non-phagocytic uptake of intravenously injected microspheres in rat spleen: influence of particle size and hydrophilic coating. Biochem Biophys Res Commun 1991; 177:861–6.

21. Porter CJ, Moghimi SM, Illum L, et al. The polyoxyethylene/polyoxypropylene block copolymer-407 selectively redirects intravenously injected microspheres to sinusoidal endothelial cells of rabbit bone marrow. FEBS Lett 1992; 305:62–6.

22. Kreuter J. Nanoparticulate systems for brain delivery of drugs. Adv Drug Del Rev 2001; 47:65–81.

23. Gulyaev AE, Gelperina SE, Skidan IN, et al. Significant transport of doxorubicin into the brain with polysorbate 80 coated nanoparticles. Pharm Res 1999; 16:1564–9.

24. Calvo P, Gouritin B, Chacun H, et al. Long circulating PEGylated polycyanoacrylate nanoparticles as new drug carrier for brain delivery. Pharm Res 2001; 18:1157–66.

25. Michaelis K, Hoffmann MM, Dreis S, et al. Covalent linkage of apolipoprotein E to albumin nanoparticles strongly enhances drug transport into the brain. J Pharmacol Exp Ther 2006; 317:1246–53.

26. Fenart L, Casanova B, Dehouck C, et al. Evaluation of effect of charge and lipid coating on ability of 60 nm nanoparticles to cross and in vitro model of the blood brain barrier. J Pharmacol Exp Ther 1999; 291:1017–22.

27. Lee HJ, Pardridge WM. Pharmacokinetics and delivery of Tat and Tat–protein conjugates to tissues in vivo. Bioconj Chem 2001; 12:995–9.

28. Hawley AE, Davis SS, Illum L. Targeting of colloids to lymph nodes: influence of lymphatic physiology and colloidal characteristics, Adv Drug Del Rev 1995; 17:129–48.

29. Moghimi SM, Bonnemain B. Subcutaneous and intravenous delivery of diagnostic agents to the lymphatic system: application in lymphoscintigraphy and indirect lymphography. Adv Drug Del Rev 1999; 37:295–312.

30. Lind K, Kresse M, Debus NP, et al. A novel formulation for superparamagnetic iron oxide (SPIO) particle enhancing MR lymphography: comparison of physicochemical properties and the in vivo behavior. J Drug Targ 2002; 10:221–30.

31. Morgan DML, Larvin, VL, Pearson JD. Chemical characterisation of polycation-induced cytotoxicity to human vascular endothelial cells. J Cell Science 1989; 94:553–9.

32. Lam KH, Schakenraad JM, Esselbrugge H, et al. The effect of phagocytosis of poly(L-lactic acid) fragments on cellular morphology and viability. J Biomed Mat Res 1993; 27:1569–77.

33. Vellodi A. Lysosomal storage disorders. Br J Haematol 2004; 128:413–31.

7

Nanoparticle Interactions with Biological Membranes: Dendrimers as Experimental Exemplars and a Proposed Physical Mechanism

James R. Baker, Jr.

Department of Internal Medicine and Michigan Nanotechnology Institute for Medical and Biological Sciences, University of Michigan, Ann Arbor, Michigan, U.S.A.

Bradford G. Orr

Department of Physics and Michigan Nanotechnology Institute for Medical and Biological Sciences, University of Michigan, Ann Arbor, Michigan, U.S.A.

Mark M. Banaszak Holl

Department of Chemistry and Michigan Nanotechnology Institute for Medical and Biological Sciences, University of Michigan, Ann Arbor, Michigan, U.S.A.

INTRODUCTION

A great variety of nanoparticles have been synthesized and characterized over the last several decades including metal and metal oxide (1–3), semiconductor (4), and organic nanoparticles (5). These materials show promise for many kinds of applications such as catalysis (6), medical diagnosis and therapy (7,8), sensors (9–13), cosmetics (14), and coatings (15). These synthetic nanoparticles are similar in size to the major classes of biologically active materials (also nano in scale) used to effect chemical change (proteins), store and process information (DNA and RNA), and provide structure and transport (membranes, actin, microtubules). The similarity in size has prompted concern regarding how synthetic particles might interact with naturally occurring particles within biological systems. Thus, the toxicology of synthetic nanoparticles has become a pressing question. A flurry of reviews has appeared in the literature discussing these concerns and summarizing studies performed to date (16–20).

A number of studies on widely varying systems indicate that nanoparticles can have substantial mobility in a variety of biological tissues. C_{60} in bass (21), metal oxides in rats (22,23), and quantum dots in ex vivo pig skin (24) are examples of studies that have prompted substantial concern. These studies raise the question of the physical mechanism(s) by which the nanoparticle transport occurs. Transport of a wide range of types of nanoparticles via the respiratory tract, the gastrointestinal tract, and the skin has been recently reviewed (25).

Nanoparticles have been shown to be toxic in a number of published studies. This is not surprising, or necessarily even related to the nanoscale nature of the material, if the nanoparticle is made from normally toxic elements and these elements leach into the biological matrix (26,27). Other recent studies indicate that even when the nanoparticles themselves show little acute toxicity they can enhance the toxicity of other materials. For example, Inoue et al. have recently reported that 14 nm carbon black particles make mice substantially more susceptible to bacterial endotoxin (28).

It has long been recognized that nanoparticles cause permeability of biological membranes. This has been particularly recognized by the community of researchers interested in cell transfection who used nanoscale polymers or other particles to complex DNA and transport it into the cell (29–35). In order to understand this process, a variety of studies on lipid vesicles and cells have been performed (33,36–43). Despite considerable interest in this mechanism, a detailed molecular- or nanoscale mechanism has not emerged and considerable debate about the mechanism of membrane permeation, and how the nanoparticles themselves enter cells, still exists. This chapter will focus on studies that have directly probed nanoparticle/membrane interactions on the nanometer scale and assess the mechanistic clues that such studies provide for those working on a cellular or organism level understanding of nanoparticle toxicity.

Many of the experiments discussed in this chapter employ poly (amidoamine) (PAMAM) dendrimers (44–49). PAMAM dendrimers are organic-based macromolecules synthesized by the Michael addition of methyl acrylate to ethylene diamine followed by reaction of the resulting ester with additional ethylene diamine. Each time these two steps are carried out, the size of dendrimer is said to increase by one "generation" and there is an accompanying doubling of the number of terminal surface groups (primary amines) and roughly a doubling of molecular weight. These materials have several properties, which make them particular interesting as exemplar nanoparticles for mechanistic studies. First, they can be synthesized with polydispersity indexes as low as 1.01 giving a control of size that far exceeds most other classes of nanoparticle. Second, the chemical structure of these materials is well-defined at the molecular scale including the surface chemistry. The as-synthesized macromolecules have primary amines as the terminal groups. The primary amines are readily modified to provide a wide array of different surface chemistries including the acetamide and carboxylic acid termination discussed in this chapter. Lastly, the tree-like architecture of these nanoparticles allows them to deform in a manner that allows a large percentage of the particle surface to come in contact with any surface upon which they adsorb (50). This property is of particular interest for nano-particles in biology given the substantial importance of multivalent and polyvalent interactions (51).

THE INTERACTION OF NANOPARTICLES WITH SUPPORTED LIPID BILAYERS

In order to test the mechanism by which membrane permeability occurs, the interactions of PAMAM dendrimers and other polymers with supported lipid bilayers (SLBs) and living cells in tissue culture have been examined (52–55). These studies initially focused on scanning probe microscopy (SPM) studies of the interactions of the nanoscale polymers with SLBs in order to obtain a direct nanoscale view of the interactions leading to membrane permeability. PAMAM dendrimers were employed because of their well-defined size and surface chemistry (47,48). The effect of decreasing dendrimer generation (size) on the ability to form holes in lipid bilayers is illustrated in Figure 1. Adding ~10 nM generation 7 amine-terminated (G7-NH$_2$) PAMAMs to the lipid bilayer panels (a–c) caused the formation of small, isolated holes (typical diameters range from 15–40 nm) in previously intact parts of the bilayer. Once the holes had formed, their position and size changed very little up to 1 h. Some erosion of the bilayer was observed at the edges of existing defects. The effect of ~100 nM G5-NH$_2$ dendrimers is highlighted in panels (d–f). Although G5-NH$_2$ dendrimers removed lipids, they did so more slowly and mostly from the edges of existing bilayer defects. This resulted primarily in the growth of existing defects rather than the formation of isolated small holes as in the case of G7. When the size of the dendrimers was reduced still further, they were no longer able to remove lipids from the surface panels (g–i). G3-NH$_2$ PAMAMs added at ~100 nM adsorbed preferentially to bilayer edges forming a layer approximately 1.5 nm in height along the boundary of the lipid bilayer as indicated by arrows in panel (i). However, the preexisting holes in the dimyristoylphosphatidyl (DMPC) bilayer were not expanded and no additional holes were created.

In order to test the generality of these observations, other nanoscale polycationic polymers were also tested. Polyethyleneimine (PEI) and poly-L-lysine (PLL) also induced the formation of holes in supported DMPC bilayers, although concentrations of ~1–2 µg/mL (~100 nM) were required (56). This is roughly a ten-fold increase in concentration as compared to the amount of G7-NH$_2$ needed to form holes. Diethylaminoethyl-dextran (DEAE-dextran) showed both a membrane thinning effect, roughly similar

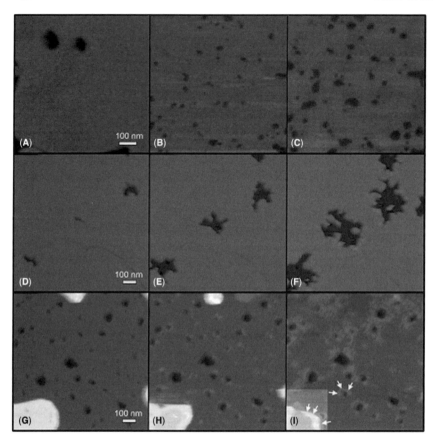

Figure 1 SPM images of interaction of G7, G5, and G3 PAMAM dendrimers with a DMPC bilayer. *Abbreviations*: DMPC, dimyristoylphosphatidyl; PAMAM, poly (amidoamine); SPM, scanning probe microscopy. *Source*: From Ref. 54.

to what is observed for antimicrobial peptides (57), as well as hole formation. As a control experiment for the PAMAM, PEI, PLL, and DEAE-dextran studies, the charge neutral, water soluble polymers polyethylene glycol (PEG) and polyvinyl alcohol (PVA) were employed. Neither polymer perturbed the bilayers up to a concentration of 6 μg/mL. These experiments demonstrate that the experimental methods do not induce hole formation and that the polycationic nature of the particle is important for the induction of holes in the lipid bilayers.

Other nanoparticles have also been observed to interact directly with SLBs. Sayes et al. noted that single-walled carbon nanotubes interact strongly with 1,2-dioleoyl-*sn*-glycero-3-phosphocholine (DOPC) bilayers on mica (58).

These interactions can be thought of using the general models of Israelachvili (59,60) and this has been independently suggested by two groups (54,61). Another interesting approach to the problem proposed by Tribet focuses on the balance of hydrophobic and hydrophilic interactions (62). Recent simulations of PAMAM dendrimers/lipid bilayers interactions provided detailed molecular level data consistent with the overall theoretical constructs of Israelachvili and Tribet (63). Other interesting papers on lipid or particle assembly have been published by Ladaviere et al. (64,65).

The Role of Membrane Phase

Studies with PAMAM dendrimers also exhibited a strong dependence on the phase of the SLB. Lipid bilayers can exist in several structural states including a liquid crystalline fluid phase and a gel phase. These are commonly referred to as L_α and L_β^* phase, respectively (66). Since the two phases differ in the thickness of the lipid bilayer, temperature-induced phase changes of bilayers can be observed by SPM (67,68). G7-NH_2 dendrimers are observed to disrupt and form holes only in the liquid crystalline phase L_α (Fig. 2) (53). No evidence of interaction is observed with gel-phase L_β^*. This strong dependence on lipid phase is important when considering how the hole-forming data presented in this chapter may be relevant to living cells and tissue. Broadly speaking, the experimental data implies that nano-particles could more easily disrupt and/or penetrate cells and tissues with liquid-phase membranes as opposed to gel-phase membranes. For example, the skin, which has an outer layer consisting mostly of dead, gelled membranes, would not be expected to be readily made permeable by nanoparticles in the absence of dermal abrasion or other stress (25,69,70). Portals of entry such as respiratory and gastrointestinal tracts, which include regions where fluid-phase membranes can more readily come into contact with the environment, are expected to be made permeable by exposure to cationic nanoparticles.

CELL-LEVEL STUDIES OF NANOPARTICLE-INDUCED MEMBRANE PERMEABILITY

The effects of G7 and G5 PAMAM dendrimers as well as PEI, PLL, and DEAE-dextran on the membrane permeability of KB and Rat2 cells were investigated using lactate dehydrogenase (LDH) and Luciferase (Luc) assays (55,56). All of the LDH and Luc studies described below were performed at noncytotoxic concentrations. The KB cell line, a variant of the human HeLa line, was selected because it overexpresses the folic acid receptor (FAR) and thus can be used in conjunction with folic acid (FA)-conjugated dendrimers to give authentic receptor-mediated endocytosis data for comparison

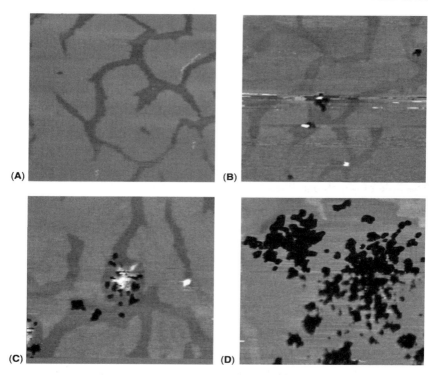

Figure 2 SPM height images of supported DMPC bilayer during phase transition before and after addition of 25 nM G7 PAMAM dendrimers. (**A**) Before adding dendrimers. The height difference between gel-phase (lighter shade) and liquid-phase (darker shade) is approximately 0.5 nm. (**B**) 3 min, (**C**) 8 min, and (**D**) 17 min after adding dendrimers. Defects (black areas) caused by dendrimers are approximately 5 nm deep. Scan size 1 μm, color height scale 0 to 5 nm. *Abbreviations*: DMPC, dimyristoylphosphatidyl; PAMAM, poly (amidoamine); SPM, scanning probe microscopy.

purposes. This makes it possible to test if the transport of the nanoparticle across the cell membrane is an intrinsically leaky process. The Rat2 fibroblast cell line was selected to provide a complement to the KB line in terms of species and tissue origin.

For both G7 and G5 PAMAM dendrimer, PLL, PEI, and DEAE-dextran, LDH release was proportionate to concentration for ∼10 to 500 nM exposures. By way of contrast, neither cell line released a significant amount of LDH as a result of exposure to G5 PAMAM dendrimer that had been acylated (G5-Ac). G5-Ac is neutral in aqueous solution. Similarly, treating the cells with similar concentrations of the neutral nanoscale polymers PVA and PEG did not result in LDH leakage. Consistent with the trends noted for SLBs as imaged by SPM (Fig. 1), G7-NH$_2$ induces substantially more release than G5-NH$_2$. Identical trends were noted when employing the Luc assay.

In order to test if internalization of a ~5 nm particle was an intrinsically leaky process, a G5-Ac sample to which FA groups had been conjugated was tested. This material has been shown to enter KB cells via FA-mediated endocytosis. Since neutral G5-Ac does not enter cells, cause holes in SLBs, or cause LDH leakage, this system appeared ideal to test if endocytosis of dendrimers necessarily caused LDH leakage. Endocytosis of G5-Ac-FA does NOT cause LDH leakage when it internalizes into cells via the FA-mediated endocytosis process. Thus, a nanoparticle without substantial positive surface charge can enter a cell without causing substantial cytosolic leakage. The leakage process appears correlated to the interaction of the positively charged nanoparticle with the cell membrane and not the entry of the nanoparticle into the cell (55).

The permanence of nanoparticle-induced permeabilization was tested by washing away the nanoparticles after 1 h exposure and then comparing to cells exposed for 3 h. For 100 to 500 nM concentrations using G5 PAMAM, LDH release ceased after removal of the dendrimer. Thus, the permeabilization of the membranes is reversible consistent with observations that the nanoparticles do not induce acute cytotoxicity at these concentrations.

To study passive diffusion in and out of the cell, propidium iodide (PI) and fluorescein diacetate (FDA) were used according to a modification of a previous literature method (71). PI is readily internalized into cells with disrupted membranes, but is excluded from cells with intact membranes. On the other hand, FDA, a nonfluorescent compound, readily enters intact cells and then undergoes hydrolysis by endogenous esterase, resulting in release of fluorescein into the cytosol. The cytosolic fluorescein is not able to transverse a normal cell membrane. Thus, FDA is used as a marker for diffusion through a membrane, which has been made permeable. Consequently, it is predicted that fluorescence intensity of PI should increase and that of fluorescein should decrease if the presence of the cationic nanoparticles makes the membrane permeable to these dyes.

Upon adding G7 PAMAM dendrimer, PLL, PEI, or DEAE-dextran to the cells, both dyes were observed to diffuse across the membrane (55). The charge neutral nanoparticles, G5-Ac, PVA, and PEG, did not induce dye diffusion across the cell membrane.

The induction of cell membrane permeability has been noted for a variety of other nanoparticle systems. Rotello et al. observed the induction of membrane permeability for cationic gold nanoparticles but a much reduced effect for anionic particles (31). Sayes et al. observed LDH release for nano-TiO_2 (anatase, 3–5 nm, varied degree of aggregation) when 3000 μg/mL was applied to HDF and A549 cells (72). However, the increased permeability was tentatively assigned to chemical oxidation of lipids and not a direct physical disruption process. Monteiro-Riviere et al. noted that CdSe core/ZnS shell quantum dots coated with PEG, amine-PEG, and carboxylic acid all entered human epidermal keratinocytes (skin cells) but that only the amine and carboxylic acid-coated materials showed signs of toxicity with the carboxylic acid-coated dots exhibiting the greatest amount of cytokine release (73). Nel et al. also recently reported studies on oxidative stress for atmospheric ultrafine particles, cationic polystyrene, TiO_2, carbon black and fullerol but did not perform studies of cell membrane permeability (74). The relationship between the physical disruption mechanism, membrane permeability, and oxidative stress in cells and tissue is not clear and needs additional studies.

INTERNALIZATION OF CATIONIC NANOPARTICLES INTO CELLS

To investigate the binding and internalization mechanism of dendrimers (SA1), confocal laser scanning microscopy (CLSM) images of Rat2 cells were taken after incubation with dendrimer-fluorescein (dendrimer-FITC) conjugates at different temperatures. Rat2, a fibroblast cell line, was chosen in

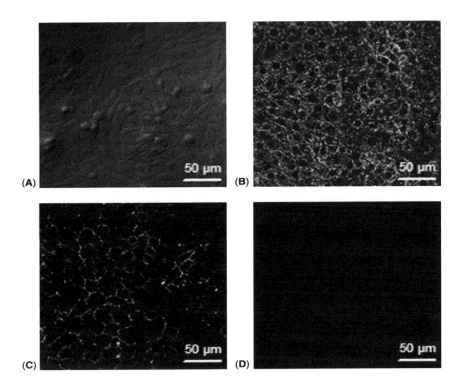

Figure 3 Differential interference contrast image of (**A**) untreated Rat2 cells (control). CLSM image of (**B**) Rat2 cells incubated with 200 nM G5-NH$_2$-FITC at 37°C, (**C**) Rat2 cells incubated with 200 nM G5-NH2-FITC at 6 C, and (**D**) Rat2 cells incubated with 200 nM G5-Ac-FITC at 37°C for 1 hour.

this experiment due to its stable surface adherence. Figure 3A shows a fluorescence image of Rat2 cells incubated with 200 nM of G5-NH$_2$-FITC at 37℃ for 1 h. Dendrimers are apparent both inside the cells as well as associated with the membrane. This indicates that the G5-NH$_2$-FITC dendrimers (a polycationic material at pH 7 with ~128 positive charges) interact with the cell membrane and enter the cell at physiological temperature (37℃). However, at 6℃ the dendrimers associated with the cell membrane, but no significant amount of internalization was observed (Fig. 3C). Identical experiments employing G5-Ac-FITC at 200 nM concentration indicate neither association with the cell membrane nor internalization into the cell (Fig. 3D). G5-Ac-FITC has all of the surface primary amines converted to acetamide groups so the particle does not protonate at pH 7 and is therefore not charged. Similar data to that shown in Figure 3 was obtained upon incubation of 6 µg/mL of PLL-FITC or 200 nM G7-NH$_2$-FITC with RAT2 cells for 1 h at 37℃ (56). Both of these materials are also polycationic in aqueous solution at pH 7.

These studies highlight the importance of understanding the role of surface charge when exploring the mechanism of nanoparticle uptake into cells. For many materials, the details of the surface chemistry, and therefore the surface charge, are not known. As the field moves forward it will be important to correlate the information that has been obtained, for example regarding cytotoxicity generally or oxidative stress specifically (74–76), to the mechanism by which nanoparticles enter the cell. Different mechanisms of entering, and the nature of the vesicle in which the nanoparticles are contained, may well have substantial impact on the toxicity of the materials once inside the cell.

Rothen-Rutishauser et al. recently reported a study following the uptake of polystyrene and TiO$_2$ particles in red blood cells and pulmonary macrophages (61,77). These studies were particularly interesting because red blood cells lack the typical cellular machinery for endoctyosis or phagocytosis, yet the particles still penetrated the cell. The authors conclude that particles enter the cells via an adhesive or diffusive mechanism and not the typically invoked endocytosis or phagocytosis mechanisms (43). This mechanistic proposal is roughly consistent with the mechanistic suggestions developed from the PAMAM nanoparticle-based studies (20,54,55). However, Rothen et al. have not observed the strong dependence on surface charge. Additional experiments are needed to clarify the importance of such nonphagocytic mechanisms and the importance of particle size and surface charge. An interesting experiment by Javier et al. combined SPM measurements (force–distance) of micron-size particle adhesion to the cell membrane with particle uptake demonstrating a clear correlation (78). The effect of changes in particle size upon adhesion and uptake mechanism still needs further exploration. It is not clear the data on 5 µm particles can or should be extrapolated to the behavior of 5 nm particles. Lai et al. have measured K_D values for G4 and G6 PAMAM dendrimers binding to cell surfaces using fluorescence microscopy (79).

CONCLUSIONS

Polycationic organic nanoparticles ~5 to 7 nm in size have been shown to induce a variety of effects at noncytotoxic concentrations including: (1) inducing nanoscale holes in fluid-phase SLBs, (2) inducing permeability in lipid vesicles, (3) inducing permeability in cell plasma membranes, and (4) readily penetrating cell plasma membranes and internalizing into cells. Similar concentrations of neutral organic nanoparticles ~5 to 7 nm in size do not induce permeability in SLBs, do not induce permeability in cell plasma membranes, and do not readily internalize into cells. The induction of nanoscale holes or pores in biological membranes, and the resulting increase in membrane permeability, provides a possible mechanism for nanoparticle transport in biological systems. The relationship of nanoscale hole formation and other possible adhesive and/or diffusive mechanisms to transport of nanoparticles in vivo, and the relationship to active transport mechanisms such as endocytosis or phagocytosis by which nanoparticles hijack normal cellular mechanisms, requires further study.

REFERENCES

1. Daniel MC, Astruc D. Gold nanoparticles: assembly, supramolecular chemistry, quantum-size-related properties, and applications toward biology, catalysis, and nanotechnology. Chem Rev 2004; 104:293–346.
2. Fernandez-Garcia M, Martinez-Arias A, Hanson JC, Rodriguez JA. Nanostructured oxides in chemistry: characterization and properties. Chem Rev 2004; 104:4063–104.
3. Bonnemann H, Richards RM. Nanoscopic metal particles—synthetic methods and potential applications. Eur J Inorg Chem 2001:2455–80.
4. Trindade T, O'Brien P, Pickett NL. Nanocrystalline semiconductors: synthesis, properties, and perspectives. Chem Mater 2001; 13:3843–58.
5. Horn D, Rieger J. Organic nanoparticles in the aqueous phase—theory, experiment, and use. Angew Chem Int Ed 2001; 40:4331–61.
6. Schlogl R, Abd Hamid SB. Nanocatalysis: mature science revisited or something really new? Angew Chem Int Ed 2004; 43:1628–37.
7. Mornet S, Vasseur S, Grasset F, Duguet E. Magnetic nanoparticle design for medical diagnosis and therapy. J Mater Chem 2004; 14:2161–75.
8. Brannon-Peppas L, Blanchette JO. Nanoparticle and targeted systems for cancer therapy. Adv Drug Deliver Rev 2004; 56:1649–59.
9. Buck SM, Koo YEL, Park E, Xu H, Philbert MA, Brasuel MA, Kopelman R. Optochemical nanosensor PEBBLEs: photonic explorers for bioanalysis with biologically localized embedding. Curr Opin Chem Biol 2004; 8:540–6.
10. Haes AJ, Van Duyne RP. Preliminary studies and potential applications of localized surface plasmon resonance spectroscopy in medical diagnostics. Expert Rev Mol Diag 2004; 4:527–37.
11. Katz E, Willner I, Wang J. Electroanalytical and bioelectroanalytical systems based on metal and semiconductor nanoparticles. Electroanalysis 2004; 16:19–44.

12. West JL, Halas NJ. Engineered nanomaterials for biophotonics applications: improving sensing, imaging, and therapeutics. Annu Rev Biomed Eng 2003; 5: 285–92.

13. Shipway AN, Katz E, Willner I. Nanoparticle arrays on surfaces for electronic, optical, and sensor applications. Chemphyschem 2000; 1:18–52.

14. Somasundaran P, Cakraborty S, Qiang Q, Deo P, Wang J, Zhang R. Surfactants, polymers, and their nanoparticles for personal care applications. J Cosmet Sci 2004; 55:S1–17.

15. Parker JC, Brotzman RW, Ali MN. Coating opportunities for nanoparticles made from the condensation of physical vapors. Mater Manufact Process 1996; 11:263–70.

16. Donaldson K, Stone V, Tran CL, Kreyling W, Borm PJA. Nanotoxicology. Occup Environ Med 2004; 61:727–8.

17. Dreher KL. Health and environmental impact of nanotechnology: toxicological assessment of manufactured nanoparticles. Toxicol Sci 2004; 77:3–5.

18. Lippmann M, Frampton M, Schwartz J, Dockery D, Schlesinger R, Koutrakis P, Froines J, Nel A, Finkelstein J, Godleski J, Kaufman J, Koenig J, Larson T, Luchtel D, Liu LJS, Oberdorster G, Peters A, Sarnat J, Sioutas C, Suh H, Sullivan J, Utell M, Wichmann E, Zelikoff G. The US Environmental Protection Agency particulate matter health effects research centers program: a midcourse report of status, progress, and plans. Environ Health Persp 2003; 111:1074–92.

19. Wiesner MR, Lowry GV, Alvarez P, Dionysiou D, Biswas P. Assessing the risks of manufactured nanomaterials. Environ Sci Technol 2006; 40:4336–45.

20. Hong S, Hessler JA, Banaszak Holl MM, Leroueil PR, Mecke A, Orr BG. Physical interactions of nanoparticles with biological membranes: the observation of nanoscale hole formation. Chem Health Safety 2006; 13:16–20.

21. Oberdorster E. Manufactured nanomaterials (Fullerenes, C-60) induce oxidative stress in the brain of juvenile largemouth bass. Environ Health Persp 2004; 112:1058–62.

22. Oberdorster G, Sharp Z, Atudorei V, Elder A, Gelein R, Kreyling W, Cox C. Translocation of inhaled ultrafine particles to the brain. Inhal Toxicol 2004; 16:437–45.

23. Elder A, Gelein R, Silva V, Feikert T, Opanashuk L, Carter J, Potter R, Maynard A, Finkelstein J, Oberdorster G. Translocation of inhaled ultrafine manganese oxide particles to the central nervous system. Environ Health Persp 2006; 114:1172–8.

24. Ryman-Rasmussen JP, Riviere JE, Monteiro-Riviere NA. Penetration of intact skin by quantum dots with diverse physicochemical properties. Toxicol Sci 2006; 91:159–65.

25. Oberdorster G, Oberdorster E, Oberdorster J. Nanotoxicology: an emerging discipline evolving from studies of ultrafine particles. Environ Health Persp 2005; 113:823–39.

26. Derfus AM, Chan WCW, Bhatia SN. Probing the cytotoxicity of semiconductor quantum dots. Nano Lett 2004; 4:11–8.

27. Kirchner C, Liedl T, Kudera S, Pellegrino T, Javier AM, Gaub HE, Stolzle S, Fertig N, Parak WJ. Cytotoxicity of colloidal CdSe and CdSe/ZnS nanoparticles. Nano Lett 2005; 5:331–8.

28. Inoue K, Takano H, Yanagisawa R, Hirano S, Sakurai M, Shimada A, Yoshikawa T. Effects of airway exposure to nanoparticles on lung inflammation induced by bacterial endotoxin in mice. Environ Health Persp 2006; 114: 1325–30.

29. Reineke TM, Grinstaff MW. Designer materials for nucleic acid delivery. MRS Bull 2005; 30:635–9.

30. Luo D. Nanotechnology and DNA delivery. MRS Bull 2005; 30:654–8.

31. Goodman CM, McCusker CD, Yilmaz T, Rotello VM. Toxicity of gold nanoparticles functionalized with cationic and anionic side chains. Bioconjugate Chem 2004; 15:897–900.

32. Sandhu KK, McIntosh CM, Simard JM, Smith SW, Rotello VM. Gold nanoparticle-mediated transfection of mammalian cells. Bioconjugate Chem 2002; 13:3–6.

33. Fischer D, Li YX, Ahlemeyer B, Krieglstein J, Kissel T. In vitro cytotoxicity testing of polycations: influence of polymer structure on cell viability and hemolysis. Biomaterials 2003; 24:1121–31.

34. Moghimi SM, Symonds P, Murray JC, Hunter AC, Debska G, Szewczyk A. A two-stage poly(ethyleneimine)-mediated cytotoxicity: implications for gene transfer/therapy. Mol Ther 2005; 11:990–5.

35. Chen H-T, Neerman MF, Parrish AR, Simanek EE. Cytotoxicity, hemolysis, and acute in vivo toxicity of dendrimers based on melamine, candidate vehicles for drug delivery. J Am Chem Soc 2004; 140:10044–8.

36. Ottaviani MF, Matteini P, Brustolon M, Turro NJ, Jockusch S, Tomalia DA. Characterization of starburst dendrimers and vesicle solutions and their interactions by CW- and pulsed-EPR, TEM, and dynamic light scattering. J Phys Chem B 1998; 102:6029–39.

37. Zhang Z-Y, Smith BD. High-generation polycationic dendrimers are unusually effective at disrupting anionic vesicles: membrane bending model. Bioconjugate Chem 2000; 11:805–14.

38. Karoonuthaisiri N, Titiyevskiy K, Thomas JL. Destabilization of fatty acid-containing liposomes by polyamidoamine dendrimers. Coll Surf B Biointerfaces 2003; 27:365–75.

39. Malik N, Wiwattanapatapee R, Klopsch R, Lorenz K, Frey H, Weener JW, Meijer EW, Paulus W, Duncan R. Dendrimers: relationship between structure and biocompatibility in vitro, and preliminary studies on the biodistribution of I-125-labelled polyamidoamine dendrimers in vivo. J Control Release 2000; 65:133–48.

40. Tajarobi F, El-Sayed M, Rege BD, Polli JE, Ghandehari H. Transport of poly amidoamine dendrimers across Madin–Darby canine kidney cells. Int J Pharm 2001; 215:263–7.

41. Behr JP. Synthetic gene-transfer vectors. Acc Chem Res 1993; 26:274–8.

42. Boussif O, Lezoualch F, Zanta MA, Mergny MD, Scherman D, Demeneix B, Behr JP. A versatile vector for gene and oligonucleotide transfer into cells in culture and in vivo—polyethylenimine. Proc Natl Acad Sci USA 1995; 92:7297–301.

43. Kopatz I, Remy JS, Behr JP. A model for non-viral gene delivery: through syndecan adhesion molecules and powered by actin. J Gene Med 2004; 6: 769–76.

44. Tomalia DA, Huang B, Swanson DR, Brothers HM, Klimash JW. Structure control within poly(amidoamine) dendrimers: size, shape and regio-chemical mimicry of globular proteins. Tetrahedron 2003; 59:3799–813.

45. Tomalia DA, Naylor AM, Goddard WA. Starburst dendrimers—molecular-level control of size, shape, surface-chemistry, topology, and flexibility from atoms to macroscopic matter. Angew Chem Int Ed 1990; 29:138–75.

46. Tomalia DA, Baker H, Dewald J, Hall M, Kallos G, Martin S, Roeck J, Ryder J, Smith P. A new class of polymers—starburst-dendritic macromolecules. Polym J 1985; 17:117–32.

47. Eichman JD, Bielinska AU, Kukowska-Latallo JF, Donovan BW, Baker JR. Bioapplications of PAMAM dendrimers. In: Frechet JMJ, Tomalia DA, eds. Dendrimers and Other Dendritic Polymers. New York: John Wiley & Sons, 2001: 441–61.

48. Duncan R, Izzo L. Dendrimer biocompatibility and toxicity. Adv Drug Deliver Rev 2005; 57:2215–37.

49. Zeng F, Zimmerman SC. Dendrimers in supramolecular chemistry: from molecular recognition to self-assembly. Chem Rev 1997; 97:1681–712.

50. Mecke A, Lee I, Baker JR, Banaszak Holl MM, Orr BG. Deformability of poly(amidoamine) dendrimers. Eur Phys J E Soft Mater 2004; 14:7–16.

51. Hong S, Leroueil PR, Majoros I, Orr BG, Baker JR, Banaszak Holl MM. The binding avidity of a nanoparticle-based multivalent targeted drug delivery platform. Chem Biol 2007; 14:107–15.

52. Mecke A, Uppuluri S, Sassanella TJ, Lee DK, Ramamoorthy A, Baker JR, Orr BG, Banaszak Holl MM. Direct observation of lipid bilayer disruption by poly(amidoamine) dendrimers. Chem Phys Lipids 2004; 132:3–14.

53. Mecke A, Lee D-K, Ramamoorthy A, Orr BG, Banaszak Holl MM. Synthetic and natural polycationic polymer nanoparticles interact selectively with fluid-phase domains of DMPC bilayers. Langmuir 2005; 21: 8588–90.

54. Mecke A, Majoros I, Patri AK, Baker JR, Banaszak Holl MM, Orr BJ. Lipid bilayer disruption by polycationic polymers: the roles of size and chemical functional group. Langmuir 2005; 21:10348–54.

55. Hong S, Bielinska AU, Mecke A, Keszler B, Beals JL, Shi X, Balogh L, Orr BG, Baker JR, Banaszak Holl MM. The interaction of polyamidoamine (PAMAM) dendrimers with supported lipid bilayers and cells: hole formation and the relation to transport. Bioconjugate Chem 2004; 15:774–82.

56. Hong SP, Leroueil PR, Janus EK, Peters JL, Kober MM, Islam MT, Orr BG, Baker JR, Holl MMB. Interaction of polycationic polymers with supported lipid bilayers and cells: nanoscale hole formation and enhanced membrane permeability. Bioconjugate Chem 2006; 17:728–34.

57. Mecke A, Lee DK, Ramamoorthy A, Orr BG, Banaszak Holl MM. Membrane thinning due to antimicrobial peptide binding—an AFM study of MSI-78 in DMPC bilayers. Biophys J 2005; 89:4043–50.

58. Sayes CM, Liang F, Hudson JL, Mendez J, Guo WH, Beach JM, Moore VC, Doyle CD, West JL, Billups WE, Ausman KD, Colvin VL. Functionalization density dependence of single-walled carbon nanotubes cytotoxicity in vitro. Toxicol Lett 2006; 161:135–42.

59. Israelachvili JN, Mitchell DJ, Ninham BW. Theory of self-assembly of hydrocarbon amphiphiles into micelles and bilayers. J Chem Soc Faraday Trans II 1976; 72:1525–68.

60. Israelachvili JN, Mitchell DJ, Ninham BW. Theory of self-assembly of lipid bilayers and vesicles. Biochim Biophys Acta 1977; 470:185–201.

61. Rothen-Rutishauser BM, Schurch S, Haenni B, Kapp N, Gehr P. Interaction of fine particles and nanoparticles with red blood cells visualized with advanced microscopic techniques. Environ Sci Technol 2006; 40:4353–9.

62. Tribet C. Hydrophobically driven attachments of synthetic polymers onto surfaces of biological interest: lipid bilayers and globular proteins. Biochimie 1998; 80:461–73.

63. Lee H, Larson RG. Molecular dynamics simulations of PAMAM dendrimer-induced pore formation in DPPC bilayers with a coarse-grained model. J Phys Chem B 2006; 110:18204–11.

64. Troutier AL, Veron L, Delair T, Pichot C, Ladaviere C. New insights into self-organization of a model lipid mixture and quantification of its adsorption on spherical polymer particles. Langmuir 2005; 21:9901–10.

65. Troutier AL, Delair T, Pichot C, Ladaviere C. Physicochemical and interfacial investigation of lipid/polymer particle assemblies. Langmuir 2005; 21:1305–13.

66. Janiak MJ, Small DM, Shipley GG. Temperature and compositional dependence of the structure of hydrated dimyristoyl lecithin. J Biol Chem 1979; 254:6068–78.

67. Tokumasu F, Jin AJ, Dvorak JA. Lipid membrane phase behaviour elucidated in real time by controlled environment atomic force microscopy. J Electron Microsc 2002; 51:1–9.

68. Xie AF, Yamada R; Gewirth AA, Granick S. Materials science of the gel to fluid phase transition in a supported phospholipid bilayer. Phys Rev Lett 2002; 89:246103.

69. Tinkle SS, Antonini JM, Rich BA, Roberts JR, Salmen R, DePree K, Adkins EJ. Skin as a route of exposure and sensitization in chronic beryllium disease. Environ Health Persp 2003; 111:1202–8.

70. Rouse JG, Yang JZ, Ryman- Rasmussen JP, Barron AR, Monteiro-Riviere NA. Effects of mechanical flexion on the penetration of fullerene amino acid-derivatized peptide nanoparticles through skin. Nano Lett 2007; 7: 155–60.

71. Umebayashi Y, Miyamoto Y, Wakita M, Kobayashi A, Nishisaka T. Elevation of plasma membrane permeability on laser irradiation of extracellular latex particles. J Biochem 2003; 134:219–24.

72. Sayes CM, Wahi R, Kurian PA, Liu YP, West JL, Ausman KD, Warheit DB, Colvin VL. Correlating nanoscale titania structure with toxicity: a cytotoxicity and inflammatory response study with human dermal fibroblasts and human lung epithelial cells. Toxicol Sci 2006; 92:174–85.

73. Ryman-Rasmussen JP, Riviere JE, Monteiro-Riviere NA. Surface coatings determine cytotoxicity and irritation potential of quantum dot nanoparticles in epidermal keratinocytes. J Invest Dermatol 2007; 127:143–53.

74. Xia T, Kovochich M, Brant J, Hotze M, Sempf J, Oberley T, Sioutas C, Yeh JI, Wiesner MR, Nel AE. Comparison of the abilities of ambient and

manufactured nanoparticles to induce cellular toxicity according to an oxidative stress paradigm. Nano Lett 2006; 6:1794–807.

75. Brunner TJ, Wick P, Manser P, Spohn P, Grass RN, Limbach LK, Bruinink A, Stark WJ. In vitro cytotoxicity of oxide nanoparticles: comparison to asbestos, silica, and the effect of particle solubility. Environ Sci Technol 2006; 40:4374–81.

76. Limbach LK, Li YC, Grass RN, Brunner TJ, Hintermann MA, Muller M, Gunther D, Stark WJ. Oxide nanoparticle uptake in human lung fibroblasts: effects of particle size, agglomeration, and diffusion at low concentrations. Environ Sci Technol 2005; 39:9370–6.

77. Geiser M, Rothen-Rutishauser B, Kapp N, Schurch S, Kreyling W, Schulz H, Semmler M, Hof VI, Heyder J, Gehr P. Ultrafine particles cross cellular membranes by nonphagocytic mechanisms in lungs and in cultured cells. Environ Health Persp 2005; 113:1555–60.

78. Javier AM, Kreft O, Alberola AP, Kirchner C, Zebli B, Susha AS, Horn E, Kempter S, Skirtach AG, Rogach AL, Radler J, Sukhorukov GB, Benoit M, Parak WJ. Combined atomic force microscopy and optical microscopy measurements as a method to investigate particle uptake by cells. Small 2006; 2:394–400.

79. Lai JC, Yuan C, Thomas JL. Single-cell measurements of polyamidoamine dendrimer binding. Ann Biomed Eng 2002; 30:409–16.

8

Placental Biological Barrier Models for Evaluation of Nanoparticle Transfer

Margaret Saunders

Biophysics Research Unit, Department of Medical Physics and Bioengineering, United Bristol Healthcare, National Health Service Trust, Bristol, U.K.

NANOPARTICLE EXPOSURE

While human exposure to airborne nanoparticles (NP) has been ongoing since early evolution, the extent of exposure increased dramatically with the advent of the industrial revolution and will continue to rise with the rapid development of nanotechnology as human use and production of these particles increases (1). Therefore, alongside these advances, we must take account of the increase in potential for release into the environment and uptake into the human body with a currently unknown magnitude of risk. The lack of information on potential effects of NP on human and environmental health has been highlighted in over 20 international reports from agencies such as DEFRA (2), US-EPA (3) and the Royal Society and Royal Academy of Engineers working group on nanoscience and nanotechnology (4) emphasizing the requirement for a proper risk assessment of NP and the need for suitable barrier models (5).

Exposure to NP can potentially arise from therapeutic or diagnostic administration as well as from occupational and environmental exposure through manufactured sources or combustion sources in the environment and as such there is the possibility for any individual to be exposed. The novel properties of NP give them the ability to interact with their biological environment in different ways. Due to their size, they have an increased surface area per unit mass leading to greater potential for biological interactions which may be distinct from behavior of larger particles of bulk material.

The influence of the different physicochemical properties of various types of NP requires investigation and these include factors such as surface area, size distribution, chemical purity, crystallinity, charge, surface structure including reactivity, surface groups, inorganic/organic coatings, solubility, shape and aggregation/agglomeration (6). Reduction in size and increase in surface area increases the relative proportion of atoms/molecules expressed on the surface and hence increases surface reactivity (1).

Penetration of Biological Systems

Much of the preliminary work on NP took place on "ultra-fine particles" and this body of work clearly shows that NP can enter the human organism through inhalation. However, it is not currently clear whether NP have the ability to transfer across biological barriers and reach other target sites. While there is ambiguous evidence for translocation of NP into the circulation, once NP reach pulmonary interstitial sites, uptake into blood circulation could occur (1). Systemic in vivo distribution of quantum dots to major organs such as liver, kidney, lung, spleen, lymph nodes and bone-marrow has been reported in mice (7,8), but overall there is a paucity of data on uptake and more studies are required (1). The skin and the gastrointestinal tract are alternative entry portals to be considered, particularly since many engineered NP are prepared and processed in liquid (9) and transfer across the gut would facilitate systemic distribution with translocation across biological barriers such as the blood-brain barrier and the placenta feasible. Uptake via the gut has been demonstrated in oral feeding or gavage experiments (10) with NP in food reported to cross into the gut lymphatic system and redistribute to other organs more readily compared with larger particles and medical or therapeutic applications would directly introduce NP into the body (11). Outcome will depend upon the characteristics of the NP but they may act at cellular, sub-cellular and protein levels and could cause effects as diverse as oxidative stress, inflammation, protein denaturation, membrane damage, DNA damage and immune reactivity (6). Characteristics such as surface charge will affect the ability of NP to cross biological barriers (12–14) and subsequent tissue distribution. Aggregation/agglomeration of NP could lead to increased persistence with trapping in placental tissue but may actually prevent transfer to the fetus dependent upon where the aggregation/ agglomeration occurs.

WHY THE INTEREST IN THE PLACENTA?

The fetus is more sensitive to the effects of exposure to external agents or xenobiotics compared with the adult due to the rapid development occurring during gestation and the altered metabolism. Adverse events during fetal development such as growth retardation may arise from placental insufficiency or fetal exposure to hazardous compounds and such events may impact on adult health in later life (15). Therefore it is important to determine whether NP are taken up by the placenta with the potential to affect placental function and transferred to the fetal circulation where they could distribute systemically and directly affect the fetus. Exposure of the fetus arises primarily through transfer across the placenta from the mother's circulation with the placenta acting as the maternal-fetal interface although exchange may also possibly occur through the amniotic fluid (16). Therefore, there is the potential for the fetus to be exposed to anything that is taken up by the mother both during and in some cases before gestation, e.g., organochlorine pesticides which are lipophilic and accumulate in the mother's body fat.

Placental Function and Development

The placenta plays a key role during fetal development with its major function being the transfer of nutrients to support embryonic and fetal growth and development (16). Other functions include metabolism, transport, immune and endocrine secretion functions, gas exchange, and removal of waste or toxic products from the fetus, all essential for maintenance of a successful pregnancy. Problems with placental structure, position or function during pregnancy can result in a range of complications such as fetal growth retardation, premature delivery, birth defects, and in the worst case, may result in fetal or neonatal death.

The placenta begins to develop at the time of blastocyst implantation and is delivered at birth. Following fertilization, the ovum undergoes mitosis to form a solid clump of cells (morula) which then differentiates into a hollow sphere known as the blastocyst (17). The blastocyst comprises an inner cell mass (ICM) or embryoblast which will go on to form the embryo and an outer wall consisting of a single layer of uninucleate trophoblast cells surrounding the ICM which will develop into the placenta and extra-embryonic membranes (18,19). Following entry into the uterus from the fallopian tubes, the blastocyst sheds its outer coat (zona pellucida) such that its outer surface now comprises trophoblast cells (17). The trophoblast cells consist of mononuclear cells called cytotrophoblasts and multinucleated cells called syncytiotrophoblasts which form an outer layer or syncytium (20). Between day 8 and 12 postconception, fluid-filled vacuoles develop within the syncytiotrophoblast which coalesce to form larger lacunae separated by attenuated trabeculae of syncytiotrophoblast. At the end of implantation, the blastocyst is totally embedded within the uterine wall and endometrial epithelium regrows over the implantation site. The trophoblast and extraembryonic mesoderm are referred to as the chorion (19). The lacunae divide the trophoblast into three zones: the primary chorionic plate facing the embryo which becomes the chorionic plate; the lacunar system and trabeculae which becomes the intervillous space of the placenta and the trophoblastic shell adjacent to the endometrium which becomes the basal plate (19).

Cytotrophoblast proliferation after day 13 results in a considerable increase in length of the trabeculae which start to branch and form primary villi. With incorporation of extraembryonic mesoderm these transform into secondary villi and then vascularization marks the formation of tertiary villi (19). Tertiary villi form the bulk of the placenta and the bulk of the syncytiotrophoblast comes into direct contact with maternal blood following maturation of the villous structure (17). Thus the syncytiotrophoblast layer covers the villous tree and forms the placental barrier with the apical membrane facing the maternal side and the basal membrane facing the fetal side (21). Maternal tissue adjacent to the trophoblast degenerates progressively such that the fetal villi are ultimately bathed directly in maternal blood from spiral arteries which open into the intervillous chamber in the human placenta thus facilitating exchange and transport of nutrients (17,22). The maternal blood then drains into the subchorial space in the basal area of the placenta returning to the maternal circulation through venous openings in the basal plate arranged around the periphery of each villous tree (17).

At term the human placenta is discoid in shape, weighs around 500 g on average and has a diameter of around 15 to 20 cm with the majority of the placenta formed of chorionic villi with attendant blood vessels and connective tissue. Two arteries within the umbilical cord supply the fetal arterial blood with oxygenated blood returning to the fetus though a single vein. Each of these vessels branches out over the fetal surface of the placenta dividing into networks of secondary vessels and then again into tertiary vessels. Paired tertiary arteries and veins penetrate through the chorionic plate to enter the main stem villi which forms the heart of a fetal cotyledon (or villous tree). The cotyledon is a placental lobule consisting of a rounded mass of villi which forms the functional vascular unit of the placenta (22). There are up to about 30 cotyledons in the placenta (17,23) with the villous trunk and branches that form the cotyledon partitioned laterally by decidual septa. The cotyledon is limited on the maternal side by the basal plate and by the chorionic plate on the fetal side (23).

Exchange between maternal and fetal circulation occurs across the endothelio-syncytial membrane and transfer depends on a number of physical factors including surface area and thickness of the membrane, blood flow, hydrostatic pressure in the intervillous chamber, fetal capillary blood pressure, and difference in maternal and fetal osmotic pressure (22). The membrane becomes progressively thinner as term approaches potentially maximizing opportunities for transfer (22) but this is modified in the haemochorial placenta by the deposition of fibrinoid on the exchange surface at the end of gestation (23).

Comparative Structure of the Placenta

The mammalian placenta, as well as being a complex organ, is the most structurally diverse among the different species. Mammalian placentas have been classified on the basis of macroscopic appearance and shape (16) and also the extent and type of maternal-fetal contact (17,19,24). Grosser suggested a classification based on the number of layers seen to separate the circulations under light microscopy. In the sheep, for example, which is one of the most commonly used species in placental transfer studies, all three maternal layers (uterine endothelium, connective tissue, endometrial epithelium) are retained as well as the chorionic epithelium, fetal connective tissue and fetal endothelial cells (epitheliochorial placenta). Dogs and cats are examples of endothelio-chorial placentas where the maternal uterine endothelium is retained but the maternal connective tissue and endometrial epithelium disintegrate. In contrast, in human and rodents, all three maternal layers disintegrate, giving rise to a haemochorial placenta. This is further sub-divided in terms of the number of trophoblast layers between maternal blood and fetal endothelium with one layer, e.g., human and guinea pig (haemomonochorial), two layers e.g., rabbit (haemodichorial) or three layers (haemotrichorial), e.g., mouse, rat (20). The interdigitation of the maternal and fetal circulation leads to further complexity with classification as villous (e.g., human, ape), labyrinthine (e.g., rabbit, guinea pig, rat, mouse), folded (e.g., pig). A final complexity is the direction of the blood flow in each circulation which can be concurrent or counter-current (opposite direction). All these factors will affect the efficiency and rate of exchange across the placenta.

TRANSPORT ACROSS THE PLACENTAL BARRIER

A major assumption and over-simplification arising from the Grosser classification system is that the number of intervening layers between the circulations directly determines the ability of material to transfer across the placenta. However, more layers does not necessarily mean a thicker barrier as indentation by maternal and fetal capillaries significantly reduces the diffusional distance as seen in the epitheliochorial placenta of the pig, for example, Ref. 16. Also, while passive diffusion is the transport route app-licable to most chemical compounds crossing the placenta (25), there are additional transport systems that function within the placenta which include active transport, facilitated transport, and to a lesser extent phagocytosis, pinocytosis and filtration (16,26,27). These are all possible mechanisms for the uptake and transport of NP across the placenta. The upper limit for transfer is 500kDa with incomplete transfer of chemicals above this (28) and unionized drugs cross more readily than ionized (25,27). The placenta has an enormous surface available for exchange with fetal capillaries within the villi being 3000 to 5000 μm in length (17) with a minimum diffusion distance of about 4 μm (29). Diffusion will be affected by characteristics including molecular weight, pKa, lipid solubility and protein binding which will vary according to the type of NP under investigation. An extensive range of over 20 different drug transporters have been identified recently (30) and any non-physiological compounds which bear a structural similarity to the natural substrates could be recognized by these transporters (31). Within the syncytiotrophoblast there is differential expression of specific transporters in the maternal facing (apical) brush border membrane and the fetal facing basal (basolateral) membrane. The brush border is in direct contact with maternal blood and the basal membrane faces the fetal blood vessels (31). Active transporters are located either in the apical or basolateral membrane and can act to pump substrates into or out of the syncytiotrophoblast membrane (30). They may therefore take on a protective role with respect to the fetus depending upon the membrane distribution which would be important if they are implicated in NP transport.

APPROACHES FOR ASSESSMENT OF PLACENTAL TRANSFER

The ideal approach to determine placental transfer of any compound would be to evaluate it in pregnant women. However, this presents a very obvious ethical dilemma due to the potential risks associated with exposure during pregnancy. Such risks have been highlighted by the unforeseen consequences of the prescription of drugs which have turned out to be pharmaceutical teratogens such as thalidomide and diethylstilbesterol. It is possible to carry out in vivo measurements of chemicals to which pregnant women are unavoidably exposed such as those taken up from the environment e.g., heavy metals, persistent organic pollutants, and medication for conditions such as epilepsy and diabetes through the sampling of adult peripheral blood and cord blood at birth. However, the information that can be obtained from such studies is limited as this information is available for a single time-point only and provides no knowledge about the kinetics of placental transfer. In order to undertake exposure-dose determinations and risk assessments related to human exposure validated alternatives are required for the investigation of new substances such as nanoparticles.

In Vivo Animal Models

Use of in vivo animal models provides an opportunity to assess uptake through different routes of exposure and biokinetics can be determined for both adult and fetal organs, highlighting any organs that may show evidence of selective uptake. Effects of metabolism and physiology can also be determined. While a range of animals are available, careful selection is required due to the extensive variability in terms of placental structure and anatomy amongst mammalian species. In terms of similarity, primates would be most suited for evaluation, since their placental structure is most like the human but ethical concerns, length of gestation and cost are issues of concern.

The guinea pig has the advantages of a placental structure similar to that of the human, a convenient gestation period (63 days), and suitable size and development at term with the fetal period of a more similar proportion to that of the human with respect to the entire gestation period in contrast to other rodents such as rats and mice. Previous studies have demonstrated suitability for the assessment of fetal exposure to agents such as radionuclides (32). Such a model can be used for determination of biodistribution of NP thus enabling us to assess biodistribution and transfer across a range of biological barriers in vivo and will certainly provide answers about how the different characteristics of NP affect their uptake and transfer. However, the major criticism that there are species-related differences still remains. While hemomonochorial and discoid like the human placenta, the interdigitation in the guinea pig is labyrinthine and the circulation is countercurrent as opposed to concurrent in humans (27) and we cannot necessarily extrapolate the outcome to what will happen in humans.

Human Perfused Ex Vivo Placenta Model

A model which overcomes this criticism and any ethical dilemmas is the human ex vivo perfused placental cotyledon model which can be considered as a more suitable barrier model of direct human relevance. It has the advantages of being human tissue; easy availability; provides information about effects and transfer of chemicals; remains viable for some time after delivery. Experiments performed in the 1960s by Panigel and his colleagues originally involved perfusion of the complete placenta but the success rate was greatly increased by modification of the technique to perfuse an isolated cotyledon (33,34). A further refinement was the inclusion of antipyrine as a reference marker (35). Antipyrine is freely diffusible and transfer is limited only by the ratio of fetal to maternal bloodflow (22).

The human perfused placental cotyledon model is used extensively in placental transfer experiments, particularly for drug studies, with the establishment of separate maternal and fetal circulations possible using suitable perfusion media. An extensive range of substances have been evaluated including nutrients such as sugars, amino acids, fatty acids; metals such as calcium and zinc; hormones including insulin and corticosteroids; vitamins; a wide range of therapeutic agents; drugs of abuse and toxic chemicals such as cadmium (23). For perfusions of short duration it is possible to use buffered physiological salt solutions with a plasma expander and glucose but for longer experiments, it is necessary to use tissue culture medium. The duration of perfusion is variable and can range from 2 to 4 hours up to 12 to 18 hours with one report of perfusion for 48 hours but maintenance of viability is challenging and best monitored by assessment of leakage from the perfusion circuit (36). The addition of dextran and human serum albumin to the perfusate help to avoid oedema but the transfer rate of particular substances e.g., lipophilic compounds may be significantly affected by the presence of albumin (17,37). This will be significant when looking at the influence of coatings on NP behavior.

Perfusions can be established by insertion of cannulae into a suitable artery and vein on the fetal side and into the corresponding intervillous space on the maternal side which becomes evident as a blanched area once perfusate is pumped though. Recirculation of the perfusate using a closed system can be considered to mimic the in vivo situation with transfer being expressed as a percentage of the amount administered to the donor circuit. Alternatively, a non-recirculating open system can be used where the material under investigation passes through the placenta once only with a steady state being reached after a period of equilibration (23). Such a system permits the calculation of clearance and comparison between experiments and compounds is feasible through the inclusion of antipyrine (37). This is particularly well-suited to the study of substances that are strongly lipophilic as it reduces the opportunity for adsorption to apparatus and tubing which requires careful selection.

The experimental criteria for a successful perfusion are strict and success is highly dependent upon provision of placentas in good condition and in a timely fashion with the most important criteria being minimal leakage of perfusate from the fetal circulation (36). The perfusion model is technically complex and due to the experimental criteria it can take a long time before an adequate number of successful experiments have been completed to provide appropriate statistical outcomes regarding transfer and behavior of a particular compound. Given the wide variety of nanoparticle types and their multiple physicochemical properties which will all have an impact on their behavior and toxicity, it would prove advantageous to have a rapid screening technique as part of the panel of models available for assessing placental transfer and toxicity. Placental cell culture models provide such a technique. There are several possible approaches that can be considered.

Cell Culture Models

Explants of placental villus trophoblast can be excised from the placenta and maintained in culture (23) but viability is limited (36). Primary trophoblast cultures can be established from fresh placental tissue using enzymatic dispersion and the cytotrophoblast cells purified using discontinuous Percoll grandients (38) but it is difficult to isolate large numbers of cells. Another alternative is the development of immortalized choriocarcinoma cell lines. Several commercial cell lines exist and these include BeWo, JAR and JEG-3 which were derived from a malignant first trimester gestational choriocarcinoma of the placenta. While the cell lines have several characteristics in common such as the secretion of placental hormones including hCG and progesterone (39) they also differ in certain characteristics which are of importance when considering transport studies. Their proliferative activity and degree of differentiation vary with BeWo and JAR cells being less differentiated compared with JEG-3 but undergoing more rapid proliferation (40).

BeWo cells resemble normal trophoblasts with close cell apposition and microvillous projections in the apical side of the monolayer (41) but do not spontaneously differentiate into a syncytium (although this can be induced in the presence of forskolin), in contrast to JEG-3 which is derived from BeWo and forms large multinucleated syncytia (36). However, one of the most important differences for transport studies is the fact that only the BeWo cell line forms a confluent monolayer and expresses functional polarity when grown on semi-permeable membranes (41,42). Careful choice of the correct clone is important as the original cell line available through the American Type Culture Collection (ATCC) does not form a monolayer in the same way as the b30 clone held by Dr. Alan Schwartz (Washington University, St. Louis, MO) (41). BeWo cells have been shown to differentially express several enzymes and transporters such as cytochrome P450, MDR1 P-glycoprotein (P-gp), MRP1 and BCRP with responses similar to trophoblast cells in vivo (36,43,44).

BeWo cells can be grown on semi-permeable membranes in Transwell® inserts placed in tissue culture wells thus allowing access to both apical (maternal) and basolateral (fetal) chambers and the measurement of transport across the monolayer. Inserts are available in different materials and with different pore sizes and can also be coated with a matrix such as collagen. Cells are seeded at an appropriate density and formation of a tight monolayer can be evaluated by measurement of the trans-epithelial electrical resistance and the reduction in passage of sodium fluorescein (45,46).

BeWo cells have the advantages that they can be grown up quickly, usually reaching confluence within 5 to 7 days depending upon seeding density and are suitable for use as a rapid screening technique for evaluation of the effects of different properties of NP upon their transport across and toxicity to biological barriers. However, they should only form the first step of evaluation using a combination of the models available. Each individual model has certain limitations and drawbacks but in combination they will help us to obtain a complete picture of how different NP interact with the placenta as part of a risk assessment for potential fetal exposure.

REFERENCES

1. Oberdorster G, Oberdorster, E, Oberdorster J. Nanotoxicology: an emerging discipline evolving from studies of ultrafine particles. Environ Health Perspect 2005; 113:823–39.
2. DEFRA, HM Government. Characterising the potential risks posed by engineered nanoparticles: A First UK Government Research Report, London, 2005. http://www.defra.gov.uk/environment/nanotech/nrcg/pdf/nanoparticles-riskreport.pdf
3. US-EPA. U.S. Environmental Protection Agency, Draft Nanotechnology White Paper, 2005. http://www.epa.gov/osa/pdfs/EPA_nanotechnology_white_paper_external_review_draft_12-02-2005.pdf
4. The Royal Society. Nanoscience and nanotechnologies: Opportunities and uncertainties, 2004. http://www.nanotec.org.uk/finalReport.htm
5. DEFRA, HM Government. Characterising the potential risks posed by engineered nanoparticles: UK Government Research—A Progress Report, London, 2006. http://www.defra.gov.uk/environment/nanotech/research/-reports/progress-report 061019.pdf
6. Nel A, Xia T, Madler L, et al. Toxic potential of materials at the nanolevel. Science 2006; 311:622–7.
7. Hoshino A, Hanaki K, Suzuki K, et al. Applications of T-lymphoma labeled with fluorescent quantum dots to cell tracing markers in mouse body. Biochem Biophys Res Commun 2004; 314:46–53.
8. Ballou B, Lagerholm BC, Ernst LA, et al. Noninvasive imaging of quantum dots in mice. Bioconjug Chem 2004; 15:79–86.
9. Colvin VL. The potential environmental impact of engineered nanomaterials. Nat Biotechnol 2003; 21:1166–70.
10. Holsapple MP, Farland WH, Landry TD, et al. Research strategies for safety evaluation of nanomaterials, part II: toxicological and safety evaluation of nanomaterials, current challenges and data needs. Toxicol Sci 2005; 88:12–17.
11. Donaldson K, Aitken R, Tran L, et al. Carbon nanotubes: a review of their properties in relation to pulmonary toxicology and workplace safety. Toxicol Sci 2006; 92:5–22.
12. McNeil SE. Nanotechnology for the biologist. J Leukoc Biol 2005; 78:585–94.
13. Lockman PR, Koziara JM, Mumper RJ, et al. Nanoparticle surface charges alter blood-brain barrier integrity and permeability. J Drug Target 2004; 12: 635–41.
14. Fenart L, Casanova A, Dehouck B, et al. Evaluation of effect of charge and lipid coating on ability of 60-nm nanoparticles to cross an in vitro model of the blood-brain barrier. J Pharmacol Exp Ther 1999; 291:1017–22.
15. Barker DJ. The developmental origins of adult disease. J Am Coll Nutr 2004; 23:588S–95S.
16. King B. Comparative studies of structure and function in mammalian placentas with special reference to maternal-fetal transfer of iron. Amer Zool 1992; 32:331–42.
17. Page K. The Physiology of the Human Placenta. London: UCL Press Limited, 1993.

18. Dey SK, Lim H, Das SK, et al. Molecular cues to implantation. Endocr Rev 2004; 25:341–73.
19. Kaufmann P, Burton G. Chapter 8: Anatomy and Genesis of the Placenta. In: Knobil E, Neill J eds., The Physiology of Reproduction, New York: Raven Press Ltd, 1994:441–84.
20. Enders AC, Blankenship TN. Comparative placental structure. Adv Drug Deliv 1999; Rev 38:3–15.
21. Kitano T, Iizasa H, Hwang IW, et al. Conditionally immortalized syncytiotrophoblast cell lines as new tools for study of the blood-placenta barrier. Biol Pharm Bull 2004; 27:753–9.
22. Bourget P, Roulot C, Fernandez H. Models for placental transfer studies of drugs. Clin Pharmacokinet 1995; 28:161–80.
23. Sastry BV. Techniques to study human placental transport. Adv Drug Deliv 1999; Rev 38:17–39.
24. Enders AC. A comparative study of the fine structure of the trophoblast in several hemochorial placentas. Am J Anat 1965; 116:29–67.
25. Audus KL. Controlling drug delivery across the placenta. Eur J Pharm Sci 1999; 8:161–5.
26. Pacifici GM, Nottoli R. Placental transfer of drugs administered to the mother. Clin Pharmacokinet 1995; 28:235–69.
27. Reynolds F, Knott C. Pharmacokinetics in pregnancy and placental drug transfer. Oxf Rev Reprod Biol 1989; 11:89–449.
28. Myllynen P, Pienimaki P, Vahakangas K. Human placental perfusion method in the assessment of transplacental passage of antiepileptic drugs. Toxicol Appl Pharmacol 2005; 207:489–94.
29. Kaufmann P. Basic morphology of the fetal and maternal circuits in the human placenta. Contrib Gynecol Obstet 1985; 13:5–17.
30. Syme MR, Paxton JW, Keelan JA. Drug transfer and metabolism by the human placenta. Clin Pharmacokinet 2004; 3:487–514.
31. Ganapathy V, Prasad PD, Ganapathy ME, et al. Placental transporters relevant to drug distribution across the maternal-fetal interface. J Pharmacol Exp Ther 2000; 294:413–20.
32. Millard RK, Saunders M, Palmer AM, et al. Approximate distribution of dose among foetal organs for radioiodine uptake via placenta transfer. Phys Med Biol 2001; 462773–83.
33. Panigel M. Placental perfusion experiments. Am J Obstet. Gynecol 1962; 84:1664–83.
34. Panigel M. The Proceedings from the Fourth Conference on fetal homeostasis, Princeton, NJ, June 1968, In: Wynn, RM ed. Fetal Homeostasis, Vol. 4. Fourth Conference on Fetal Homeostasis, New York: Appleton-Century_Crofts, 1969:15–25.
35. Schneider H, Panigel M, Dancis J. Transfer across the perfused human placenta of antipyrine, sodium and leucine. Am J Obstet Gynecol 1972; 114:822–8.
36. Vahäkängas K, Myllynen P. Experimental methods to study human trans-placental exposure to genotoxic agents. Mutat Res 2006; 608:129–35.
37. Dancis J, Jansen V, Levitz M. Placental transfer of steroids: effect of binding to serum albumin and to placenta. Am J Physiol 1980; 238:E208–13.

38. Kliman HJ, Nestler JE, Sermasi E, et al. Purification, characterization, and *in vitro* differentiation of cytotrophoblasts from human term placentae. Endocrinology 1986; 118:1567–82.

39. Sastry BVR. Techniques: Cultured tissues and cells to study placental function. In:Sastry BVR ed. Placental Pharmacology, London: CRC Press, 1996:47–66.

40. Serrano MA, Macias RI, Briz O, et al. Expression in human trophoblast and choriocarcinoma cell lines, BeWo, Jeg-3 and Jar of genes involved in the hepatobiliary-like excretory function of the placenta. Placenta 2007; 28: 107–17.

41. Bode CJ, Jin H, Rytting E, et al. In vitro models for studying trophoblast transcellular transport. Methods Mol Med 2006; 122:225–39.

42. Cariappa R, Heath-Monnig E, Smith CH. Isoforms of amino acid transporters in placental syncytiotrophoblast: plasma membrane localization and potential role in maternal/fetal transport. Placenta 2003; 24:713–26.

43. Thadani PV, Strauss JF, 3rd, Dey SK, et al. National Institute on Drug Abuse Conference report on placental proteins, drug transport, and fetal development. Am J Obstet Gynecol 2004; 191:1858–62.

44. Jin H, Audus KL. Effect of bisphenol A on drug efflux in BeWo, a human trophoblast-like cell line. Placenta 2005; 26(Suppl A):S96–103.

45. Ampasavate C, Chandorkar GA, Vande Velde DG, et al. Transport and metabolism of opioid peptides across BeWo cells, an in vitro model of the placental barrier. Int J Pharm 2002; 233:85–98.

46. Liu F, Soares MJ, Audus KL. Permeability properties of monolayers of the human trophoblast cell line BeWo. Am J Physiol 1997; 273:C1596–604.

9

Pharmacokinetics of Nanomaterials

Jim E. Riviere

Center for Chemical Toxicology Research and Pharmacokinetics, Biomathematics Program, North Carolina State University, Raleigh, North Carolina, U.S.A.

C. Lang Tran

Institute of Occupational Medicine, Edinburgh, U.K.

INTRODUCTION

A crucial component of understanding the activity of nanomaterials and constructing realistic quantitative risk assessment models is knowledge of the rate and extent of nanomaterial absorption, distribution, metabolism and elimination (ADME), essential parameters needed to connect dose to observed effects. The evaluation of these processes, referred to in chemical and pharmaceutical disciplines as pharmacokinetics or toxicokinetics, is often referred to in the nanosciences as biokinetics or biodistribution. Whatever the term used to describe this discipline, very few classical pharmacokinetic studies have been done on nanomaterials, especially manufactured substances not designed for biomedical and therapeutic applications. A number of issues important to nanomaterial risk assessment depend on having a knowledge of dose at the target tissues and which specific tissues they become sequestered in. If these coincide with a potential target for toxicity, this knowledge is crucial to making a risk assessment.

WHAT ARE PHARMACOKINETIC STUDIES?

Pharmacokinetics is defined as the science of quantifying the rate and extent of ADME processes using various mathematical modeling approaches. Space restrictions prevent a detailed review of the design of modern ADME or pharmacokinetics studies as extensive reviews and texts exist (1–3). Fundamentally, ADME is the study of the relative rates of absorption, distribution, metabolism and elimination of drugs and chemicals in the body. Administering drugs by the intravenous route bypass all absorption pathways making material immediately accessible to tissues. This is the route to which all other data are compared.

Pharmacokinetic models are used to compute the relative rates of each process that determine overall distribution and elimination from the body. The extent of absorption and distribution are crucial factors that relate the size of the absorbed dose to that which actually results in systemic exposure. This might relate to the relative rate of absorption from a dosing formulation compared to its rate of renal excretion or hepatic metabolism. The field of controlled drug delivery is based on designing the dosage form to be the rate limiting step in ADME, thereby prolonging a drug's sojourn in the body by controlling its rate of release from the dosage formulation. For nano-materials, although rates and extent of absorption may be low by many non-parenteral routes, the corresponding rates of elimination may also be low making accumulation and retention a potential issue. Pharmacokinetics provides the tools in the form of mathematical models to assess these phenomena.

Pharmacokinetics has developed an extensive family of mathematical models that provide parameters that quantitate the rate and extent of ADME. There are numerous modeling approaches [compartmental, non-compartmental, population, physiological-based (PBPK)] in use today (1,2) that are beyond the scope of the present introduction. Absorption is assessed by estimating its rate (Ka: mass/time) and extent (Bioavailability: F%), F being the fraction of administered dose absorbed into the body. IV administration is used to calculate F (as this route is assumed to be completely absorbed) from a ratio of area under the curve (AUC) of the same dose given by both routes (extravascular/IV). A comparison of relative bioavailabilities for two different formulations of the same drug, estimated by the ratio of their AUCs, is termed as bioequivalence. The procedures and statistical approaches for ADME are well regulated and described elsewhere (4,5).

Distribution is assessed by the parameter of volume of distribution (Vd: volume/kg), which is the ratio of administered dose to the blood concentration achieved, giving one an estimate of the "volume" in the body to which a compound is distributed. Elimination from the body is assessed using clearance (Cl: volume/time-kg) that estimates the efficiency of an elimination pathway. Major paths of chemical elimination are the kidney and liver. When a compound is eliminated by metabolism, hepatic clearance will reflect this. Based on nanomaterial studies conducted to date, metabolism of carbon nanomaterials does not occur (side-chain derivatives may be metabolized) and will not be discussed further. Finally, since most pharmacokinetic processes are first-order, their rate is often described in terms of half-life $(T \frac{1}{2})$ that is a function of Vd/Cl.

Knowledge of these basic pharmacokinetic parameters (Ka, F, Vd, Cl) allows prediction of body burden, systemic exposure, and blood concentrations as a function of applied dose and time. The actual determination of parameter values is very dependent upon the pharmacokinetic model used. PBPK approaches describe the disposition of a chemical based on a mathematical model that mirrors the physiological structure of the body, with compartments linked by tissue blood flow. Such models easily incorporate in vitro data and define target doses of materials. This should be the ultimate aim of developing models for nanomaterials. However, basic ADME parameters must first be conducted before formal PBPK models can be constructed.

Issues of laboratory animal study design and how these relate to subsequent human exposure are also important since species-specific patterns of ADME processes may occur. Modeling approaches such as PBPK facilitate these comparisons, however such studies have not been conducted to date.

COULD NANOMATERIAL PHARMACOKINETICS BE DIFFERENT THAN CHEMICALS?

Before we discuss the existing literature on nanomaterial pharmacokinetics, one can pose the question if differences are expected between nanomaterials and drug or chemicals? These potential considerations would put available data in the proper context. One dimension of this question is how material size alone modifies disposition. As will be seen, existing data suggest that size is a primary determinant of disposition, both in respect to decreased absorption for large particles, and altered pattern of distribution and elimination of systemic material based on interactions with the reticuloendothelial system (RES). What has not been addressed is the precise size cutoffs that determine these patterns, or their relationship to nanomaterial shape, elemental composition or surface characteristics, the latter of which also facilitates interaction with the RES.

It is widely acknowledged that an important phenomenon that determines the "reactivity and availability" of manufactured carbon nanomaterials is their tendency to self associate and interact with molecules (proteins, salts, lipids, etc) in biological environments. Agglomeration may produce particles too large for absorption. Similarly, the same phenomenon occurring after absorption could result in tissue deposition. The impact of these potential nanomaterial interactions on ADME relates both to the relative rate of the nanomaterial interactions compared to the ADME process impacted (Ka, Cl), as well as the stoichiometry of the process (which relates to mass of particles actually involved). These rate and mass issues are crucial but have not been systematically addressed.

What animal species should be used for defining nanomaterial ADME parameters? The limited number of nano-biodistribution or translocation studies conducted to date and reviewed below have used small laboratory animals including mice, rats, and rabbits. This is fully justified as these animals provide direct comparisons with the extensive pharmacology/ toxicology databases available for drugs and chemicals, and regulatory agencies have experience interpreting them. For many compounds, they have shown good correlation to human disposition. Their smaller size results in use of smaller doses that are required in early stages of development when available test material was severely limited (e.g., most early nanomaterial experiments).

However, the smaller body mass of laboratory animals compared to humans results in these species having a higher basal metabolic rate (BMR) with resulting shorter blood circulation times. This results in much higher clearances, and thus shorter $T\frac{1}{2}$ in laboratory animals compared to humans across a wide variety of drugs and chemicals (6). In fact, this is the basis of using allometry and/or body surface area to extrapolate pharmacokinetic parameters across species to predict human disposition (7–11). If this concept holds for nanomaterials, then $T\frac{1}{2}$ data in Table 1 below may greatly underestimate human residence times. What is the potential impact of this on nanomaterial studies? Carbon nanomaterials undergo a number of time-dependent interactions with biological constituents dependent upon their material and surface characteristics (e.g., ionic interchanges with electrolytes and metals, hydrophobic binding to proteins, lipids, etc). Many interactions result in particle agglomeration with potential biological consequences. The nature of these interactions is a function of where the particles are distributed and the resulting local biological environment. All interactions are time-dependent. In order to accurately predict what their consequences would be in humans, the animal model must provide sufficient

Table 1 Intravenous Nanomaterial Pharmacokinetic Studies

Species	Material	Dose (If available)	$T\frac{1}{2}$ (hours)	Citation
Mice	f-SWNT	3 mg/kg	3	(12)
Mice	(+) f-SWNT	3 mg/kg	3.5	(12)
Mice	$C_{60}(OH)n$	–	≈17	(13)
Rats	MSAD C_{60}	15 mg/kg	6.8	(14)
Rats	TMM C_{60}	–	≈3 initial, longer >6	(15)
Rabbits	SWNT	0.02 mg/kg	1	(16)
Mice	SWNT(PL)	0.05–0.5 mg/kg	0.5–2	(17)

Abbreviations: f = functionalized; + = charge; PL = phospholipids; ≈ estimated by authors.

time for these to occur within the body before excretion. For modeling behavior in humans, this requires that compound residence times be similar. Small laboratory rodents do not provide this property. A larger animal with similar body mass (swine, larger dogs), and thus BMR and residence times as humans, might be required. This limitation of small animals has been appreciated in the pharmaceutical industry when controlled release dosage forms or devices have been developed for human and veterinary drugs (18–20). A larger species would also have similar gastrointestinal transit times, a requirement that would allow nanomaterial interactions to occur with GI contents in a time frame similar to humans (21,22). Another potential limitation of using small animals for nanomaterial research is that the stoichiometric nature of nanomaterial interactions, in that the small doses (and hence numbers) of nanomaterial used might not be sufficient for biologically significant agglomeration to occur.

NANOMATERIAL PHARMACOKINETIC STUDIES CONDUCTED TO DATE

Fullerenes

There is minimal literature on the pharmacokinetics of fullerenes (C_{60}) in laboratory animals, with that available being focused on therapeutic applications (Table 1). Physical chemical characterization using techniques applied to other nanomaterials have not been performed. Many of the approaches to derivatization employ materials designed for therapeutic targeting, rather than simply altering surface charge or solubility to specifically assess the correlation of physicochemical properties to ADME parameters.

A "classic" pharmacokinetic study was conducted in Sprague-Dawley rats using MSAD-C_{60}, a water-soluble C_{60} derivative with antiviral properties (14). Terminal $T\frac{1}{2}$ was approximately seven hours, Vd was 2 l/kg indicating extensive distribution, and there was no evidence of urinary excretion. C_{60} was 99% protein bound in plasma. There was a great variability not evident in the $T\frac{1}{2}$ data, with 2/5 rats having two fold differences in Cl and Vd parameters. This observation underlines the weakness in using $T\frac{1}{2}$ as the sole pharmacokinetic parameter, since as discussed earlier $T\frac{1}{2}$ is physiologically Vd/Cl. Yamago et al. (15) studied a ^{14}C labeled (trimethylenemethane (TMM) derived) lipophilic yet water-soluble C_{60} after IV and oral (very low absorption) administration (dosed in ethanol/PEG/albumin vehicle). After IV administration, only 5% of the compound was excreted, all by the fecal route; with most label retained in the liver after 30 hours. Some derivatives (altered side chains attached to C_{60}) were also located in the spleen, kidney and importantly the brain.

Qingnuan et al. (13) showed distribution of ^{99m}Tc labeled $C_{60}(OH)_x$ in mice and rabbits after IV dosing to primarily occur in the kidney, bone, spleen, and liver with slow elimination occurring after 48 hours, except for bone which accumulated label. T ½ in blood was 17 hours in mice. Cagle et al. (23) studied the biodistribution of endohedral metallofullerenes ($^{166}HoC_{82}(OH)_n$) in mice and reported relatively rapid blood Cl (few hours), bone accumulation, and liver localization with slow elimination. As with the $C_{60}(OH)_x$ studies above, total body Cl was slow with only 20% of intact compound being excreted by five days, a retention time much longer than when metal chelates alone were administered. The disposition of this metallofullerene was very different than reported for gold particle microcolloids. Bullard-Dillard et al. (24) using ^{14}C labeled particles in rats showed longer persistence in the circulation of water-soluble ammonium salt derivative C_{60} compared to very rapid clearance of C_{60}. Both primarily targeted the liver, although all pristine C_{60} went to and was retained in liver for at least 120 hours. For water-soluble C_{60} derivatives, Cl is low and liver is a target organ.

Carbon Nanotubes

Rigorous, "classical" pharmacokinetic studies on other manufactured nanomaterials have not been conducted to date. The few that have been done have employed indirect measures of concentration (IR) (16) PET (17) or were particles functionalized (f) with specific tracers (12). Methods using such modifications assume radiolabel or fluorescent tags remain attached to the nanomaterial throughout its sojourn through the body, as well as not impart any different physiochemical properties that would alter ADME. Although these approaches might be appropriate for studies of nano-materials used in drug targeting or radio-imaging medical applications, manufactured nanomaterials encountered in the workplace or commerce do not come with such tracer tags. Studies have been done in small numbers of laboratory animals often with insufficient time points.

Mice showed urinary excretion and accumulation in muscle, skin and kidney for neutral and (+) f-SWNTs, as well as f-MWNTs (12). Cherukuri et al. (12) using rabbits showed SWNTs had accumulated in liver after 24 hours. Nanotube length has not been rigorously controlled, nor in some cases even determined, in the studies reported to date. Liu et al. (17) studied phospholipids-coated SWNT in mice using PET. Tissue distribution (liver, spleen) and blood T ½ (0.5–2 hour) were dependent upon phospholipid constituents. Significant body burden persisted after 24 hour sacrifice. Table 1 summarizes the available T ½ kinetic data.

Other Materials

There are systemic disposition studies reported using inherently fluorescent quantum dots (QD) derivatized for medical imaging. Most studies do not rigorously determine particle concentrations using analytical techniques as is required in classic pharmacokinetic studies. However, general patterns of particle distribution can often be assessed. These studies suggest that QDs, tagged with homing peptides, can be targeted to specific tissues (e.g., lung, vessels) after IV administration of $\approx 10 \, mg/kg$ to mice. Similar to carbon materials reviewed above, they accumulate in liver and spleen (25). Coating QD with polyethylene glycol allows particles to escape detection by reticuloendothelial tissues (liver, spleen, lymph nodes). Imaging studies in mice clearly show that QD surface coatings alter their disposition and pharmacokinetic properties (26). Plasma T½ were less than 12 min for amphiphilic poly (acrylic), short chain (750 Da) methoxy-PEG or long chain (3400 Da) carboxy-PEG QD, but over an hour for long-chain (5000 Da) methoxy-PEG QD. These coatings determined the in vivo tissue localization, with retention of some QDs occurring up to four months.

Iron nanoparticles (FeNP) have been explored as novel magnetic resonance imaging agents. In a series of in vitro tissue studies, cellular uptake of anionic particles was greater compared to neutral or cationic species (27). Nanomaterial imaging studies using magnetic particles have been conducted and showed surface-specific tissue targeting, including delivery to the brain, as well as prolonged tissue retention in organs including the liver (four weeks) (28). Although such persistence may be a laudable goal for some imaging applications, they raise toxicological concern when chronic exposure to nanomaterial occurs. Takenaka et al. (29) used 16 female Fischer 344 rats that were between 150 and 200 g. This study measured the content of ultrafine silver particles (EA) in the liver and the lung over a period of seven days after six hours inhalation exposure of $133 \, \mu gEAg/m^3$ (particle number concentration of $3 \times 10^6/cm^3$, $14.6 \, nm \pm 1$ (MD) mean 17.1 ± 1.2, GSD 1.38). They also investigated the concentration of silver particles in the heart, spleen, kidney, brain and blood. For comparison purposes the rats received either $150 \, \mu L$ of aqueous solution of $7 \, \mu g$ silver nitrate, $AgNO_3$, ($4.4 \, \mu g$ Ag) or $150 \, \mu L$ aqueous solution of $50 \, \mu g$ EAg by intratracheal instillation. The ultrastructure of the Ag particles collected from the inhalation exposure or the instillation aqueous suspension was examined by a transmission electron microscope. Ventilation exchange rate was about 20 times/hour. They found that the amount of silver particles in the lungs decreased significantly after both inhalation and instillation exposure so that only 4% of the initial burden remained after seven days. They also found that the levels of silver particles in the other organs considered decreased rapidly after exposure.

Oberdörster et al. (30) investigated the translocation of inhaled ultrafine carbon particles ^{13}C to the liver and the lung by exposing male Fischer 344 rats (weight 250–600 g) for six hours in compartmentalized whole-body chambers and taking measurements over a period of 24 hours. Six rats were exposed to a concentration of $180 \, \mu L$ $^{13}C/m^3$ (CMD = 29.7 nm,

1.7 GSD), 6 were exposed to 80 μg ^{13}C/m^3 (CMD $= 22$ nm, 1.8 GSD) while six rats were unexposed and served as controls.

The retention of ^{13}C was measured by continuous-flow isotope-ratio mass spectrometry using a Carlo Erba elemental analyser coupled to a Finnigan Mat Delta Plus mass spectrometer. The results are expressed in the paper as $\delta^{13}C$ where:

$$\delta^{13}C = \frac{^{13}C/^{12}C_{sample} - ^{13}C/^{12}C_{standard}}{^{13}C/^{12}C_{standard}} \times 1000$$

They found that significant amounts of ^{13}C had accumulated in the liver half an hour post-exposure and that at 18 and 24 hours post-exposure the amount of ^{13}C in the liver was five times that in the lung. They demonstrated a significant translocation of ^{13}C particles from the lung to the liver by one day after inhalation exposure.

Oberdörster et al. (31) again used male Fischer 344 rats (weight 284 ± 9 g) to measure the translocation of ^{13}C (ultrafine carbon) particles by exposing the rats through inhalation while in a compartmentalized whole-body exposure chamber for 6 hours. This study measured the retention of ^{13}C particles in the lung, olfactory, cerebellum, and cerebrum over a period of seven days. Six rats were exposed to a concentration of 170 μg ^{13}C/m^3 (CMD $=$ 37 nm, GSD $= 1.66$), six were exposed to 150 μg ^{13}C/m^3 (CMD $= 35$ nm, GSD $= 1.66$) and three rats were unexposed and served as controls. The method of measurement was the same as the previous study by Oberdörster (30). It was found that the levels of ultrafine carbon particles in the lung decreased significantly after exposure, while the levels in the olfactory bulb increased. At day seven the levels in the olfactory bulb (μg/g) were close to that of the lung, but as the olfactory is small (only 85 mg) the levels are very small also. They noted that as the levels in the olfactory bulb did not decrease then continuous exposure would likely result in much higher levels.

Kreyling et al. (32) used male WKY/NCrl BR rats (weight 170 ± 10 g) to investigate the translocation of ^{192}Ir (ultrafine iridium) particles by measuring the fraction of particles left in the lung, feces, urine and carcass over a period of seven days after exposure. The rats were ventilated for one hour via an endotracheal tube (inhalation). The study tested two different concentrations of iridium particles; Trial 1 used a concentration of 15 nm while the second used 80 nm iridium particles. The breathing frequency was 45/min and inspiration of 75% to 80%. A complete balance of ^{192}Ir activity retained in the body and cleared by excretion out of the body was quantified by gamma spectroscopy. They also carried out a trial to determine the iridium retention after intratracheal instillation of soluble ^{192}Ir^{3+} in saline. They found that almost 20% and 10% of the 15 and 80 nm particles, respectively, was cleared into the gastrointestinal tract at six hours after exposure. After seven days 47% and 36% of 15 and 80 nm particles, respectively, were cleared to the feces, while 2% and 0.3% were cleared through the urine. At each time point they found very low fractions of translocated particles in other organs.

Semmler et al. (33) carried out an investigation into the lung retention and clearance kinetics of 12 male WKY rats that weighed about 250 g. After 1 to 1.5 hours of inhalation of between 15 and 20 nm (CMD) ^{192}Ir particles, at specific time points, a complete balance of ^{192}Ir (iridium) activity retained in the body and cleared by excretion out of the body was quantified by gamma spectroscopy. The breathing frequency was 45/min and inspiration of 75% to 80%. The particle concentration was 3×10^7 *cm*^{3} 3×10^7 cm^3 (0.2 mg/m^3). The study measured the retention/excretion in a number of organs over 180 days. The organs were spleen, liver, lung, kidney and brain. It was found that the lung contained significantly more iridium particles than any other organ at each time point. A small but detectable fraction of iridium were found translocated to the secondary organs, with a peak at about seven days. They noted that the excretion of ultrafine iridium particles occurred only through the feces and urine.

Finally, many pharmacokinetic studies have been conducted using nano-dimension drug block-copolymers. The physical chemical properties of the drug and polymer carrier (e.g., pluronic surfactant micelles) effects disposition and circulating T½ (34). A body of literature exists on nanomaterial deposition after inhalational exposure, a topic focused on local deposition within the respiratory tract (35,36). In some recent work, prolonged retention for six months of absorbed particles occurred (33). This data is consistent with the findings above of slow CL and retention of materials after systemic exposure.

LYMPHATIC TRAFFICKING

Although most ADME and pharmacokinetic studies focus on the blood circulatory system, animals and humans also have another system which traffics cells and large lipophilic molecules and proteins, the lymphatic system. The lymphatics have been extensively studied relative to their role in absorption of particulates and protein therapeutics for molecules with molecular weights greater than 16 KDa (37–39). After absorption in local lymphatic vessels, a compound moves to regional lymph nodes and ultimately re-enters the systemic circulation via the thoracic duct. An important toxicological implication of this pathway is that all such transported material has the potential for interaction with the immune system resident in regional lymph nodes.

Some nanomaterials are relatively large and possess surface modifications that could make them ideal candidates for lymphatic transport.

This is relevant since several reports have indicated that titanium dioxide particle penetration can occur through the stratum corneum layers (40) and dermis (41) of skin. Size selected fluorospheres in conjunction with motion could also penetrate through skin (42) causing potential exposure to lymph. Rouse et al. (43) has also reported similar dermal absorption with fullerenes through mechanically stressed skin. Microparticles of silica and alumino-silicates have been shown to penetrate through skin and migrate to femoral lymph nodes of barefooted people in Africa, thereby causing non-filarial elephantiasis of the lower legs known as podoconiosis (44,45) These particles found in red clay soil areas near volcanoes can cause lymphatic obstruction.

Solid lipid nanoparticles designed for magnetic resonance imaging have been shown to enter lymph after duodenal administration to rats (46). In other imaging studies conducted in pigs, intradermal injection of 400 pM of fluorescent QD targeted sentinel lymph nodes (47), a finding relevant to dermal absorption of even minute fractions of topically applied or orally dosed manufactured nanomaterials. In fact, it has been suggested that nanocapsules, ultrafine oily droplet-coated polymeric drug substances may be one of the most promising candidates for lymphatic targeting (48). Based on these data, lymphatic uptake of nanomaterials after topical dermal and oral dosing may significantly contribute to their ADME profile and not be easily studied solely by blood-based pharmacokinetic studies.

CONCLUSION

There are a few conclusions that can be drawn from the available literature on nanomaterial biodistribution and kinetics, including those of imaging compounds (QDs and other materials), therapeutic polymers, as well as available data from carbon nanomaterials. Increased water solubility results in a lower blood clearance and more extensive tissue distribution than seen with non-derivatized pristine materials. Most nanomaterials tend to accumulate in the liver, potentially because of RES cell trapping. However, particles also distribute to other tissues, including the kidney, depending on surface characteristics. The effect of size within a nano-material class has not been extensively evaluated. All classes of particles also have extensive tissue retention, a property of potential toxicological significance. Note that as tissue deposition occurs, Vd increases resulting in prolongation of T½. Available studies are difficult to directly compare (different species, doses, vehicles, different approaches to functionalized particles, lack of common characterization techniques) making interpretation problematic at best and definitely not adequate to begin risk assessment analyses for manufactured materials.

Most pharmacokinetic models are based on diffusion as the primary mode of chemical movement. Can nanoparticle movement be modeled based on these assumptions? Does Brownian motion significantly modify their behavior? Active transport processes introduce non-linearity into chemical kinetic studies. Are nanomaterials subject to transport by these systems, and more importantly do pinocytotic/phagocytotic pathways that do not modify some organic drugs play a major role in nanomaterial transport? These issues have not been specifically addressed.

REFERENCES

1. Riviere JE. Comparative Pharmacokinetics: Principles, Techniques, and Applications. Ames, Iowa: Iowa State Press, 1999.
2. Reddy MB, Yang RSH, Clewell HJ, Andersen ME. Physiologically Based Pharmacokinetic Modeling: Science and Applications. Hoboken, New Jersey: John Wiley & Sons, Inc., 2005.
3. Gibaldi M, Perrier D. Pharmacokinetics. 2nd ed. New York, New York: Marcel Dekker, Inc., 1982.
4. Chow SC, Liu JP. Design and Analysis of Bioavailability and Bioequivalence Studies. 2nd ed. New York: Marcel Dekker, 2000.
5. Patterson S, Jones B. Bioequivalence and Statistics in Clinical Pharmacology. Boca Raton, Fl: Chapman and Hall/CRC, 2006.
6. Craigmill AL, Riviere JE, Webb AI. Tabulation of FARAD Comparative and Veterinary Pharmacokinetic Data. Ames, IA: Blackwell Publishing. 2006.
7. Boxenbaum H. Interspecies scaling, allometry, physiological time, and the ground plan for pharmacokinetics, J. Pharmacokin. Biopharm 1982; 10:201–27.
8. Calabrese EJ. Principles of Animal Extrapolation. New York: John Wiley, 1983.
9. Riviere JE, Martin T, Sundlof S, Craigmill AL. Interspecies allometric analysis of the comparative pharmacokinetics of 44 drugs across veterinary and laboratory species. J Vet Pharmacol Therap 1997; 20:453–63.
10. West GB, Brown JH, Enquist BJ. A general model for the origin of allometric scaling laws in biology. Science 1997; 276:122–6.
11. Martin-Jimenez T, Riviere JE. Mixed effect modeling of the interspecies pharmacokinetic scaling of oxytetracycline. J Pharm Sci 2002; 91:331–41.
12. Singh R, Pantarotto D, Lacerda L, Pastorin G, Klumpp C, Prato M, Bianco A, Kostarelos K. Tissue biodistribution and blood clearance rates of intravenously administered carbon nanotubes radiotracers. PNAS 2006; 103:3357–62, 2006.
13. Qingnuan L, Yan X, Xiaodong Z, Ruili L, Qieqie D, Xiaoguang S, Shaoliang C, Wenxin L. Preparation of 99mTc-C60(OH)x and its biodistribution studies. Nuc Med Bio 2002; 29:707–10.
14. Rajagopalan P, Wudl F, Schinazi RF, Boudinot FD. Pharmacokinetics of a water-soluble fullerene in rats. Antimicro Agents Chemother 1996; 40:2262–5.
15. Yamago S, Tokuyama H, Nakamura E, Kikuchi K, Kananishi S, Sueki K, Nakahara H, Enomoto S, Ambe F. In vivo biological behavior of a water-miscible fullerene: 14C labeling, absorption, distribution, excretion and acute toxicity. Chem Bio1995; 2:385–9.
16. Cherukuri P, Gannon CJ, Leeuw TK, Schmidt HK, Smalley RE, Curley SA, Weisman RB. Mammalian pharmacokinetics of carbon nanotubes using intrinsic near-infrared flurorescence. PNAS 2006; 103:18882–6.

17. Liu Z, Cai W, He L, Nakayama N, Chen K, Sun X, Chen X, Dai H. In vivo biodistribution and highly efficient tumour targeting of carbon nanotubes in mice. Nat Nanotechnol 2006; 2:47–52.

18. Davies B, Morris T. Physiological parameters in laboratory animals and humans. Pharm. Res. 1993; 10:1093–586.

19. Martinez MN, Amidon G, Clarke L, Jones WW, Mitra A, Riviere JE. Applying the biopharmaceutics classification system to veterinary pharmaceutical products. Part II. Physiological considerations. Adv Drug Deliv Rev 2002; 54:825–50.

20. Martinez MN, Papich MG, Riviere JE. Veterinary application of in vitro dissolution data and the biopharmaceutics classification system. Pharmacopeial Forum 2004; 30:2295–303.

21. Aoyagi N, Ogata H, Kaniwa N, Uchiyama M, Yasuda Y, Tanioka Y. Gastric emptying of tablets and granules in humans, dogs, pigs, and stomach-emptying controlled rabbits. J Pharm Sci 1992; 81:1170–4.

22. Stevens CE, Hume ID. Comparative Physiology of the Vetebrate Digestive System, 2nd ed. Cambridge: Cambridge University Press, 1995.

23. Cagle DW, Kennel SJ, Mirzadeh S, Alford JM, Wilson LJ. In vivo studies of fullerene-based materials using endohedral metallofullerene radiotracers. Proc Natl Acad Sci USA 1999; 96:5182–7.

24. Bullard-Dillard R, Creek KE, Scrivens WA, Tour JM. Tissue sites of uptake of 14C-labeled C60. Bioorganic Chem 1996; 24:376–85.

25. Akerman ME, Chan WCW, Laakkonen P, Bhatia SN, Ruoslahti E. Nanocrystal targeting in vivo. PNAS 2002; 99:12617–21.

26. Ballou B, Lagerholm BC, Ernst LA, Bruchez MP, Waggoner AS. Noninvasive imaging of quantum dots in mice. Bioconjugate Chem 2004; 15:79–86.

27. Wilhelm C, Billotey C, Roger J, Pons JN, Bacri JC, Gazeau F. Intracellular uptake of anionic superparamagnetic nanoparticles as a function of their surface coating. Biomaterials 2003; 24:1001–11.

28. Kim JS, Yoon TJ, Yu KN, Kim BG, Park SJ, Kim HW, Lee KH, Park SB, Lee JK, Cho MH. Toxicity and tissue distribution of magnetic nanoparticles in mice. Toxicol Sci 2006; 89:338–47.

29. Takenaka, S, Karg, E, Roth, C, Schulz, H, Ziesenis, A, Heinzmann, U, Schramel, P., Heyder, J Pulmonary and systemic distribution of inhaled ultrafine silver particles in rats. EnvironHealth Perspect 2001; 109(Suppl 4): 547–51.

30. Oberdörster, G, Sharp, Z, Atudorei, V, Elder, A, Gelein, R, Lunts, A, Kreyling, W, Cox, C. Extrapulmonary translocation of ultrafine carbon particles following whole-body inhalation exposure of rats. J Toxicol Environ Health, Part A2002; 65:1531–43.

31. Oberdörster, G, Sharp, Z, Atudorei, V, Elder, A, Gelein, R, Kreyling, W. Cox, C. Translocation of inhaled ultrafine particles to the brain. Inhal Toxicol 2004; 16:43745.

32. Kreyling, WG, Semmler, M, Erbe, F, Mayer, P, Takenaka, S, Schulz, H, Oberdörster, G. Ziesenis, A. Translocation of ultrafine insoluble iridium particles from the lung epithelium to extrapulmonary organs is size dependent but very low. J Toxicol Environ Health, Part A 2002; 65:1513–30.

33. Semmler M, Seitz J, Erbe F, Mayer P, Heyder J, Oberdörster G, Kreyling WG. Long-term clearance kinetics of inhaled ultrafine insoluble iridium particles from the rat lung, including transient translocation into secondary organs. Inhal Toxicol 2004; 16:453–9.

34. Kabanov AV, Batrakova EV, Alakhov VY. Pluronic block copolymers as novel polymer therapeutics drug and gene delivery. J Control Rel 2002; 82: 189–212.

35. Oberdörster G, Oberdörster E, Oberdörster J. Nanotoxicology: an emerging discipline evolving from studies of ultrafine particles. Environ Health Perspect 205; 113:823–39.

36. Oberdörster G, Maynard A, Donaldson K, Castranova V, Fitzpatrick, Ausman K, Carter J, Karn B, Kreyling W, Lai D, Olin S, Monteiro-Riviere N, Warheit D, Yang H. Principles for characterizing the potential human health effects from exposure to nanomaterials: elements of a screening strategy. Part. Fibre Toxicol 2005; 2:8:1–35.

37. Porter CJH, Edwards GA, Charman SA. Lymphatic transport of proteins after s.c. injection: implications of animal model selection. Adv Drug Deliv Rev 2001; 50:157–71.

38. McLennan DN, Porter CJH, Edwards GA, Brumm M, Martin SW, Charman SAPharmacokinetic model to describe the lymphatic absorption of r-metHu-Leptin after subcutaneous injection to sheep. Pharm Res (NY) 2003; 20: 1156–62.

39. McLennan DN, Porter CJH, Edwards GA, Martin SW, Heatherington AC, Charman SA. Lymphatic absorption is the primary contributor to the systemic availability of epoetin alfa following subcutaneous administration to sheep. J Pharmacol Exp Ther 2005; 313:345–51.

40. Lademann J, Weigmann HJ, Rickmeyer C, Barthelmes H, Schaefer H, Mueller G, Sterry W. Penetration of titanium dioxide microparticles in a sunscreen formulation into the horny layer and the follicular orifice. Skin Pharmacol Appl Skin Physiol 1999; 12:247–56.

41. Tan MH, Commens CA, Burnett L, Snitch PJ. A pilot study on the percutaneous absorption of microfine titanium dioxide from sunscreens. Australas J Dermatol 1996; 37:185–7.

42. Tinkle SS, Antonini JM, Rich BA, Roberts JR, Salmen R, DePree K, Adkins EJ. Skin as a route of exposure and sensitization in chronic beryllium disease. Environ Health Perspect 2003; 111:1202–8.

43. Rouse JG, Yang J, Ryman-Rasmussen, Barron AR, Monteiro-Riviere NA. Effects of mechanical flexion on the penetration of fullerene amino acid-derivatized peptide nanoparticles through skin. Nano Lett 2007; 7:155–60.

44. Corachan M, Tura JM, Campo E, Soley M, Traveria A. Podoconiosis in aequatorial guinea. Report of two cases from different geological environments. Trop Geogr Med 1988; 40:359–64.

45. Blundell G, Henderson WJ. Soil particles in the tissues of the foot in endemic elephantiasis of the lower legs. Ann Trop Med Parasitol 1989; 83:381–5.

46. Peira E, Marzola P, Podio V, Aime S, Sbarbati A, Gasco MR. In vitro and in vivo study of solid lipid nanoparticles loaded with superparamagnetic iron oxide. J Drug Targeting 2003; 11:19–24.

47. Kim S, Lim YT, Soltesz EG, De Grand AM, Lee J, Nakayama A, Parker JA, Mihaljevic T, Laurence RG, Dor DM, Cohn LH, Bawendi MG, Frangioni JV. Near-infrared fluorescent type II quantum dots for sentinel lymph node mapping. Nat Biotechnol 2004; 22:93–7.
48. Nishioka Y, Yoshino H. Lymphatic targeting with nanoparticulate system. Adv Drug Deliv Rev 2004; 47:55–64.

10

Estimating Nanoparticle Dose in Humans: Issues and Challenges

Eileen D. Kuempel

National Institute for Occupational Safety and Health, Cincinnati, Ohio, U.S.A.

OVERVIEW

Quantitative estimation of internal dose is a key step in the risk assessment of nanoparticles. Lung dosimetry models describe the deposition and clearance of inhaled particles in the respiratory tract, but these models have not been fully validated for the disposition of nanoparticles, which may include translocation beyond the respiratory tract. The current models and methods will be discussed, along with the data needs and challenges to validate and extend these models to better estimate nanoparticle dose.

INTRODUCTION

Workers historically have been among those in the human population most likely to be exposed to hazardous substances. With new technologies comes the potential for worker exposures to new substances such as nanoparticles.[*] Of particular concern to understanding the health risk to workers are the limited data available to evaluate the potential toxicity of new engineered nanoparticles and the lack of standardized methods for measuring and characterizing exposures to nanoparticles in the workplace (2). In addition, the potential for exposure outside the workplace exists when nanoparticles

---

[*]The term "nanoparticle" refers here to any nanometer-sized structure with at least one dimension <100 nm, including spherical, fibrous, or other shapes; nanoparticle refers to the primary structure, but aggregates or agglomerates of nanoparticles also occur (1).

are released into the environmental (either by disposal or intentional use in environmental remediation) or used in consumer products (such as cosmetics or sunscreens). The existing scientific literature on the physical and biological factors influencing particle and fiber toxicity in animals and humans provides information and data to develop interim risk estimates and health protection strategies. These studies indicate that the particle characteristics (including size, shape, and chemical composition), the internal dose in the respiratory tract, and the fate and persistence of the particles in the body are key factors influencing the risk of developing adverse health effects (2–5).

Workers may be exposed to nanoparticles by various routes including inhalation, ingestion, and dermal exposure. Inhalation exposure to various airborne particles and fibers continues to be associated with increased morbidity and mortality from work-related lung diseases (6). Nanoparticles may become airborne during production and use, particularly when present in dry powders or liquid sprays (2). This chapter focuses on airborne nanoparticle exposures and the estimation of internal nanoparticle dose in workers.

BIOMATHEMATICAL LUNG MODELS

To estimate the risk of disease in humans exposed to nanoparticles, it is necessary to understand the relationship between the external exposure and the internal dose. Biomathematical models are used to quantitatively describe the physical and physiological factors that influence the uptake and retention of substances in the body, as well as the biological responses to a given dose. Biomathematical models that describe the exposure-dose relationship are variously called dosimetric, toxicokinetic, or physiologi-cally-based pharmacokinetic (PBPK) models, while those that describe the dose-response relationship are called toxicodynamic or pharmacodynamic models.

Biomathematical models have applications in both experimental design and risk assessment. In experimental studies, biomathematical models may be used to generate and test hypotheses of biological mechanisms. For example, by evaluating whether a dosimetric model validated for respirable particles also adequately describes the disposition of nanoparticles, hypotheses about the factors influencing the deposition and retention of particles of various characteristics can be evaluated. Biomathematical models are also used to estimate doses for toxicological study. For example, a lung dosimetry model can be used to estimate the airborne particle concentration that will result in a target dose in the lungs over a given duration of exposure. In quantitative risk assessment, validated biomathe-matical models are used to: (1) provide estimates of the biologically-effective dose; (2) extrapolate exposure, dose, and response data from one species to another, from one dose to another, or from one route of exposure to another; and (3) describe the sources of variability in the factors that influence internal dose in a population. Obtaining the data required to calibrate and validate biomathematical models can be facilitated by collaboration among experimenters and modelers and by consideration of quantitative modeling needs in the experimental design.

Current biomathematical models pertaining to particles and fibers generally focus on particle deposition and/or clearance and retention processes (7–2), although some models in rats quantitatively describe the relationships between exposure, dose, and markers of adverse biological responses (11,12). For poorly-soluble particles and fibers, these models are typically limited to the respiratory tract; yet data from animal studies indicate that additional paths need to be considered to accurately estimate nanoparticle dose in humans. To the extent that particles are soluble, uptake of their elemental constituents into the blood from the lungs or gut may also determine their systemic distribution and potential toxicity (e.g., soluble forms of various metals such as manganese, nickel, or chromium). For poorly-soluble nanoparticles, additional pathways beyond the lungs include nerve axon transport to the brain (13) and entry into the blood circulation and transport to nonpulmonary organs (14,15). Intra-cellular organelles (e.g., mitochondria) in the lungs and other organs may also be target sites for nanoparticles (16,17). Models to estimate nanoparticle dose by non-inhalation routes of exposures, such as dermal (18, see Chapter 9), may also be required to adequately describe nanoparticle dose in humans.

Deposition of Nanoparticles in Human Lungs

Particle size is a key factor determining whether and in what location inhaled particles are likely to deposit in the respiratory tract. Human studies using radiolabeled particles have shown that the total fraction of particles depositing in the respiratory tract increases to greater than 90% as particle size decreases into the nanoparticle size range (1–100 nm) (7). The fractional deposition of nanoparticles in the alveolar and tracheobronchial regions can be several times higher than that for larger respirable particles.[†] Total nanoparticle deposition increases with exercise (19) and among individuals with chronic obstructive lung disease or asthma (20). Nanoparticle deposition in exercising individuals was shown to be underpredicted by several human lung deposition models (21). Current human lung models have had limited evaluation of the deposition of the smallest

---

[†]The term respirable refers to particles that are capable of depositing in the alveolar (gas-exchange) region of the lungs (7).

nanoparticles (e.g., <10 nm) (9) and of charged particles including nanoparticle sizes (22).

Clearance and Retention of Nanoparticles in Human Lungs

Limited human data are available on the clearance and retention of inhaled particles and fibers. Recent studies have measured the short-term retention of nanoparticles based on low dose, short-term exposure to radiolabeled carbon nanoparticles ("Technegas"; ~25–100 MBq dose achieved in a few breaths). Most of the deposited nanoparticles remained in the lungs up to two days following exposure, although the measured amount varied (~65% at 24 hours (20); 95% at six hours (23); 99% at 46 hours (24)). These studies did not find evidence for the rapid translocation of nanoparticles to the blood circulation or accumulation in the liver, as had been reported earlier (25). The findings of the Nemmar et al. study (25) may have been influenced by the instability of the radiolabel-nanoparticle complex (20,24).

Long-term clearance and retention data of nanoparticles in humans are not available. For larger, respirable particles (~1–5 μm), the long-term retention half-time in humans is on the order of months to years (7). Human studies of retained particle dose are rare, and coal miners have been the most studied. One study of coal miners found black pigment in liver and spleen tissues, and the amount of pigment was associated with both lung disease severity and years worked in coal mining (although no pigment-related pathology was observed in these nonpulmonary organs) (26). This study suggests that both lifetime cumulative exposure and lung disease status can influence the translocation of particles into the blood circulation—even for larger (micrometer size) coal particles. Another possible route by which particles can enter the blood circulation is via the digestive tract (e.g., from ingestion of particles following mucociliary clearance from the lungs). Particle characteristics (e.g., surface reactivity) can also influence the disposition of inhaled particles. Tran and Buchanan (27) showed that respirable quartz, which is cytotoxic, was cleared less effectively from coal miners' lungs and was transported more readily to the lung-associated lymph nodes than was coal dust, which has relatively low inherent toxicity.

Translocation of Nanoparticles in Rats

Studies in rats have shown that nanoparticles can enter the blood circulation and translocate to nonpulmonary organs. This translocation appears to be influenced by the particle dose; particle size; and chemical composition. Oberdörster et al. (14) showed significant accumulation of ^{13}C nanoparticles in the liver of rats within 18 and 24 hours of inhalation. At the higher dose of 180 μg/m^3, increased ^{13}C was detected in the rat liver within 0.5 hour of exposure, but not until 18 hour at the $80 \mu g/m^3$ dose. In contrast to ^{13}C nanoparticles, iridium nanoparticles had very low translocation from the lungs (15). The ^{192}Ir in the blood was close to the level of detection and had very low accumulation in other organs (<1%); yet, the fraction of the 15-nm nanoparticles translocating to other organs was nearly 10 times greater than that for the 80-nm particles—indicating that smaller nanoparticles are more easily transported from the lungs (15). Geiser et al. (17) observed the rapid translocation of titanium dioxide nanoparticles from the lungs in rats; within one hour after inhalation, 24% of the nanoparticles were observed within and beyond the epithelial cell barrier of the lungs, including within blood capillaries and red blood cells.

Limited data are available on the long-term clearance and retention of nanoparticles in rat lungs. Semmler et al. (28) reported similar long-term retention of iridium nanoparticles compared to micrometer-size particles. Kuempel et al. (29) found that the long-term retained lung burdens of ultrafine and fine titanium dioxide, carbon black, and diesel exhaust particles in rats were similar to those predicted from several rat lung dosimetry models. While these studies suggest that the long-term clearance of respirable particles may be similar for micrometer- and nanometer-size particles, they do not explain the systemic translocation observed in short-term studies of nanoparticles (14,15) or the potential role of particle characteristics in addition to size.

Biological Mechanisms of Nanoparticle Disposition

Our understanding of the mechanisms of particle clearance and retention comes largely from animal studies. Nanoparticles have been shown to be less effectively phagocytized by alveolar macrophages than larger respirable particles (30,31). Nanoparticles are also taken up and retained in the lung interstitium to a greater extent (32–34). If the epithelium is damaged, such as by pulmonary inflammation, particles can more easily penetrate the lung epithelial barrier (35). A possible mechanism for the adverse cardiovascular events associated with increased particulate air pollution in human studies (36) may be related (either directly or indirectly) to combustion-derived nanoparticles through inflammatory and prothrombic processes (4).

Nanoparticles that deposit in the nasal region in rats have been shown to translocate to the brain via olfactory and trigeminal nerve axons (13,37) and have been associated with inflammation in specific brain regions (37). Nanoparticles have also been shown to localize in or near cell organelles, including mitochondria and nuclei, and have been associated with oxidative stress and cell damage (16,17). The extent these pathways and processes may occur in humans exposed to nanoparticles is not known.

Use of Lung Dosimetry Models in Risk Assessment

Several chronic inhalation studies of nanoparticles (poorly-soluble ultrafine particles) in rats provide quantitative dose-response data that can be used to develop initial risk estimates for nanoparticles. The steps to using animal inhalation bioassay data in developing quantitative risk estimates include (29):

1. Select the animal model, dose metric, and disease response.
2. Analyze the dose-response relationship (e.g., statistical model) and estimate the internal dose associated with a specified risk of disease (target dose).
3. Extrapolate the target dose from animals to humans (e.g., normalize on lung mass or lung surface area)—assuming equal response to equivalent doses (if no data otherwise).
4. Determine the human-equivalent airborne exposure concentration and duration associated with the target lung dose (e.g., using a human lung dosimetry model).

This approach is illustrated in Fig. 1. It has been used in quantitative risk assessment of occupational exposure to poorly-soluble particles (ultrafine or fine titanium dioxide, ultrafine carbon black, diesel exhaust particulate) (29). Two current human lung dosimetry models (8,9) were used to estimate the working lifetime exposure associated with the lung doses identified in the rat dose-response modeling. Although all the particles analyzed are considered to be poorly-soluble with low inherent toxicity (38), the rat-based lung cancer risk estimates were higher for the ultrafine particles compared to the same airborne mass concentration of fine particles (29). This finding reflects the greater pulmonary inflammation and lung tumor response that have been observed in rats exposed to nanoparticles compared to an equal mass of larger particles of similar composition. Other dose metrics including particle surface area (39,40) or particle size and volume (41) have been shown to better predict these adverse responses to either nanoparticles or larger respirable particles in the rat lungs.

ISSUES AND CHALLENGES TO NANOPARTICLE DOSE ESTIMATION IN HUMANS

In the absence of human data, animal models are often used in risk assessment (as described above). One of the major challenges in using animal data is extrapolating from animals to humans. It is often not clear to what extent observed differences in dose and response are due to qualitative versus quantitative differences across species. For example, rat studies have shown that nanoparticles can translocate from the lungs to the blood circulation and other organs (14,15,17), while most of the human studies of

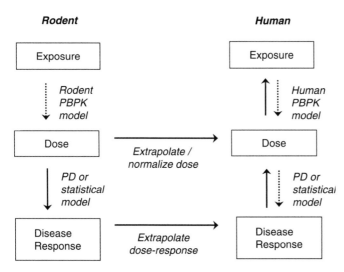

Figure 1 Schema for using rodent exposure-dose-response data and biomathematical models in risk assessment of nanoparticles. The steps are as follows: The internal dose associated with an adverse effect is estimated from rodent data using a dose-response model. The target dose is extrapolated to humans by normalization (e.g., equivalent dose per unit of tissue mass, volume, or surface area). The rodent dose-response relationship is also extrapolated to humans, typically by assuming equal response to an equivalent dose in both species if no other data are available. A human PBPK or dosimetry model is used to estimate the exposure scenarios (concentration and duration) that are expected to lead to the target dose in a given population (by age, exercise level, breathing pattern, etc.). Alternatively, if human exposure data are available, then the internal dose can be predicted and evaluated with the dose-response model in rodents (or humans, if available) to estimate the associated disease risk. Also, if a rodent study does not include internal dose data, a relevant PBPK model could be used to estimate it. *Abbreviations*: PBPK, physiologically-based pharmacokinetic model (also called dosimetry model); PD, pharmacodynamic model.

short-term exposure to carbon nanoparticles have not (20,23,24). From these studies alone it is not possible to determine whether the differences are qualitative (e.g., nanoparticles do not translocate across human lung epithelium into the blood, but do so in rats); quantitative (e.g., translocation is dose-dependent and the doses in humans were too low or of too short a duration to detect an effect); or some combination (e.g., various translocation processes exist and operate to different extents across species). A challenge for dosimetry modeling of nanoparticles is to determine what physical and biological factors allow nanoparticles to translocate beyond the lungs (e.g., by blood circulation or axonal transport) and at what rates in humans and animals, since these pathways and processes are not considered in the current particle and fiber lung dosimetry models.

Additional challenges to estimating nanoparticle dose relate to both general model validation issues and nanoparticle-specific issues (Table 1). Many biomathematical models of particle and fiber deposition and clearance have been developed in rodents and humans; however, before such models are extended to nanoparticle-specific processes, evaluation of the model structure and validation is needed. Harmonization of the various respiratory tract models and features would help to reduce uncertainties pertaining to model structure. A major limitation in any of these investigations is the sparse human data. New tools and techniques are promising to provide alternative approaches to obtaining useful data. For example the use of human lung casts with simulated air flow allows measurement of fiber deposition fractions (42), a technique which could be applied to nanoparticles of varying size and shape. New applications of labeling techniques to nanoparticles (e.g., using gold-label or quantum dots) are also promising for detecting and quantifying nanoparticles dose in the body in experimental animal studies (43). In vivo and in vitro studies can also provide the scientific basis for determining the appropriate dose metric (e.g., particle mass, number, surface area) (39) to predict exposure, dose, and response relationships for nanoparticles in animals and humans. Collaboration among biomathematical modelers and experimental scientists is critical to identifying and filling data gaps for improved model development and prediction of nanoparticle dose in humans. As with any biomathematical modeling, additional challenges include determining the sensitivity of the model predictions to alternative assumptions and parameter values, and accounting for population variability in key parameter values (44).

The development and validation of human lung dosimetry models for nanoparticles would provide an improved tool for risk assessment, by reducing uncertainty in estimating what exposures are likely—or unlikely—

Table 1   Challenges and Data Needs for Estimating Nanoparticle Dose in Humans

Validation of Current Lung Models	Extension of Models for Nanoparticles
Harmonize the various respiratory tract models	Include pathways for particle translocation beyond the lungs
Validate model predictions by particle size and type	Identify uptake by routes other than inhalation
Evaluate and validate extrapolation methods from animals to humans	Determine appropriate particle dose metric (e.g., surface area, mass, number)
Perform sensitivity analysis of model parameter values	Determine role of nanoparticle shape and agglomeration
Include population variability in key parameters and pathways	Identify target tissues for nanoparticle disposition
	Determine association between internal dose and adverse biological responses

to result in internal doses associated with adverse effects. Questions remain concerning the adequacy of current lung dosimetry models to adequately describe the inhalation and retention of nanoparticles. It is also not known what exposures to nanoparticles occur in workers and whether the exposures present a health concern. Given these uncertainties, research is needed to fill the key data gaps to improve the risk estimates in workers, consumers, and the environment. In the meantime, strategies are needed to minimize nanoparticle exposures in workers producing or using these materials (including engineering controls, work practices, and personal protective equipment) (1,45,46).

CONCLUSIONS

Dose estimation is an important element in evaluating the potential toxicity of nanoparticles and estimating the risk of exposure. The extent to which current models and methods accurately predict the internal dose of nanoparticles from occupational or environmental exposures is not fully understood. Compared to larger particles, inhaled nanoparticles may translocate within the body much more readily. They may enter previously unrecognized pathways (e.g., olfactory nerve transport to the brain) and retention sites in cells (e.g., mitochondria). Ingestion and dermal pathways are potential routes of exposure to nanoparticles but have had limited study. Studies to date suggest that the traditional focus on the lungs as the primary route of exposure and target organ of inhaled particles will need to be expanded to consider all the possible pathways and organs that may receive nanoparticle doses. New experimental methods for tracking and measuring nanoparticles dose in vivo provide potential tools for obtaining quantitative dose data that are essential for dosimetry model validation and refinement.

REFERENCES

1. Maynard AM, Kuempel ED. Airborne nanostructured particles and occupational health. J Nanoparticle Res 2005; 7(6):587–614.
2. ISO. Workplace atmospheres—ultrafine, nanoparticle and nano-structured aerosols—exposure characterization and assessment. International Standards Organization Document No. ISO/TR 27628:2007. Geneva: Switzerland: International Standards Organization.
3. Oberdörster G, Oberdörster E, Oberdörster J. Nanotoxicology: an emerging discipline evolving from studies of ultrafine particles. Environ Health Perspect 2005; 113(7):823–39.
4. Donaldson K, Tran L, Jimenez LA, et al. Combustion-derived nanoparticles: a review of their toxicology following inhalation exposure. Part Fibre Toxicol 2005; 2(10).
5. Kreyling WG, Semmler-Behnke M, Möller W. Ultrafine particle-lung interactions: Does size matter? J Aerosol Med 2006; 19(1):74–83.

6. NIOSH. Work-related lung disease surveillance report, 2002. DHHS (NIOSH) Publication No. 2003-11. Cincinnati, OH: U.S. Department of Health and Human Services, Centers for Disease Control and Prevention, National Institute for Occupational Safety and Health, 2003.

7. ICRP. Human respiratory tract model for radiological protection. International Commission on Radiological Protection Publication No. 66. Oxford, England: Pergamon, Elsevier Science Ltd., 1994.

8. Kuempel ED, O'Flaherty EJ, Stayner LT, et al. A biomathematical model of particle clearance and retention in the lungs of coal miners: Part I. Model development. Reg Toxicol Pharmacol 2001; 34(1):69–88.

9. CIIT, RIVM. Multiple-path particle deposition (MPPD V 1.0): A model for human and rat airway particle dosimetry. Research Triangle Park, NC: Centers for Health Research (CIIT), Bilthoven, The Netherlands: National Institute for Public Health and the Environment (RIVM), 2002.

10. Martonen TB, Rosati JA, Isaacs KK. Modeling deposition of inhaled particles. In: Ruzer LS, Harley NH, eds. Aerosols Handbook: Measurement, Dosimetry, and Health Effects. Boca Raton, FL: CRC Press, 2005:113–55.

11. Tran CL, Kuempel ED, Castranova V. A model of exposure, dose and response to inhaled silica. Ann Occup Hyg 2002; 46 (Suppl. 1):14–17.

12. Stöber W, Morrow PE, Morawietz G. Alveolar retention and clearance of insoluble particles in rats simulated by a new physiology-oriented compartmental kinetics model. Fund Appl Toxicol 1990; 15:329–49.

13. Oberdörster G, Sharp Z, Atudorei V, et al. Translocation of inhaled ultrafine particles to the brain. Inhal Toxicol 2004; 16(6–7):437–45.

14. Oberdörster G, Sharp Z, Atudorei V, et al. Extrapulmonary translocation of ultrafine carbon particles following whole-body inhalation exposure of rats. J Toxicol Environ Health 2002; 65 Part A(20):1531–43.

15. Kreyling WG, Semmler M, Erbe F, et al. Translocation of ultrafine insoluble iridium particles from lung epithelium to extrapulmonary organs is size dependent but very low. J Toxicol Environ Health 2002; 65(20):1513–30.

16. Li N, Sioutas C, Cho A, et al. Ultrafine particulate pollutants induce oxidative stress and mitochondrial damage. Environ Health Perspect 2003; 111(4):455–60.

17. Geiser M, Rothen-Rutishauser B, Kapp N, et al. Ultrafine particles cross cellular membranes by nonphagocytic mechanisms in lungs and in cultured cells. Environ Health Perspect 2005; 113(11):1555–60.

18. Riviere JE, Tran CL. Pharmacokinetics of Nanomatcrials. In: Nanotoxicology: Characterization, Dosing, and Health Effects. Monteriro-Riviere NA and Tran CL, eds., New York: Informa Healthcare, 2007.

19. Daigle CC, Chalupa DC, Gibb FR, et al. Ultrafine particle deposition in humans during rest and exercise. Inhal Toxicol 2003; 15(6):539–52.

20. Brown JS, Zeman KL, Bennett WD. Ultrafine particle deposition and clearance in the healthy and obstructed lung. Am J Respir Crit Care Med 2002; 166:1240–7.

21. Frampton MW, Stewart JC, Oberdorster G, et al. Inhalation of ultrafine particles alters blood leukocyte expression of adhesion molecules in humans. Environ Health Perspect 2006; 114(1):51–8.

22. Jeffers DE. Relative magnitudes of the effects of electrostatic image and thermophoretic forces on particles in the respiratory tract. Radiat Protect Dosimetr 2005; 113(2);189–94.

23. Mills NL, Amin N, Robinson SD, et al. Do inhaled carbon nanoparticles translocate directly into the circulation in humans? Am J Respir Crit Care Med 2006; 173:426–31.

24. Wiebert P, Sanchez-Crespo A, Seitze J, et al. Negligible clearance of ultrafine particles retained in healthy and affected human lungs. Eur Respir J 2006; 28: 286–90.

25. Nemmar A, Hoet PHM, Vanquickenborne B, et al. Passage of inhaled particles into the blood circulation in humans. Circulation 2002; 105:411–14.

26. LeFevre ME, Green FH, Joel DD, et al. Frequency of black pigment in livers and spleens of coal workers: correlation with pulmonary pathology and occupational information. Hum Pathol 1982; 13(12):1121–6.

27. Tran CL, Buchanan D. Development of a biomathematical lung model to describe the exposure-dose relationship for inhaled dust among U.K. coal miners, Institute of Occupational Medicine Research Report TM/00/02. Edinburgh, UK: Institute of Occupational Medicine, 2000.

28. Semmier M, Seitz J, Erbe F, et al. Long-term clearance kinetics of inhaled ultrafine insoluble iridium particles from the rat lung, including transient translocation into secondary organs. Inhal Toxicol 2004; 16(6–7):453–9.

29. Kuempel ED, Tran CL, Castranova V, et al. Lung dosimetry and risk assessment of nanoparticles: Evaluating and extending current models in rats and humans. Inhal Toxicol 2006; 18(10):717–24.

30. Renwick LC, Donaldson K, Clouter A. Impairment of alveolar macrophage phagocytosis by ultrafine particles. Toxicol Appl Pharmacol 2001; 172(2): 119–27.

31. Renwick LC, Brown D, Clouter A, et al. Increased inflammation and altered macrophage chemotactic responses caused by two ultrafine particles. Occup Environ Med 2004; 61:442–7.

32. Ferin J, Oberdörster G. Translocation of particles from pulmonary alveoli into the interstitium. J Aerosol Med 1992; 5(3):179–87.

33. Oberdörster G, Ferin J, Lehnert BE. Correlation between particle-size, in-vivo particle persistence, and lung injury. Environ Health Perspect 1994; 102(S5): 173–9.

34. Takenaka S, Karg D, Roth C, et al. Pulmonary and systemic distribution of inhaled ultrafine silver particles in rats. Environ Health Perspect 2001; 109 (Suppl. 4):547–51.

35. Adamson IY, Prieditis HL. Response of mouse lung to carbon deposition during injury and repair. Environ Health Perspect 1995; 103(1):72–6.

36. Pope CA, Burnett RT, Thurston GD, et al. Cardiovascular mortality and long-term exposure to particulate air pollution: epidemiological evidence of general pathophysiological pathways of disease. Circulation 2004; 109(1): 71–4.

37. Elder A, Gelein R, Silva V, et al. Translocation of inhaled ultrafine manganese oxide particles to the central nervous system. Environ Health Perspect 2006; 114:1172–8.

38. ILSI(International Life Sciences Institute Working Group). The relevance of the rat lung response to particle overload for human risk assessment: a workshop consensus report. Inhal Toxicol 2000; 12:1–17.
39. Driscoll KE. Role of inflammation in the development of rat lung tumors in response to chronic particle exposure. In: Mauderly JL, McCunney RJ, eds. Particle Overload in the Rat Lung and Lung Cancer: Implications for Human Risk Assessment. Philadelphia, PA: Taylor & Francis, 1996:139–52.
40. Duffin R, Tran CL, Clouter A, et al. The importance of surface area and specific reactivity in the acute pulmonary inflammatory response to particles. Ann Occup Hyg 2002; 46:242–5.
41. Pott F, Roller M. Carcinogenicity study with nineteen granular dusts in rats. Eur J Oncol 2005; 10(4):249–81.
42. Su W-C, Cheng YS. Fiber deposition pattern in two human respiratory tract replicas. Inhal Toxicol 2006; 18(7–10):749–60.
43. Mercer RR, Scabilloni J, Wang L, et al. Distribution and response due to deposition of single-walled carbon nanotubes in the lungs, 1st International Conference on Nanotoxicology: Biomedical Aspects, Miami, FL, Jan 29–Feb 1, 2006.
44. Kuempel ED, Tran CL, Smith RJ, et al. A biomathematical model of particle clearance and retention in the lungs of coal miners: Part II. Evaluation of variability and uncertainty. Regul Toxicol Pharmacol 2001; 34:89–102.
45. NIOSH. Approaches to safe nanotechnology: An information exchange with NIOSH. Version 1.1. Cincinnati, OH: U.S. Department of Health and Human Services, Centers for Disease Control and Prevention, National Institute for Occupational Safety and Health, 2006. (Available at: http://www.cdc.gov/niosh/topics/nanotech/safenano/).
46. Schulte PA, Salamanca-Buentello F. Ethical and scientific issues of nanotechnology in the workplace. Environ Health Perspect 2007; 115(1):5–12.

11

Dispersion of Nanoparticles in Pulmonary Surfactants for In Vitro Toxicity Studies: Lessons from Ultrafine Diesel Exhaust Particles and Fine Mineral Dusts

William E. Wallace

Health Effects Laboratory Division, National Institute for Occupational Safety and Health and College of Engineering and Mineral Resources, University of West Virginia, Morgantown, West Virginia, U.S.A.

Michael J. Keane

Health Effects Laboratory Division, National Institute for Occupational Safety and Health, Morgantown, West Virginia, U.S.A.

Mridul Gautam

College of Engineering and Mineral Resources, West Virginia University, Morgantown, West Virginia, U.S.A

Xiao-Chun Shi, David Murray, and Tong-man Ong

Health Effects Laboratory Division, National Institute for Occupational Safety and Health, Morgantown, West Virginia, U.S.A.

INTRODUCTION

Nanostructured materials including nanoparticles (NP) are generally defined as having at least one dimension smaller than 100 nm (1). Ultrafine particles are similarly defined as having diameters less than 100 nm; the general convention being that NP are manufactured or engineered materials in contrast to incidental or natural ultrafine particles. NPs are of special interest to the health effects researcher. They are not merely smaller forms of particulate matter; they can profoundly differ in their toxicological proper-ties from fine-sized respirable particles, i.e., particles between 0.1 and 2.5 μm in size. For example, fine-sized respirable TiO_2 particles are typically inert when studied in vitro and in vivo and are typically used as particle negative controls; while in contrast, nanoparticulate TiO_2, when used in animal model inhalation studies, causes lung injury (2). The basis for change in health effects associated with decreasing particle size is not necessarily size per se. There are other physical factors that change very strongly with decreasing particle size: one is particle number per unit mass; another is specific surface area (surface area per unit mass).

Because of their submicrometer sizes, NP or ultrafine particles have high specific surface areas. For example, ultrafine diesel exhaust particulate materials (DPM) can have specific surface areas in the range of 100 to $1000 \, m^2/g$, in contrast to many fine-sized mineral dusts with values in the $10 \, m^2/g$ range. In some cases, ultrafine particle surface area has provided an effective metric-relating exposure and response: TiO_2 ultrafine particles and carbon black dust were active for tumor induction in the rat with toxicity increasing with dust surface area (1). And surface area in some cases provides a measure of comparability between different ultrafine dusts, e.g., for some clearance or inflammation processes in vivo (3).

However, not all respirable particulate materials are equally toxic when concentration or exposure dose are normalized by surface area. The composition or structure of the particle surface can greatly affect toxicity. For fine-sized respirable particles, surface structural properties which are submicrometer or ultrafine in dimension can be determinants of health hazard and disease risk. For instance, unexpected morbidity and mortality in the workforce of a hard metal fabrication plant using a new process were related to subtle surface structural features of the generated fine respirable dusts: ultrathin cobalt coatings on the tungsten carbide particles were strongly catalytic in aqueous media for toxic reactive oxygen species generation (4–6). Anomalous differences in silicosis risk between two worker cohorts in China, identified in a 20,000 worker medical registry, were largely resolved by quantitatively normalizing exposures to respirable silica dust that was free from submicrometer aluminosilicate surface contamination (7–9). Such surface ultrafine structural effects on health hazard, albeit for fine-sized respirable particles, suggest the need for a thorough characterization of surface physicochemical and toxicological properties of new NP respirable materials with their very large specific surface areas.

Expression of toxic activities associated with respirable particle surfaces can be significantly modified by the initial interaction of particles depositing in the acinar region of the lung. After inhalation, the first contact of respired particles is with the lung's rich surfactant-coated hypophase lining of the air–tissue interface of the alveoli or respiratory bronchioles. Insoluble particles can adsorb components of that pulmonary hypophase surfactant, resulting in fundamental changes in the particles' biological disposition and expression of toxicity. In vitro toxicology studies can be designed to retain particle surface structure and composition and to model the conditioning of those surfaces upon particle deposition in the deep lung in order to analyze consequent effects on toxicity. Ultrafine or fine respirable particulate materials have been dispersed into phospholipid components of lung surfactant as preparation for in vitro cytotoxicity and genotoxicity studies. Pragmatically, this overcomes laboratory handling problems innate in attempting aqueous system preparations of insoluble hydrophobic particulate materials, by permitting their dispersion in a physiologically reasonable manner. More profoundly, this provides a model of their surface conditioning as would occur upon deposition in the lung; of their in vivo biological availability; and of potential nanostructural synergisms for the expression of surface-associated toxicant activity. Some in vitro studies of phospholipid surfactant-conditioned ultrafine or fine respirable particles are reviewed here to illustrate testing procedures and their limitations for identification of NP toxic activities and potential respiratory hazard.

LUNG SURFACTANT AND INSOLUBLE RESPIRABLE PARTICLE IN VITRO TESTING

Lipid and lipoprotein surfactants synthesized and secreted by pulmonary alveolar II cells coat the air interface of the hypophase surface of the deep lung. Phospholipids constitute about three-quarters of the mass of pulmonary surfactant, with diacyl phosphatidylcholines (DAPC) accounting for over half of them (10,11). When spread upon the aqueous–air interface, phospholipids lower surface tension about 50-fold, down to the order of 1 dyne/cm; and they make surface tension a function of surfactant surface concentration, closely modeling those physiologically important properties of the pulmonary alveolar hypophase (12). A specific DAPC, dipalmitoyl phosphatidylcholine (DPPC), dispersed into physiologic saline has been used frequently as a simple model of lung surfactant in physiology studies; and more complex mixtures derived from animal lung lavage containing DAPC have been used in research, and have been used clinically, e.g., as therapy for infants' respiratory distress.

Hydrophobic or hydrophilic respirable fine or ultrafine particles can adsorb components of lung surfactant from aqueous dispersion. That results in prompt modification of the expression of some particle surface-associated toxicities; and subsequent cellular enzymatic digestive processing of that particle surface-adsorbed surfactant can determine the evolution of a particle's expression of toxicity. These surfactant interactions can significantly affect the biological availability or activity of particle-surface-borne toxicants or surface chemical functional groups. Such particle surface– surfactant interactions have been researched to address two general concerns for respirable particulate material toxicity: (1) the question of the physiological significance and interpretability of conventional in vitro assays of diesel exhaust or other hydrophobic ultrafine particulate genotoxicants as conventionally performed on organic solvent extracts of collected DPM; and (2) the question of the failures of in vitro cytotoxicity assays to predict and distinguish pneumoconiosis hazard of fine-sized respirable mineral dusts.

Genotoxicity of Ultrafine Diesel Exhaust Particulate Materials

Diesel exhaust has been evaluated to be a potential or probable human carcinogen by the Centers for Disease Control and Prevention—National Institute for Occupational Safety and Health (13), the International Agency for Research on Cancer (14), and the U.S. Environmental Protection Agency (15). DPM is ultrafine carbonaceous hydrophobic particulate material, frequently containing complex polycyclic aromatic hydrocarbon (PAH) compounds which, separately, are known carcinogens, and sometimes containing a number of proven toxic species, including polar hetero- and polycyclic aromatics, radical species, entrained metal species, and other organic species (16). Being hydrophobic and insoluble in water, DPM typically have been prepared for chemical study or in vitro bioassay by dissolution and extraction in organic solvents. It has long been observed that in vitro genotoxic activities are expressed by organic solvent extracts of some filter-collected DPM, e.g., using acetone or dichloromethane (DCM) solvent (17–24). In vitro mutagenicity of solvent extract of DPM can vary systematically with operating conditions for a given engine, e.g., with engine speed, torque, and fuel (25).

One question of the role of DPM genotoxicants for in vivo tumorogenicity is this: are hydrophobic particle-borne genotoxicants biologically available for activity under conditions of particle deposition in the lung? Testing organic solvent extracts of DPM does not provide, a priori, a physiologically reasonable model of genotoxicant biological availability from intact DPM particles deposited in the lung aqueous hypophase. It was found that attempting to extract DPM with principal components of lung surfactant released few or no organic genotoxicants from the particles, and the surfactant extract expressed little or no in vitro genotoxic activity (26–29). That is, the hydrophobicity of the organic genotoxicants carried by the carbonaceous DPM particles prevented their extraction or release from the particles under conditions modeling their deposition on the surface lining of the deep lung.

Instead, a different paradigm—distinct from an extraction mechanism—was observed that could result in biological availability and activity of hydrophobic ultrafine particle-borne genotoxicants: if DPM were simply mixed into aqueous phospholipid surfactant dispersion, then the resultant dispersion expressed genotoxic activity in vitro. Those activities were shown to be associated with the nondissolved but surfactant-dispersed particulate phase material (29–34). That is, phospholipid surfactant adsorbs to the DPM surface, providing a hydrophilic coating, and permitting dispersion of the surfactant-coated DPM as particles in aqueous media; and those particles can express genotoxic activities.

Such dispersion of DPM into components of lung surfactant in part models possible in vivo particle surface conditioning, disaggregation, and particulate-bound toxicant bioavailability, while avoiding the destruction of particle size, structure, and compositional properties that would result from organic solvent extraction of DPM. Surfactant dispersion also provides a convenience in preparatory handling of DPM for aqueous in vitro test systems or in vivo studies using instillation of collected NP materials.

The basis for the ability of DPPC to disperse DPM or other hydrophobic particles is the combination of hydrophobic and hydrophilic moieties of the DPPC molecule. One end of the molecule consists of hydrophilic choline and phosphate: a trimethyl ammonium cationic group is bound through a two-carbon chain to an acidic phosphate, forming a zwitterionic dipole and providing a hydrophilic end of the molecule. The phosphate then is esterified to the first carbon of a glycerol, which is esterified at the other two carbons to two long-chain fatty acid residues; palmitate in the case of DPPC. These provide two hydrophobic, lipophilic long tails to the molecule. When dispersed into aqueous media, the phospholipid molecules aggregate into multimolecular structures such that the hydrophilic zwitterionic head groups of the molecules are oriented to face into the surrounding water, while the hydrophobic fatty acid tails cluster among themselves, minimizing contact with water or with the hydrophilic heads of other phospholipids. This gives rise to spherical or lamellar structures made up of bilayers of surfactant molecules. The zwitterionic head groups are on the outer aqueous-side surfaces of the bilayer, with the lipid tails "sandwiched" between in order to minimize hydrophobic lipid tail contact with water. This structure also is the general basis for the bilayer phospholipid underlying all cell membrane structure.

Dry, waxy DPPC can be dispersed into aqueous media by ultrasonication, forming a pale milky and relatively stable dispersion. When dry or oily filter-collected DPM is mixed into this aqueous DPPC dispersion then the agglomerates of soot particles are observed to disperse. The DPM is "solu-bilized," that is, dispersed as small surfactant-coated particles, rather than dissolved. In this state, long-chain lipophilic/hydrophobic tails of the DPPC molecule associate with the organic DPM particle surfaces, while the zwitterionic hydrophilic trimethyl ammonium and phosphate head of the DPPC molecule orients outward to face the surrounding aqueous medium. A simplified picture is that of a DPM particle as a tar "pin-cushion" covered by DPPC soap molecule "pins" with their tails adsorbed to the tarry DPM particle and their heads oriented outward, providing a hydrophilic outer coating, in turn permitting the structure to act as a water-wet but nondissolved particle, which disperses in water. Filter-collected DPM mixed into an aqueous DPPC dispersion then can challenge cells effectively to express genotoxic activities for mammalian cell DNA and clastogenic damage, as well as for bacterial cell mutagenicity.

Order of magnitude estimate of the amounts of DPPC needed to fully disperse DPM or other ultrafine or NP material, and so to permit bioassay of full activity, can be estimated from the specific surface areas of the particulate materials. For fine mineral particulate matter a measure was made of the amount of DPPC mass adsorption per unit dust surface area as necessary to fully passivate the membranolytic toxicity of two silicate dusts (see below). Using that so-derived value of about 5 mg DPPC/m^2 surface area as an approximate general measure independent of particle composition, then ultrafine particles with specific surface areas of 100 to 1000 m^2/g would require, respectively, on the order of 500 mg DPPC to 5000 mg DPPC/g of particulate material. As a caveat to this estimate for hydrophobic NP materials: the minimal coating may be a monolayer of DPPC for hydrophobic particles, e.g., diesel soot, in contrast to a bilayer for mineral dusts. On the other hand, if the sample is collected on a filter from the aerosol state or otherwise aggregate collected, then agglomeration in the sample may require surfactant multilayers for physical disaggregation to proceed to completion. Bacterial mutagenic activity was measured versus DPPC concentration for three concentrations of DPM from a diesel truck exhaust-pipe deposit over a range from 1/1 to 10/1 mass ration DPPC/DPM. At any DPM concentration the mutagenic activity increased with DPPC concentration up to a DPPC/ DPM ratio of about 7/1, i.e., 7000 mg DPPC/g DPM (29).

In Vitro Genotoxicity Assays of DPM Dispersed in Surfactants

In vitro genotoxic activities have been compared on organic solvent extraction versus surfactant dispersion preparations of parallel DPM samples. Several assays were performed upon DPM that had been filter-collected from the exhaust of a 1980-commercial 5.7 liter V-8 diesel engine operated on a dynamometer test stand under a Federal Test Procedure urban duty cycle, the material graciously supplied by the Lovelace Inhalation Toxicology Institute. Organic solvent extraction was prepared by dissolution of DPM in DCM or acetone and evaporative exchange into dimethylsulf-oxide (DMSO). In some experiments, DMSO was used as the organic solvent for extraction. For the surfactant dispersion sample, the surfactant was prepared by ultrasonically dispersing DPPC into physiological saline solution (PSS); then DPM was mixed (not sonicated) into that dispersion. The Ames *Salmonella typhimurium* histidine reversion assay was used for the detection of gene mutation in bacteria. The assays for mammalian cells include sister chromatid exchange (SCE), micronucleus induction (MN), unscheduled DNA synthesis (UDS), chromosomal aberration (CA), gene mutation, and the single cell gel electrophoresis for single- or double-strand DNA damage. These comparison studies have been recently reviewed (35).

Both solvent and surfactant total preparations showed positive activity increasing with DPM concentration, for gene mutation in *S. typhimurium*

TA98 without microsomal S9 activation, with the 1980-engine soot somewhat more active as a surfactant dispersion compared to its preparation in DMSO. The extract of the solvent preparation was mutagenic, while the particulate residue of the solvent extraction was not. For the surfactant preparation of the DPM, the dispersion of whole DPM into surfactant was mutagenic, while its filtrate was not. When the surfactant-dispersed DPM was centrifuged rather than filtered, then some mutagenic activity was expressed by the supernatant suggesting a very fine particulate-active fraction, which could be filtered out but not centrifuged out of the surfactant dispersion (29–31).

The Chinese hamster pulmonary fibroblast-derived cell line (V79) was used for the SCE and UDS assays. Both DMSO organic solvent and DPPC surfactant dispersion total preparations of the 1980-diesel DPM expressed comparable activity, increasing SCEs with DPM concentration. Induction of SCE activity was found to reside in the supernatant fraction of the DMSO solvent-extracted samples, and in the sedimented (particulate) fraction for DPPC surfactant-dispersed samples (31). Using a DPM collected from a diesel truck exhaust-pipe deposit, both DPPC surfactant dispersion and DMSO solvent total preparations were active for the induction of SCE, with the DMSO solvent preparation about twice as strong as the surfactant preparation (30). Both DPPC dispersion and DMSO solvent preparations of the 1980-diesel DPM were also active in the UDS assay with the dispersion preparation about 50% stronger per mass of soot extracted. Induction of UDS was found in the supernatant fraction of the DMSO-extracted sample and in the sediment (particulate) fraction of the surfactant-dispersed sample (33).

In the study of MN induction in V79 cells by the 1980-diesel DPM, samples in DMSO solvent or DPPC surfactant preparation showed increasing positive concentration-response activity with the surfactant preparation about twice the strength of the solvent preparation. For CA induction by the same DPM and cells, DPPC surfactant-dispersed DPM was active, increasing with DPM concentration; CA comparison was not made with solvent extract samples. The 6-thioguanine-resistant gene mutation assay for a forward gene mutation using this DPM and V79 cells did not show a significant positive response as either DMSO solvent or DPPC dispersion preparations (34). In a separate MN study of the same DPM, the DPPC surfactant sediment and DMSO supernatant of preparations were comparably active in Chinese hamster ovary (CHO) cells; however, in V79 cells the DMSO solvent extract was active while the DPPC surfactant sediment was only marginally active (32). In contrast, MN assay of a National Institute of Standards and Technology standard DPM obtained from a fork-lift diesel exhaust expressed significantly greater activity for DPPC surfactant sample preparation versus that expressed by acetone solvent extract of an equal mass of soot. The same sample showed similar behavior of heightened activity for surfactant-dispersed particles in single cell gel electrophoresis assay for single- or double-strand DNA break; but both preparations were comparably active in YG1024 bacterial mutagenicity assays (36). That is, in this case there appeared to be a synergistic increase in mammalian cell genotoxic activity for genotoxicants carried by ultrafine particles.

Surfactant Effects on Mineral Particle Toxicity

Fine-sized respirable mineral particle surface interactions with pulmonary surfactants significantly affect the dusts' expression of toxicities in vitro; and those findings can provide some semiquantitative design information for similar studies of ultrafine or NP respirable materials. Respirable fine-sized crystalline silica dust, e.g., quartz dust, is an exposure agent for pulmonary fibrosis; and it is promptly cytotoxic or membranolytic in numerous short-term in vitro bioassays (37). However, in vitro cellular bioassays cannot be used with specificity to distinguish quartz-associated fibrosis hazard in many mixed dusts. That is because it was found that kaolin dust, a common aluminosilicate clay dust, is as cytotoxic as quartz dust (38), despite the fact that kaolin dust exposures are associated with only limited risk of pneumoconioses in contrast with quartz dust (41–43). The two dusts expressed comparable in vitro cytotoxic activities on a surface area basis, as measured by mammalian cell release of lactate dehydrogenase (LDH) and lysosomal enzymes or by erythrocyte membranolysis (38–40). This fails to distinguish the strong pathogenic potential of quartz dust for fibrosis from kaolin dusts' far weaker hazard.

In vitro investigations of possible bases for the anomaly of equal cytotoxicities but different disease risks found that dust surface adsorption of components of lung surfactant can be prophylactic against otherwise prompt cytotoxic activities of both quartz and clay dust; and subsequent cellular enzymatic processes can modify that prophylaxis and permit expression of particle surface toxic interactions, in some cases with mineral specificity. Respirable particles can be conditioned by pulmonary surfactants (44). Adsorbed phospholipid can suppress silica particle cytotoxicity (45,46). Kaolin can adsorb surfactant (47) with suppression of membranolytic and cytotoxic activity in a number of short-term in vitro bioassays (48). That is, short-term in vitro assays of native quartz or kaolin dusts provide a "false-positive" prediction for native kaolin dust; but they result in a "false-negative" prediction for quartz dust when the dusts are surfactant-coated.

Assays of membranolytic activity versus adsorption of DPPC surfactant indicate that the amount of DPPC needed for full suppression of toxicity of quartz or kaolin dusts is proportional to the dust surface area. It was found that about 4 to 5 mg DPPC adsorbed per square meter of quartz surface and about 5 to 6 mg DPPC adsorbed per square meter of kaolin surface were the minimum amounts needed to provide complete prophylaxis of otherwise prompt membranolytic activity (40,49,50). For comparison, a computational model of the surface area of DPPC at the aqueous interface of a bilayer suggests a value of about 62 square angstroms per molecule, which would be about 4 mg DPPC per square meter for a bilayer (51).

Significant quartz dust fibrogenic activity is observed following in vivo animal model or human exposures, suggesting loss with time of the surfactant prophylaxis. Cellular lysosomes contain enzymes, which digest components of pulmonary surfactant, including phospholipases. Quartz or kaolin dusts passivated by surface-adsorbed DPPC can be taken into the cell, e.g., by phagocytosis, and subjected to phagolysosomal phospholipase activity. In some cases the dust particles can be subjected in the extracellular environment to phospholipase released by cells.

In acellular studies, dusts were incubated in DPPC dispersion, rinsed to remove loosely held surfactant; and then were incubated with three different levels of porcine pancreatic neutral pH-optimum phospholipase A2 (PLA2). DPPC and lysolecithin remaining adsorbed and erythrocyte membranolytic activity of the preparations were measured at times out to 72 h of PLA2 incubation. Half the DPPC was rapidly hydrolyzed to lysolecithin within the 1-h first time point; and the second half of the DPPC was digested much more slowly, and with mineral specificity. Kinetics of the cell-free process were well-modeled mathematically with a two-exponential function for DPPC remaining adsorbed with time under enzymatic digestion; the exponential rate constant was fivefold greater for removal of DPPC from quartz than from kaolin. Membranolytic activity of the dusts was restored in parallel with the removal of the DPPC (50,52).

The same free energy considerations responsible for phospholipid bilayer conformation in cell membranes also suggests that DPPC surfactant is adsorbed to some hydrophilic-surfaced mineral dusts as such a bilayer, with one surface of the bilayer in contact with the particle mineral surface, and the other side oriented to the surrounding aqueous medium. PLA2 hydrolyzes the ester linkage of the fatty acid at the middle carbon of the glycerol moiety that links the hydrophilic "head" of the molecule to the two long-chain fatty acid hydrophobic "tails." The rapid loss of half the surfactant from both dusts, the slower removal of the second half, and the mineral specificity for the rate of digestive removal of the second half of the surfactant can be modeled as enzymatic digestion of an adsorbed bilayer of surfactant: A surfactant bilayer remains on the particle after DPPC incubation and rinsing. Subsequent incubation with PLA2 permits rapid hydrolysis of the outer aqueous-side face of the bilayer. The inner DPPC layer, in direct contact with the mineral surface, is digested more slowly due to more restricted access of the PLA2 enzyme. The mineral-specificity of the rate of enzymatic digestion of the second half of the adsorbed surfactant suggests a further mineral-specific hindrance to activity of the PLA2 for the

DPPC in contact with the particle mineral surface. The silica surface consists of silanol groups with their surface hydroxyls weakly acidic. The kaolin surface has both silanol and aluminol groups; and the surface aluminol hydroxyl groups are weakly basic or amphoteric. Thus, different interactions can occur on the surfaces of the two dusts with differences in the strengths or conformation of the adsorbed DPPC. The additional aluminol groups on the kaolin surface provide sites distinct from the quartz surface for interactions e.g., with DPPC phosphate or carbonyls. Consequent mineral-specific steric hindrance to PLA2 enzymatic activity and rates of digestive removal of prophylactic DPPC could then result in distinct rates or levels of expression of particle toxicity. There is limited infrared and nuclear magnetic resonance spectroscopic data indicating quartz versus kaolin mineral-specific differences in the adsorption of cationic trimethylammonium at the hydrophilic end of the DPPC molecule and of the phosphate near the carbonyl ester bonds in the DPPC (49,52–56).

Quartz or kaolin loss of adsorbed surrogate lung surfactant has been measured for cellular systems. Silica dust preincubation with a commercial multicomponent surrogate lung surfactant derived from bovine lung surfactant was used for in vitro challenge of lung macrophages lavaged from male Fischer 344 rats. It protected cell viability at 1 h; but the prophylaxis was significantly reduced at 24 h. Preincubation with Survanta of a high dose of silica instilled in vivo in the animals resulted in significant reduction in biochemical and cellular response parameters in bronchiolar lavage at 1 day but not at 14 days after challenge (37,57). Digestion of C-13 radiolabeled DPPC on quartz or kaolin after in vitro challenge of the P388D1 macrophage-like cell line found half the surfactant was digested for both dusts in the first 3 days; and approximately half of that remainder was digested at 9 days for both dusts. That is, no mineral specificity was seen for this system with cellular acidic phagolysosomal digestion conditions. In addition to digestion within the cell, phospholipase exudate of the cells was identified, which was active at pH 7 but not at pH 5 in the extracellular medium. Incubation of the DPPC-coated dusts with cellular-conditioned culture medium containing this pH-neutral phospholipase resulted in digestion of DPPC on quartz at the same rates effected by cellular digestion; however, half of the original amount of DPPC remained undigested on the kaolin after 14 days (58). In vitro cellular digestion was measured over 7 days for a fluorescent probe-labeled analog of DPPC from quartz and kaolin dust by pulmonary macrophages lavaged from male Fischer 344 rats. No difference was observed between quartz and kaolin for the decay of fluorescence intensity from labeled surfactant on cell-ingested particles; a single exponential fit was fit with a $T_{1/2}$ of about 40 h for both dusts (59). A similar fluorescent-labeled phospholipid preparation of quartz and kaolin dust was used to challenge alveolar macrophages lavaged from

Sprague–Dawley male rats. Quantitative fluorescence microscopy of label intensity on particles within cells at times from 1 to 10 days showed two exponential behavior with half or more surfactant removed at 1 day; and loss was more rapid from quartz compared to kaolin (60).

A SUMMARY OF METHODS AND CAVEATS

Different genetic endpoints in bacteria and in mammalian cells all showed genotoxic activity for DPM dispersed into DPPC surfactant for cases where the DPM also express activity as solvent extract. The activities in surfactant dispersion were associated with the nondissolved particulate phase material that were coated and solubilized, i.e., given a hydrophilic coating, by a major component of lung surfactant. In this way, DPM inhaled into the lung may be made bioavailable by virtue of the solubilization and dispersion properties of pulmonary surfactant components. This suggests that other insoluble hydrophobic ultrafine or NP materials depositing in the deep lung may effectively carry and deliver genotoxicants as particulate phase materials, which can there express their genotoxic activities as lung surfactant-dispersed particles.

In vitro assays, in general, are inexpensive and useful test systems for detection of genotoxic agents and potential carcinogens. Surfactant conditioning appears to permit the extension of such in vitro bacterial and mammalian cell testing to insoluble NP materials. DPM studies indicate dispersion in phospholipid surfactant of 5 to 10 mg $DPPC/m^2$ particulate material surface area can permit full expression of genetic toxicity in mammalian cell assays. In vivo, pulmonary surfactant is well in excess of amounts needed to provide such adsorption and solubilization of respired NP. By calculation from the amount of lavagable lung surfactant from the rat of about 7 ug phospholipid per mg dry lung weight (61), and the half life time of surfactant replacement of about 14 h (12), lung surfactant is in sufficient quantity to disperse some 100 times or more of the DPM that would be respired per workday under occupational exposures at the NIOSH recommended exposure limit of 0.05 mg DPM/m^3 (34).

A concern for the interpretation from in vitro genotoxic activity to disease risk, including the case of surfactant-dispersed DPM, is that DPM induction of lung tumors in animal models has been reported for conditions of "particle overload" exposures rather than under conditions representative of occupational exposures (62–64). Conditions of in vitro cell challenge leading to induction of genotoxic activities have usually been at DPM-to-cell concentrations far exceeding doses estimated for 1 day of exposure at the NIOSH recommended DPM exposure limit (13). However, incomplete lung clearance or sequestration of DPM within pulmonary cells can lead to increasing lung loads of DPM with increasing exposure times. This has been observed in inhalation exposures of the rat to 0.25 to 6 mg DPM/m^3 of air, which resulted in residual lung burdens after 7 to 112 days of 0.2 to 12 mg retained DPM (65). These would be modeled for in vitro study by concentrations in the range of 1 to 10 µg DPM/cm^2 of plated cells, which are within concentrations used for in vitro mammalian cell studies of surfactant-dispersed DPM showing clastogenic and DNA damage (34).

Short-term in vitro cytotoxicity assays fail in the simplest comparison of quartz versus kaolin dusts to predict the great difference seen in vivo, e.g., for pulmonary fibrosis. In vitro assays for cytotoxicity risk false-positive interpretation for native particles and false-negative interpretation for surfactant-treated particles. Research implicates but does not clearly establish digestive removal of particle-adsorbed surfactant as a basis for distinguishing mineral-specific expression of toxicity that predicts disease risk with specificity. In vitro cellular systems using phospholipid surfactant and phagocytic cell systems are limited in several ways.

Firstly, DPPC is a limited model of lung surfactant. Other surfactants and other biological molecules are found in the lung alveolar hypophase; and mineral specificity of level of prophylaxis or of rate of restoration of toxicity may differ for them. Lipoprotein fractions of cell test system media serum can reduce the expression of crystalline silica cytotoxicity (66–68), with reactivation following trypsin digestion (69). Quartz and kaolin dust prompt in vitro induction of LDH release from macrophage was suppressed in 10% fetal bovine serum medium; however, quartz but not kaolin activity was restored at 6 h (70–72). This cautions that short-term in vitro results can be affected by assay system nutrients that are not necessarily representative of in vivo pulmonary hypophase exposures. Some typical components of nutrient serum, e.g., albumin, are increased in the alveolar hypophase by in vivo acute inflammatory reactions causing increased permeability of the microvasculature with transudation of plasma protein (73–75) into the lung alveoli. Thus, nonmineral specific retoxification of surfactant-conditioned particles by acidic processes in alveolar macrophages with subsequent inflammatory response might evoke a secondary round of prophylaxis, by plasma protein leaked into the alveolar hypophase interactions.

Secondly, the use of macrophage or phagocytic cell lines may not well-model the phagolysosomal digestive processes for primary cells involved in lung fibrosis. Some research has indicated that epithelial or interstitial cells of the pulmonary alveolus rather than macrophages are the target cells for silica dust-induced in vivo interactions that signal the pulmonary fibroblasts to upregulate collagen synthesis and produce lung fibrosis (76). Interstitial cells have pH neutral phagolysosomal conditions (77), similar to the pH conditions of the cell-free PLA2 tests, in contrast to lung macrophages and cell lines with pH acidic-optimum lysosomal phospholipases. The difference in rates of surfactant removal and restoration of dust toxicity seen for these in vitro macrophage-like cell systems with acidic phagolysosomal conditions for enzymatic digestion does not appear sufficient to account for the differences of in vivo induction of fibrosis between quartz and clay dusts.

That is, development of in vitro cytotoxicity assays for endpoints other than genotoxic effects, e.g., for fibrosis, might require additional features to better model in vivo conditions, including (1) the use of additional constituents of the deep lung hypophase; (2) other cells or cell lines representative of structural cells of the lung acinus; and (3) incubation times consistent with rates of cellular metabolic processing of NP surface-adsorbed prophylactic biomolecules. Validity of resultant assays might then be tested by complementary in vivo measures of labeled surfactant loss from particles in tissue (60) correlated with histopathology measures of the onset of fibrogenic activity.

Conventional in vitro cellular assays for first-tier screening of potentially genotoxic compounds can be extended to ultrafine or NP materials by surrogate lung surfactant solubilization of the particulate sample, using adequate amounts of surfactant based on sample-specific surface area, as demonstrated for diesel exhaust particulate samples. In vitro cytotoxicity assays for particulate material performed without consideration of surfactant conditioning of particle surfaces can give false-positive results for the prediction of some lung disease, as demonstrated by aluminosilicate kaolin dust samples. But in vitro cytotoxicity assays of surfactant-treated mineral dusts require further development and validation to clearly distinguish disease hazard with specificity, as seen in comparisons of quartz and clay surfactant modified in vitro toxicities versus their in vivo fibrogenic activities. In vitro short-term assays for genotoxic or cytotoxic activities by ultrafine or nanoparticulate materials must be interpreted with caution until such time as bioassay systems considering NP surface properties and physiological conditioning are demonstrated to clearly distinguish respirable particulate materials of known differing disease risk.

DISCLAIMER

The findings and conclusions in this report are those of the authors and do not necessarily represent the views of the National Institute for Occupational Safety and Health.

ACKNOWLEDGMENT

Research on surfactant-dispersed diesel exhaust particulate genotoxicity was supported in part by the U.S. Department of Energy—FreedomCar and Vehicle Technologies Activity.

REFERENCES

1. Maynard AD, Kuempel ED. Airborne nanoparticles and occupational health. J Nanoparticle Res 2005; 7:587–614.
2. Oberdörster G. Toxicology of ultrafine particles: in vivo studies. Phil Trans R Soc London Series A 2000; 358:2719–40.
3. Tran CL, Buchanan D, Cullen RT, Searl A, Jones AD, Donaldson K. Inhalation of poorly soluble particles. II. Influence of particle surface area on inflammation and clearance. Inhal Toxicol 2000; 12:1113–26.
4. Stephens JW, Harrison JC, Wallace WE. Correlating Auger electron spectroscopy with scanning electron microscopy–energy dispersive spectroscopy for the analysis of respirable particles. Scanning 1998; 20:302–10.
5. Keane MJ, Hornsby-Myers JL, Stephens JW, Harrison JC, Myers JR, Wallace WE. Characterization of hard metal dusts from sintering and detonation coating processes and comparative hydroxyl radical production in vitro. Chem Res Toxicol 2002a; 15:1010–6.
6. Keane MJ, Martin J, Hornsby-Myers J, Stephens J, Harrison J, Myers J, Ong T, Wallace W. Particle characterization, free radical generation, and genotoxicity of hard metal and detonation coating dusts. In: Proceedings of Inhaled Particles IX, Cambridge, UK. Ann Occup Hyg 2002b; 46:402–5.
7. Chen W, Hnizdo E, Chen J-Q, Attfield MD, Gao P, Hearl F, Lu J, Wallace WE. Risk of silicosis in cohorts of Chinese tin and tungsten miners and pottery workers (I): an epidemiological study. Am J Ind Med 2005; 48:1–9.
8. Harrison J, Chen J-Q, Miller W, Chen W, Hnizdo E, Lu J, Chisholm W, Keane M, Gao P, Wallace WE. Risk of silicosis in cohorts of Chinese tin and tungsten miners and pottery workers (II): workplace-specific silica particle surface composition. Am J Ind Med 2005; 48:10–5.
9. Wallace WE, Harrison J, Keane MJ, Bolsaitis P, Epplesheimer D, Poston J, Page SJ. Clay occlusion of respirable quartz particles detected by low voltage scanning electron microscopy—X-ray analysis. Ann Occup Hyg 1990b; 34: 195–204.
10. Bourbon JR, ed. Pulmonary Surfactant: Biochemical, Functional, Regulatory, and Clinical Concepts. Boca Raton, FL: CRC Press, 1991:438.
11. Hagwood S. Surfactant: composition, structure, and metabolism. In: Crystal RG, West JB, eds. The Lung: Scientific Foundations. New York: Raven Press, 1991:249–61.
12. Scarpelli EM. The Surfactant System of the Lung. Philadelphia: Lea & Febiger, 1968:97.
13. National Institute for Occupational Safety and Health. Carcinogenic effects of exposure to diesel exhaust. NIOSH Current Intelligence Bulletin 50, 1988. DHHS (NIOSH) Publication #88-116. Centers for Disease Control and Prevention, Atlanta, GA.
14. International Agency for Research on Cancer. Diesel and Gasoline Engine Exhausts and Some Nitroarenes. Vol. 46. Monographs on the Evaluation of Carcinogenic Risks to Humans. Lyon, France: World Health Organization, IARC, 1989.
15. US Environmental Protection Agency. Health Assessment Document for Diesel Engine Exhaust. USEPA EPA/600/8-90/057F, 2002. U.S. EPA, Office

of Research and Development, National Center for Environmental Assessment, Washington, DC.

16. Morimoto K, Kitamura M, Kondo H, Korizumi A. Genotoxicity of diesel exhaust emissions in a battery of in-vitro short-term and in-vivo bioassays. Dev Toxicol Environ Sci 1986; 13:85–101.

17. Huisingh J, Bradow R, Jurgens R, Claxton LD, Zweiding R, Tejada S, Bumgarner J, Duffield F, Simmon VF, Hare C, Rodriguez C, Snow L, Waters MD. Application of bioassay to characterization of diesel particle emissions. In: Waters MD, Nesnow S, Huisingh JL, Sandhu SS, Claxton LD, eds. Application of Short-Term Bioassays in the Fractionation and Analysis of Complex Environmental Mixtures. New York: Plenum Press, 1979:381–418.

18. Claxton LD. Mutagenic and carcinogenic potency of diesel and related environmental emissions: salmonella bioassay. In: Pepelko WE, Danner RM, Clarke NA, eds. Health Effects of Diesel Emissions: Proceedings of an International Symposium, December 3–5, 1979. Cincinnati, OH: U.S. Environmental Protection Agency, EPA-600/9-80-057b, 1980:801–9.

19. Pepelko WE, Danner RM, Clarke NA. Health effects of diesel engine emissions. Proceedings of an International Symposium, December 3–5, 1979, Vols. 1 and 2. Cincinnati, OH: U.S. Environmental Protection Agency, 1980: 45268.

20. Claxton LD, Kohan M. Bacterial mutagenesis and the evaluation on mobile source emissions. In: Waters MD, Sandhu SS, Lewtas-Huisingh J, Claxton LD Nesnow S, eds. Short-Term Bioassays in the Analysis of Complex Environmental Mixtures II. New York: Plenum Press, 1981:299–317.

21. Lewtas J. Evaluation of the mutagenicity and carcinogenicity of motor vehicle emissions in short-term bioassays. Environ Health Persp 1983; 47:141–52.

22. Lewtas J, Williams K. A retrospective view of the value of short term genetic bioassays in predicting the chronic effects of diesel soot. In: Ishinishi N, Koizumi A, McClellan RO Stober W, eds. Carcinogenic and Mutagenic Effects of Diesel Engine Exhaust. Elsevier Science Publishers, Amsterdam, The Netherlands, 1986:119–40.

23. Rosenkranz HS. Diesel emissions revisited: is the carcinogenicity due to genotoxic mechanism? Mutat Res 1987; 182:1–4.

24. McClellan RO, Mauderly JL, Jones RK, Cuddihy RG. Health effects of diesel exhaust. A contemporary air pollution issue. Postgrad Med 1985; 78(6): 199–201, 204–207.

25. McMillian MH, Cui M, Gautam M, Keane M, Ong T, Wallace W, Robey E. Mutagenic potential of particulate matter from diesel engine operation on Fischer–Tropsch fuel as a function of engine operating conditions and particle size. Society of Automotive Engineers Technical Paper 2002-01-1699, 2002: 1–18.

26. Brooks AL, Wolff RK, Royer RE, Clark CR, Sanchez A, McClellan RO. Deposition and biological availability of diesel particles and their associated mutagenic chemicals. Environ Int 1981; 5:263–8.

27. King LC, Kohan MJ, Austin AC, Claxton LD, Hunsingh JL. Evaluation of the release of mutagens from diesel particles in the presence of physiological fluids. Environ Mutag 1981; 3:109–29.

28. McClellan RO, Brooks AL, Cuddihy RG, Jones RK, Mauderly JL, Wolff RK. Inhalation toxicology of diesel exhaust particles. Dev Toxicol Environ Sci 1982; 10:99–120.

29. Wallace WE, Keane MJ, Hill CA, Xu J, Ong T. Mutagenicity of diesel exhaust particles and oil shale particles dispersed in lecithin surfactant. J Toxicol Environ Health 1987; 21:163–71.

30. Wallace WE, Keane M, Xing S, Harrison J, Gautam M, Ong T. Mutagenicity of diesel exhaust soot dispersed in phospholipid surfactants. In: Seemayer NH, Hadnagy W, eds. Environmental Hygiene II. Berlin, Heidelberg: Springer-Verlag, 1990a:7–10.

31. Keane MJ, Xing SG, Harrison J, Ong T, Wallace WE. Genotoxicity of diesel exhaust particles dispersed in simulated pulmonary surfactant. Mutat Res 1991; 260:233–8.

32. Gu ZW, Zhong BZ, Nath B, Whong WZ, Wallace WE, Ong T. Micronucleus induction and phagocytosis in mammalian cells treated with diesel emission particles. Mutat Res1992; 279:55–60.

33. Gu ZW, Zhong BZ, Keane MJ, Whong WZ, Wallace WE Ong T. Induction of unscheduled DNA synthesis in V79 cells by diesel emission particles dispersed in simulated pulmonary surfactant. Ann Occup Hyg 1994; 38:345–9.

34. Gu ZW, Keane MJ, Ong T, Wallace WE. Diesel exhaust particulate matter dispersed in a phospholipid surfactant induces chromosomal aberrations and micronuclei but not 6-thioguanine-resistant gene mutation in V79 cells in vitro. J Toxicol Environ Health 2005; 68:431–44.

35. Wallace W, Keane M, Murray M, Chisholm W, Maynard A, Ong T. Phospholipid lung surfactant and nano-particle surface toxicity: lessons from diesel soots and silicate dusts. J Nanoparticle Res 2007; 9:23–38.

36. Shi XC, Keane M, Ong T, Harrison J, Gautam M, Bugarski A, Wallace W. In vitro mutagenic and DNA and chromosomal damage activity by surfactant dispersion or solvent extract of a reference diesel exhaust particulate material. 12th Diesel Engine Efficiency and Emissions Reduction Conference 2006. http://www.cemamerica.com/doeevents/DEER/presentations.html

37. Green HYF, Vallyathan V. Pathologic responses to inhaled silica. In:Castranova V, Vallyathan V, Wallace W, eds. Silica and Silica-Induced Lung Disease: Current Concepts. Boca Raton, FL: CRC Press, 1995:163–85.

38. Vallyathan V, Schwegler D, Reasor M, Stettler L, Clere J, Green FHY. Comparative in vitro cytotoxicity and relative pathogenicity of mineral dusts. Ann Occup Hyg 1988; 32:279–89.

39. Wallace WE, Keane MJ, Vallaythan V, Hathaway P, Regad ED, Castranova V, Green FHY. Suppression of inhaled particle cytotoxicity by pulmonary surfactant and re-toxification by phospholipase. Ann Occup Hyg 1988a; 32:291–8.

40. Wallace WE, Keane MJ, Hill CA, Vallyathan V, Saus F, Castranova V, Bates D. The effect of lecithin surfactant and phospholipid enzyme treatment on some cytotoxic properties of respirable quartz and kaolin dusts. In: Frantz RL, Ramini RV, eds. Respirable Dust in the Mineral Industries: Health Effects, Characterization, and Control. ACGIH Monograph: ISBN 0-936712-76-71988b. American Conference of Governmental Industrial Hygienists, Cincinnati, OH, 1988.

41. Lynch K, McIver FA. Pneumoconiosis from exposure to kaolin dust: kaolinosis. Am J Pathol 1954; 30:1117–22.
42. Sheers G. Prevalence of pneumoconiosis in Cornish kaolin workers. Br J Ind Med 1964; 21:218–25.
43. Schulz CO. Silicon and silicates including asbestos. In: Clayton GD, Clayton FE, eds. Patty's Industrial Hygiene and Toxicology. Vol. II, Part A. New York: Wiley, 1993.
44. Emerson RJ, Davis GS. Effect of alveolar lining material-coated silica on rat alveolar macrophages. Environ Health Persp 1983; 51:81–4.
45. Marks J. The neutralization of silica toxicity in vitro. Br J Ind Med 1957; 14:81–84.
46. Allison AC, Harrington JS, Birbeck M. An examination of the cytotoxic effects of silica on macrophages. J Exp Med 1966; 124:141–54.
47. Wallace WE, Headley LC, Weber KC. Dipalmitoyl lecithin adsorption by kaolin dust in vitro. J Coll Interface Sci 1975; 51:535–7.
48. Wallace WE, Vallyathan V, Keane MJ, Robinson V. In vitro biological toxicity of native and surface modified silica and kaolin. J Toxicol Environ Health 1985; 16:415–24.
49. Keane MJ, Wallace WE, Seehra M, Hill C, Vallyathan V, Raghootama P, Mike P. Respirable particulate interactions with the lecithin component of pulmonary surfactant. In: VII International Pneumoconiosis Conference. DHHS (NIOSH) Publication #90-108 Part 1, 1990:231–44.
50. Wallace WE, Keane MJ, Mike PS, Hill CA, Vallyathan V, Regad ED. Contrasting respirable quartz and kaolin retention of lecithin surfactant and expression of membranolytic activity following phospholipase A2 digestion. J Toxicol Environ Health 1992; 37:391–409.
51. Nagle JF. Area/lipid of bilayers from NMR. Biophys J 1993; 64:1476–81.
52. Wallace WE, Keane MJ, Harrison JC, Stephens JW, Brower PS, Grayson RL, Vallyathan V, Attfield MD. Surface properties of respirable silicate and aluminosilicate dusts affecting bioavailability. In: Davis JMG, Jaurand MC, eds. Cellular and Molecular Effects of Mineral and Synthetic Dusts and Fibres. NATO ASI Series. Vol. H85. Berlin, Heidelberg: Springer-Verlag, 1994:369–79.
53. Wallace WE, Keane MJ, Mike PS, Hill CA, Vallyathan V. Mineral surface-specific differences in the adsorption and enzymatic removal of surfactant and their correlation with cytotoxicity. In: Mossman BT, Begin RO, eds. Effects of Mineral Dusts on Cells. NATO ASI Series. Vol. H30. Berlin, Heidelberg: Springer-Verlag, 1989:49–56.
54. Liu X, Keane MJ, Zhong BZ, Ong T, Wallace WE. Micronucleus formation in V79 cells treated with respirable silica dispersed in medium and in simulated pulmonary surfactant. Mutat Res 1996; 361:89–94.
55. Liu X, Keane MJ, Harrison JC, Cilento EV, Ong T, Wallace WE. Phospholipid surfactant adsorption by respirable quartz and in vitro expression of cytotoxicity and DNA damage. Toxicol Lett 1998; 96:77–84.
56. Murray D, Harrison J, Wallace W. A ^{13}C CP/MAS and ^{31}P NMR study of the interactions of dipalmitoylphosphatidylcholine with respirable silica and kaolin. J Colloid Interface Sci 2005; 288:166–70.

57. Antonini JM, Reasor MJ. Effect of short-term exogenous pulmonary surfactant treatment on acute lung damage associated with the intratracheal instillation of silica. J Toxicol Environ Health 1944; 43:85–101.

58. Hill CA, Wallace WE, Keane MJ, Mike PS. The enzymatic removal of a surfactant coating from quartz and kaolin by P388D1 cells. Cell Biol Toxicol 1995; 11:119–28.

59. Das A, Cilento E, Keane MJ, Wallace WE. Intracellular surfactant removal from phagocytized minerals: development of a fluorescent method using a BODIPY labelled phospholipid. Inhal Toxicol 2000; 12:765–81.

60. Keane M, Wallace W. A quantitative in vitro fluorescence imaging method for phospholipid loss from respirable mineral particles. Inhal Toxicol 2005; 7: 287–92.

61. Godish D, Rhoades RA. Quantitative recovery of phospholipids from alveolar wash. Respir Physiol 1970; 10:396–404.

62. Heinrich U, Muhle H, Takenaka S, Ernst E, Fuhst R, Mohr U, Pott F, Stober W. Chronic effects on the respiratory tract of hamsters, mice, and rats after long-term inhalation of high concentrations of filtered and unfiltered diesel engine emissions. J Appl Toxicol 1986; 6:383–95.

63. Heinrich U, Dungworth DL, Pott F, Peters L, Dasenbrock C, Levsen K, Koch W, Creutzenberg O, Schulte AT. The carcinogenic effects of carbon black particles and tar-pitch condensation aerosol after inhalation exposure of rats. Ann Occup Hyg 1994; 38:351–6.

64. Nikula KJ, Snipes MB, Barr EB, Griffith WC, Henderson RF, Mauderly JL. Comparative pulmonary toxicities and carcinogenicities of chronically inhaled diesel exhaust and carbon black in F344 rats. Fund Appl Toxicol 1995; 25: 80–94.

65. Cheng YS, Yeh HC, Mauderly JL, Mokler BV. Characterization of diesel exhaust in a chronic inhalation study. Am Ind Hyg Assoc J 1984; 45: 547–55.

66. Kozin F, McCarty BJ. Protein binding to monosodium urate monohydrate, calcium pyrophosphate dihydrate, and silicon dioxide crystals. I. Physical characteristics. J Lab Clin Med 1977; 89:1314–25.

67. Barrett EG, Johnston C, Oberdorster G, Finkelstein JN. Silica binds serum proteins resulting in a shift of the dose-response for silica-induced chemokine expression in an alveolar type II cell line. Toxicol Appl Pharmacol 1999a; 161: 111–22.

68. Barrett EG, Johnston C, Oberdorster G, Finkelstein JN. Antioxidant treatment attenuates cytokine and chemokine levels in murine macrophages following silica exposure. Toxicol Appl Pharmacol 1999b; 158:211–20.

69. Fenoglio F, Gillio F, Ghiazza M, Fubini B. Modulation of free radical generation at the surface of quartz by albumin adsorption/digestion. [Abstract]. In: Mechanisms of Action of Inhaled Fibres, Particles, and Nanoparticles in Lung and Cardiovascular Disease, Research Triangle Park, NC; October 26–28, 2005.

70. Gao N, Keane MJ, Ong T, Wallace WE. Effects of simulated pulmonary surfactant on the cytotoxicity and DNA-damaging activity of respirable quartz and kaolin. J Toxicol Environ Health 2000; 60:153–67.

71. Gao N, Keane MJ, Ong T, Ye J, Miller WE, Wallace WE. Effects of phospholipid surfactant on apoptosis induction by respirable quartz and kaolin in NR 8383 rat pulmonary macrophages. Toxicol Appl Pharmacol 2001; 175:217–25.
72. Gao N, Keane MJ, Ong T, Martin J, Miller W, Wallace WE. Respirable quartz and kaolin aluminosilicate expression of in vitro cytotoxicity and apoptosis in the presence of surfactant or serum: caveats to bioassay interpretation. In: Proceedings of Inhaled Particles IX, Cambridge, UK. Ann Occup Hyg 2002; 46:50–2.
73. Slauson DO, Cooper BJ. Mechanisms of Disease. 2nd ed. Baltimore: Williams & Wilkins, 1990:192–3.
74. Driscoll KE. Macrophage inflammatory proteins: biology and role in pulmonary inflammation. Exp Lung Res 1994; 20:473–90.
75. Driscoll KE. Role of inflammation in the development of rat lung tumors in response to chronic particle exposure. In: Mauderly JL, McCunney RJ, eds. Particle Overload in the Rat Lung and Lung Cancer: Implications for Human Risk Assessment. Philadelphia: Taylor & Francis, 1996:139–53.
76. Adamson IYR, Letourneau HL, Bowden DH. Enhanced macrophage-fibroblast interactions in the pulmonary interstitium increases after silica injection to monocyte-depleted mice. Am J Physiol 1989; 134:411–7.
77. Johnson NF, Maples KR. Fiber-induced hydroxyl radical formation and DNA damage. In: Cellular and Molecular Effects of Mineral Dusts and Fibres. NATO ASI Series H, Cell Biology. Vol. 85. Berlin, Heidelberg: Springer-Verlag, 1994:23–37.

12

Gene–Cellular Interactions of Nanomaterials: Genotoxicity to Genomics

Mary Jane Cunningham

Houston Advanced Research Center, The Woodlands, Texas, U.S.A.

INTRODUCTION

Nanotechnology is a new technology field with a wealth of promise. Nanomaterials are defined as materials with at least one dimension of 100 nm or less (1,2). This definition was initially set by the National Nanotechnology Initiative of the United States. In some instances, this definition has been broadened to include materials with at least one dimension within the *entire nanometer scale* (3–5).

Nanomaterials vary greatly in their size, their composition, and their structure. Recently, these materials were organized into three large classes: (*i*) naturally occurring, (*ii*) anthropogenic-unintentional, and (*iii*) anthropogenic-intentional (2). The first class includes viruses, biogenic magnetite, and ashes and particles from forest fires and active volcanoes. The second class, unintentional anthropogenic materials, includes asbestos, silica (SiO_2), titanium dioxide (TiO_2), carbon black (CB), metal or welding fume particles, and combustion by-products such as diesel exhaust particulate (DEP) and ultrafine particles (UFP).

UNINTENTIONAL ANTHROPOGENIC NANOMATERIALS

The safety of these anthropogenic materials has been studied for many years. DEP and UFP are used as model substances to investigate air pollution. Air pollutants occur as complex mixtures and may include gases, transition metals, organic chemicals, and particulate matter (PM) (6). The PM is classified by what size particles can be captured on a filter and has been divided into three designations: coarse (PM_{10} or particles 2.5 to 10 µm in diameter), fine ($PM_{2.5}$ or particles less than 2.5 µm in diameter), and ultrafine ($PM_{0.1}$ or particles less than 0.1 µm in diameter) (7,8). By this definition, UFP are sometimes included in the narrower definition of nanomaterials described above.

Epidemiology studies first pointed to the adverse effects associated with these unintentional anthropogenic materials. Air pollutant PM has been correlated with several respiratory ailments, such as asthma and chronic obstructive pulmonary disease, cardiovascular disease, and in some cases, mortality (9–11). Welding fumes are the cause of metal fume fever, increased susceptibility to infection, decreased lung function, pneumonia and may be carcinogenic (12). Asbestos is linked with mesothelioma (13). A specific form of SiO_2, alpha-quartz, is associated with silicosis, emphysema, bronchitis, and an increased risk for lung cancer (14–16). These particulate materials and their adverse effects have been the subject of decades of research.

ENGINEERED NANOMATERIALS

The third class listed above, intentional anthropogenic nanomaterials, includes engineered nanomaterials. These nanomaterials (e.g., nanotubes, nanowires, nanospheres, nanocrystals, fullerenes) offer more desirable attributes than their micron-sized counterparts (17–19). New or additional characteristics attributed to nanometer-scale materials are enhanced mechanical and tensile strength (20,21), increased electrical mobility and conductance (22–24), enhanced heat resistance (25,26), improved catalysis (27), and tunable wavelength-sensing ability (28). For example, quantum dots (QD) or semiconductor nanocrystals can be excited by several wavelengths to give a range of fluorescence emission (28–30). This attribute allows these nano-materials to be extremely versatile in medical imaging and diagnostics (31). Carbon nanotubes are being manufactured for applications in energy and communications (32–34). Their tensile strength is in excess of what is now available with other technologies (34).

However, early reports raised the possibility that these engineered materials may be toxic, although these reports were not always in agreement. Two citations found that single-walled carbon nanotubes (SWNT) caused granulomas in rodents. One citation concluded that SWNT was more toxic than alpha-quartz while the other citation found the presence of granulomas inconclusive of the toxicity of SWNT (35,36). Another study showed that fullerenes or "bucky balls" caused oxidative stress in the brains of an aquatic species (37). Additional studies are now being performed in a more comprehensive way to see if this caution is deserved.

Unintentional anthropogenic nanomaterials have been the subject of several investigations as to their genetic toxicity or genotoxicity. Several review articles summarize these results (38–42). This chapter will first focus on the issues that arose in these genotoxicity investigations of unintentional anthropogenic nanomaterials. Most experiments used materials whose dimensions were on the low micron to upper nanometer scale. The tools to be able to capture and investigate materials with smaller dimensions were not available until recently. However, what questions were asked at this low micron to upper nanometer size level may be pertinent to investigations of materials on the lower nanometer scale. Second, this chapter will present a summary of genetic toxicity investigations of engineered nanomaterials and nanoparticles manufactured on the low nanometer scale. Finally, this chapter will conclude with the newest reports of genetic and cellular interactions of engineered nanomaterials, including studies using OMICs technologies.

GENOTOXICITY ASSAYS

Genetic toxicology aims to determine adverse effects on the molecular and genetic level. Most assays use three major endpoints: (*i*) gene mutation, (*ii*) clastogenicity, and (*iii*) aneuploidy (43). These endpoints are focused on discovering damage to the DNA-a genotoxic event (44–46). Current genotoxicity tests (both regulatory and exploratory) include assays, which detect DNA breaks, bacterial mutations, chromosomal aberrations (CA), sister chromatid exchanges (SCE), micronuclei (MN), unscheduled DNA synthesis (UDS) as well as the formation of 8-OHdG and DNA adducts (43). This chapter will not review the description of each of these assays but will instead focus on the issues resulting from testing unintentional anthropogenic nanomaterials using these assays.

ISSUES FROM GENOTOXICITY STUDIES OF UNINTENTIONAL ANTHROPOGENIC NANOMATERIALS

Tested Substance: Form, Size, Manufacturing, and Preparation

The physical form of the tested substance may dictate whether or not it gives a positive result in a genotoxicity assay. For example, SiO_2 can be present as two different physical forms: amorphous and crystalline (47). The fibrogenic and tumor-inducing crystalline form causes more DNA damage (i.e., DNA breaks) in the comet assay, increased mutation frequency in the HPRT assay and increased MIP-2 gene expression than the nonfibrogenic amorphous form (48,49). Similarly, the anatase form of TiO_2 resulted in significantly more single-strand DNA breaks than the rutile form during an assay to determine photocatalytic ability (50).

Size can also make a difference. Ultrafine nickel (Ni) with a mean diameter of 20 nm was shown to increase TNF-alpha at a higher level than fine Ni (mean diameter of 5000 nm) after intratrachael instillation in rats (51). Ultrafine CB (14 nm) generated more reactive oxygen species (ROS) and increased MIP-2 mRNA expression compared to fine CB (260 nm) (52,53). In addition, ultrafine TiO_2 (20 nm) showed more free radical activity, as detected by the strand break assay using supercoiled plasmid DNA, than with normal-sized (500 nm) TiO_2 (54). Fisher et al. investigated the genotoxicity of different sized fractions of fly ash collected from a coal-burning power plant using the bacterial mutagenicity assay. The fraction containing the finest particles was found to be the most mutagenic (55).

UFPs, while having a very small particle diameter, tend to exist as agglomerates or aggregates of larger sizes. In a study by Johnston et al. significantly greater values of cytotoxic damage by lactic dehydrogenase (LDH) and beta-glucuronidase assays were observed with freshly prepared Teflon fume particles with a mean diameter of 15 nm versus coagulated particles with mean diameters of greater than 100 nm (56).

In addition, how the test substance is manufactured for testing can influence the genotoxic outcome. For example, several types of fume particles can result by welding different types of materials. Welding using stainless steel creates vaporized particles consisting of mostly chromium and Ni while welding using mild steel creates particles almost entirely of iron (57). In bacterial mutagenicity assays, fumes from stainless steel were positive for mutagenicity while fumes from mild steel were not (58,59). Another study showed that coal mine dust made fresh resulted in an increase in ROS due to the "fresh" surface versus coal mine dust, which had been stored for a while (60). The grinding and cleaving of the dust particles seemed to result in a more active surface. In addition, fly ash made from fluidized bed combustion was more mutagenic than fly ash made by conventional combustion (61).

To discuss this point further, how a test substance is prepared for testing also may make a difference in the genotoxicity result. A study investigated two different preparations of DEP (62). What was interesting was that the method of production did not determine the result of toxicity using the bacterial mutagenicity assay but how they were extracted to be used in the assay. The preparations were either extracted with an organic solvent or with phospholipids. They were then separated into supernatants and pellets (sediments). The supernatant of the solvent extract was much more active in the bacterial mutagenicity assay than the supernatant using the phospholipid extraction. In the case of the pellets, the exact opposite relationship existed. The surfactant extracts were more mutagenic than the solvent extracts.

Cocomponents

Several particulate materials tend to exist as complex mixtures, which include metal and organic components as well as the particles themselves.

In a DNA-strand break assay, SiO_2 caused double-strand breaks (63). However, when etched with hydrofluoric acid to remove the trace iron, this same preparation of SiO_2 was retested and was found to be negative. In a study by Ball et al. DEP and PM were extracted with phosphate-buffered saline. The extracts gave dose–response curves for ROS but the main cause seemed to be traced to the transition metals present (64). Another study investigated the presence of transition metals further by exposing human T-lymphocytes and macrophages to synthetic carbon (C) and carbon/iron particles (C/Fe) (65). Both particles were phagocytized by macrophages but the C/Fe particles resulted in organelle lysis as well as a positive result in a luminol bioassay and electron spin resonance spectroscopy, two methods, which monitor the presence of ROS.

Several studies looked to resolve the issue of organic components associated with particulates. One study investigated the ability of DEP to cause DNA adduct formation (66). The DEP preparation was extracted with organics and cleaned to leave only the carbonaceous core. When this core particle was retested, it did not cause a significant level of DNA adduct formation and was nontoxic. Several genotoxicity assays cited positive results with the organic extractable portions of DEP and foundry fume particulates (67,68). Similar studies were done with air pollutant particles but resulted in conflicting conclusions. Fly ash was found to be mutagenic by itself but not when it was tested after being extracted with water (69). Another study showed that the core particles of air pollutants after extraction with organic solvents resulted in significantly more DNA-strand breaks (70). However, in the study by Fisher et al. cited above with fly ash collected from a coal-burning plant, the fractions which were most mutagenic were those collected after the electrostatic precipitator step through the sampling of the stack (55). Collecting the fraction at this point allowed for other pollutant materials to condense onto the particles causing them to be positive in the bacterial mutagenicity assay.

Gene–Cellular Interactions: Primary vs. Secondary Genotoxicity

Interactions of unintentional anthropogenic nanomaterials with cells have been shown to lead to changes in the expression of several cellular macromolecules. The most frequently affected macromolecules are those genes or proteins, which have roles in oxidative stress and DNA damage or produce inflammation or injury to the immune system (39). Low micron- to nanometer-sized preparations of SiO_2 increased arachidonic acid metabolism (eventually leading to lung inflammation and pulmonary disease) as well as expression in genes directly related to inflammation: MIP-2, CINC, MCP-1, RANTES (49,71–73). Similar findings were found for TiO_2 nanometer particles and TiO_2 whiskers (width of 140 nm) (74).

By analyzing studies, which investigated the mechanisms of these adverse effects, the theory of primary versus secondary genotoxicity was put forth by several reviews (16,39,42,75). Genotoxicity directly related to the exposure of the substance is referred to as primary genotoxicity. Secondary genotoxicity is the result of the substance interacting with cells or tissues and releasing factors, which cause the adverse effects, such as inflammation and oxidative stress. The most common mechanistic scenario is that the particles interact with cells to induce ROS, which in turn lead to a cascade of effects, such as lysosomal membrane damage causing leakage of lytic enzymes, more ROS, recruitment of inflammatory cells, increased expression and release of proinflammatory mediators and cytokines, all of which amplify the immune and inflammatory response.

GENOTOXICITY OF ENGINEERED NANOMATERIALS

Investigations of genotoxicity and cellular interactions of engineered nanomaterials and nanoparticles manufactured on the low nanometer scale have been limited so far and the majority of the studies have screened for cytotoxicity (Table 1). Cytotoxicity has been measured using different methods: tetrazolium dye assays (e.g., MTT, XTT, WST-1), viability markers (e.g., trypan blue, neutral red, thymidine uptake), apoptotic and necrotic markers with immunocytochemistry and flow cytometry staining (e.g., propidium iodide) and cell growth by counting cells, subpassages and population doubling levels. Several investigations have focused on the photocatalytic activity of nanomaterials. The remaining studies have screened for biocompatibility of those molecules slated for use in medical imaging and bioengineering applications. Table 2 is a preliminary list of studies using standardized assays to assess the genotoxicity of nanomaterials. As can be noted, no material has been tested with a complete battery of assays and the results for the same type of material using the same test sometimes differed.

The studies cited in these tables do show a trend toward addressing the issues discussed in the early particulate studies. Varied results have been obtained with different forms, sizes, and the manufacturing process of the nanomaterials. Studies with different functionalized forms of QD showed mixed results in the comet assay (104). CdSe/ZnS nanocrystals functionalized with –COOH groups showed definite DNA damage whereas QD functionalized with –OH, –NH$_2$, –OH/COOH, and –NH$_2$/OH were negative. Nanoscale TiO$_2$ composed of anatase showed more ROS than nanoscale TiO$_2$ composed of rutile (122). Two different studies focused on particle size and found that the size of a particle and its surface area did not seem to be a major determining factor. Nanoscale Ni and cobalt (20 nm diameter each) were found to be more cytotoxic than nanoscale TiO$_2$ (28 nm) (108). A comparison of nanoscale TiO$_2$ rods, dots, and particles found that the cytotoxic response did not change whether the materials were on the low- or high-nanometer scale (124).

Table 1   Cytotoxicity Assays of Engineered Nanomaterials and Low Nanoscale Materials

Authors and date	Ref.	Result	Particle type
A. Fullerenes and their functionalized counterparts			
Moussa et al. (1995)	(76)	neg	C_{60}
Baierl et al. (1996)	(77)	sl pos	C_{60}
Nakajima et al. (1996)	(78)	pos	$C_{60}PEGNH_2$; $C_{60}EDPEGCOOH$
Tsuchiya et al. (1996)	(79)	pos	$C_{60}PVP$
Moussa et al. (1997)	(80)	neg	C_{60}
Sakai et al. (1999)	(81)	pos[a]	C_{60}
Fumelli et al. (2000)	(82)	neg	$C_{60}(OH)n$
Babynin et al. (2002)	(83)	pos	$C_{60}COOHCH_3$; $C_{60}COOHC_2H_5$; C_{60}pyrrolidine derivative
Cusan et al. (2002)	(84)	pos	Triamino-C_{60}
Rancan et al. (2002)	(85)	neg	C_{60}malonic acid; Dendro-C_{60}
Yang et al. (2002)	(86)	pos[a]	C_{60}malonic acid derivatives
Mikata et al. (2003)	(87)	pos[a]	C_{60}sugar-pendant derivatives
Bosi et al. (2004)	(88)	pos	Water-soluble C_{60} derivatives
Burlaka et al. (2004)	(89)	pos[a]	Water-soluble C_{60}
Jia et al. (2005)	(90)	neg	C_{60}
Lyon et al. (2005)	(91)	pos	nanoC_{60}
Sayes et al. (2005)	(92)	pos	nanoC_{60}
Rancan et al. (2005)	(93)	pos[a]	C_{60}pyropheophorbide derivatives
Fiorito et al. (2006)	(94)	sl pos	C_{60}
Isakovic et al. (2006)	(95)	pos	nanoC_{60}; $C_{60}(OH)n$
Rouse et al. (2006)	(96)	pos	C_{60}amino acid derivatives
Xiao et al. (2006)	(97)	neg	$C_{60}PVP$
Yamawaki and Iwai (2006)	(98)	pos	$C_{60}(OH)_{24}$
B. Nanocomposites			
Lesniak et al. (2005)	(99)	pos	Ag/dendrimers
C. Nanocrystals (quantum dots) and their functionalized counterparts			
Derfus et al. (2004)	(100)	pos	TOPO-coated Cd/Se QDs
Chen and Gerion (2004)	(101)	sl pos	CdSe/ZnS QDs
Hoshino et al. (2004a)	(102)	pos-HD	CdSe/ZnS QDs
Hoshino et al. (2004b)	(103)	pos; neg	CdSe/ZnS-COOH, CdSe/ZnS-OH/COOH; CdSe/ZnS-OH
Kirchner et al. (2005)	(104)	pos; neg	Polymer CdSe and CdSe/ZnS; $PEGSiO_2$-CdSe

(*Continued*)

Table 1 Cytotoxicity Assays of Engineered Nanomaterials and Low Nanoscale Materials (*Continued*)

Authors and date	Ref.	Result	Particle type
			and -CdSe/ZnS
Lovric et al. (2005)	(105)	pos	CdTe QDs
Shiohara et al. (2004)	(106)	pos-HD	CdSe/ZnS MUA derivatives
D. Nanohorns			
Isobe et al. (2006)	(107)	pos	amino-nanohorn aggregate
E. Nanoparticles and their functionalized counterparts			
Zhang et al. (1998)	(108)	pos	20 nm Ni and 20 nm Co
Gupta et al. (2003)	(109)	pos; neg	SPION; insulin coated SPION
Goodman et al. (2004)	(110)	Pos; sl pos	cationic Au NP; anionic Au NP
Braydich-Stolle et al. (2005)	(111)	pos	Ag, MoO_3, Al NP
Cheng et al. (2005)	(112)	neg	Fe_3O_4 NP
Gupta and Gupta (2005)	(113)	pos; neg	SPION; pullulan coated SPION
Hussain et al. (2005)	(114)	pos	CdO, Ag, W, MnO_2, MoO_3, Fe_3O_4, Al NP
Lu et al. (2005)	(115)	pos	QD-conjugated nanoTiO_2 films
Petri-Fink et al. (2005)	(116)	pos; neg	amino SPION; PVA-, carboxy-, thiol-SPION
Shukla et al. (2005)	(117)	neg	Au NP
Auffan et al. (2006)	(118)	pos	DMSA-coated maghemite NP
Dufour et al. (2006)	(119)	pos	< 200 nm ZnO
Hussain et al. (2006)	(120)	pos	Mn and Ag NP
Qi et al. (2007)	(121)	pos	chitosan NP
Sayes et al. (2006)	(122)	pos-HD	nano-TiO_2 (3-5 nm)
Wang et al. (2006)	(123)	pos	nano-Zn and micro-Zn
Warheit et al. (2006)	(124)	pos-HD; neg	nano-TiO_2 rods; nano-TiO_2 dots
F. Nanospheres			
Ameller et al. (2004)	(125)	pos	PEG-polymers w/antiestrogen
De et al. (2005)	(126)	pos	paclitaxel loaded nanospheres
Park et al. (2005)	(127)	sl pos	paclitaxel loaded nanospheres
G. Nanotubes (SWNT, MWNT) and their functionalized counterparts			
Shvedova et al. (2003)	(128)	pos	SWNT
Kam et al. (2004)	(129)	neg	SWNT

(Continued)

Table 1 Cytotoxicity Assays of Engineered Nanomaterials and Low Nanoscale Materials (*Continued*)

Authors and date	Ref.	Result	Particle type
Pantarotto et al. (2004a)	(130)	neg	*f*-SWNT, up to 10 μM
Pantarotto et al. (2004b)	(131)	neg	*f*-SWNT
Warheit et al. (2004)	(36)	pos	SWNT (24 h only)
Bianco et al. (2005a)	(132)	pos; neg	MWNT, *f*-MWNT
Bianco et al. (2005b)	(133)	pos; neg	SWNT, *f*-SWNT
Cunningham et al. (2005)	(134)	neg	SWNT, up to 0.5 mg/mL
Cui et al. (2005)	(135)	pos	SWNT
Ding et al. (2005)	(136)	pos	MWNT > MWNO
Jia et al. (2005)	(90)	pos	SWNT > MWNT
Manna et al. (2005)	(137)	pos	SWNT
Monteiro-Riviere et al. (2005a)	(138)	pos	MWNT, MWNT-Pluronic F127
Monteiro-Riviere et al. (2005b)	(139)	pos	MWNT
Muller et al. (2005)	(140)	pos-HD	MWNT
Murr et al. (2005)	(141)	pos	SWNT, MWNT
Shvedova et al. (2005)	(142)	pos	SWNT
Bottini et al. (2006)	(143)	pos	MWNT
Dumortier et al. (2006)	(144)	neg	*f*-SWNT
Fiorito et al. (2006)	(94)	sl pos	SWNT
Magrez et al. (2006)	(145)	pos	MWNT, nanofibers
Nimmagadda et al. (2006)	(146)	pos	SWNT
Sayes et al. (2006)	(147)	neg; pos	*f*-SWNT; SWNT-PluronicF108
Tian et al. (2006)	(148)	pos	SWNT > MWNT
Worle-Knirsch et al. (2006)[b]	(149)	neg; pos	SWNT
Zanello et al. (2006)	(150)	pos	SWNT, *f*-SWNT, MWNT
Zhu et al. (2006)	(151)	pos	MWNT
Pulskamp et al. (2007)	(152)	neg	SWNT
Wick et al. (2007)	(153)	pos	SWNT

[a] Irradiated solutions or cells, photoactivation was involved
[b] The varied cytotoxicity response was due to different assays used (WST-1 and LDH=neg; MTT=pos).
Abbreviations: pos, positive; neg, negative; sl pos, slightly positive; QD, quantum dot; HD, high dose; SPION, superparamagnetic iron oxide nanoparticles; NP, nanoparticles; *f*, functionalized; SWNT, single-walled carbon nanotubes; MWNT, multiwalled carbon nanotubes; MWNO, multiwalled carbon nano-onions.

Purity and the presense of cocomponents have become general issues. The presence of metals and contaminants associated with carryover from the manufacturing process may be the cause of the observed oxidative stress. SWNT manufactured with a large residual of Fe (possibly 30%) gave rise to free radical formation (128). Fullerenes caused oxidative stress in

Table 2 Standard Genotoxicity Assays of Engineered Nanomaterials and Low Nanoscale Materials

Authors and date	Ref.	Dros.[a]	BMT[b]	SB[c]	MN[d]	CA[e]	ROS[f]
A. Fullerenes and their functionalized counterparts							
Zakharenko et al. (1994)	(154)	neg					
Baierl et al. (1996)	(77)						neg
Nakajima et al. (1996)	(78)						pos[g]
Sera et al. (1996)	(155)			pos[g]			pos[g]
Tsuchiya et al. (1996)	(79)						pos
Zakharenko et al. (1997)	(156)	sl pos					
Lin et al. (1999)	(157)						neg
Kamat et al. (2000)	(158)						pos[g]
Babynin et al. (2002)	(83)		neg				
Cusan et al. (2002)	(84)						neg
Rancan et al. (2002)	(85)						pos
Mikata et al. (2003)	(87)						pos[g]
Burlaka et al. (2004)	(89)						pos[g]
Sayes et al. (2005)	(92)						pos
Isakovic et al. (2006)	(95)						pos
Mori T et al. (2006)	(159)		neg			neg	
Xia et al. (2006)	(160)						pos
B. Nanocrystals (quantum dots) and their functionalized counterparts							
Green and Howman (2005)	(161)				pos		
Hoshino et al. (2004b)	(103)				pos		
C. Nanoparticles and their functionalized counterparts							
Zhang et al. (1998)	(108)				pos		
Ye et al. (2004)	(162)					neg	
Hussain et al. (2005)	(114)						pos
Lu et al. (2005)	(115)			pos[g]			pos
Shukla et al. (2005)	(117)						neg
Auffan et al. (2006)	(118)				neg		
Dufour et al. (2006)	(119)					pos	
Hussain et al. (2006)	(120)						pos

(*Continued*)

Table 2 Standard Genotoxicity Assays of Engineered Nanomaterials and Low Nanoscale Materials (*Continued*)

Authors and date	Ref.	Dros.[a]	BMT[b]	SB[c]	MN[d]	CA[e]	ROS[f]
Kim et al. (2006)	(163)		neg			neg	
Qi et al. (2007)	(121)			pos			pos
Sayes et al. (2006)	(122)						pos-HD
D. Nanotubes (SWNT, MWNT) and their functionalized counterparts							
Shvedova et al. (2003)	(128)						pos
Cui et al. (2005)	(136)			pos			
Manna et al. (2005)	(138)						pos
Pulskamp et al. (2007)	(154)						pos

[a] Drosophila somatic mutation test
[b] Bacterial mutagenicity test
[c] DNA strand break assays
[d] Induction of micronuclei
[e] Chromosomal aberrations
[f] Reactive oxygen species
[g] Irradiated solutions or cells, photoactivation was involved
Abbreviations: pos, positive; neg, negative; sl pos, slightly positive; QD, quantum dot; HD, high dose; SPION, superparamagnetic iron oxide nanoparticles; NP, nanoparticles.

largemouth base, as noted before (37). However, a later study showed that the mechanism may be due to fullerenes encapsulating the tetrahydrofuran (THF) used in their purification and that the toxicity may be due to degradative product of THF (164). Work is continuing on these issues and a definitive answer of toxicity as well as its mechanisms, which might cause these adverse effect is still forthcoming.

GENOMICS OF UNINTENTIONAL ANTHROPOGENIC NANOMATERIALS

Genomics is the study of gene expression profiles of cells or tissues perturbed by a substance. This new field has led to another branch of toxicology, toxicogenomics. The technologies used to investigate gene expression are varied but most studies have centered on high-throughput screening technologies of gene expression microarrays. The use of these arrays to investigate toxicity has been reviewed elsewhere (165–167). Briefly, two types of arrays have been used to monitor gene expression: macroarrays and microarrays. Macroarrays are made by spotting DNA clones onto a nitrocellulose filter and using a radioactive label for detection. Microarrays have DNA clones spotted onto glass slides or silicon wafers with the resulting signal detected by fluorescence.

Several citations have reported genomics studies of particulates. Macroarray studies have included in vivo and in vitro exposures to PM$_{10}$ particulate fraction, DEP, and SiO$_2$ (168–171). These studies have been limited in the results observed (usually between 6 and 12 genes) due to the small number, which can be printed on the filter membranes (less than 500 probes). Additional studies were performed with gene expression microarrays involving treatments with burned ash, DEP, and ultrafine CB (172–176). The arrays in these studies contained thousands of gene representatives. The most common significantly expressed genes in these studies were those involved in ROS and DNA damage as well as cytoskeletal rearrangement, copper and iron homeostasis, protein degradation, inflammation and injury.

GENOMICS OF ENGINEERED NANOMATERIALS

Using genomics to investigate the safety of engineered nanomaterials has just begun. Three studies have been done to date. Ding et al. investigated gene expression profiling of human skin fibroblasts exposed to multiwalled carbon nanotubes (MWNT) and multiwalled carbon nano-onions (MWNO) (136). Both nanomaterials activated the expression of genes involved in cell cycle regulation, cellular transport, metabolism and stress response. However, the expression profile from cells exposed to the nano-onions induced additional genes related to external stimuli whereas the expression profile for cells exposed to MWNT induced genes involved in inflammatory and immune responses. Cui et al. investigated the gene expression profile of a human embryo kidney cell line exposed to SWNT and found significantly expressed genes associated with cell cycle regulation but also with apoptosis and signal transduction (135). The most comprehensive study to date has been by Cunningham et al. (134). The gene expression profile in primary normal human keratinocytes exposed to SWNT at a noncytotoxic dose was similar to the profile obtained with the negative control, carbonyl iron. The profile for SWNT only matched the profile with the most toxic control compound, SiO$_2$, when the cells were exposed at a cytotoxic dose. The SWNT preparation in this case was highly purified and contained less than 1% heavy metal contamination. The profiles of the most highly expressed genes at both noncytotoxic and cytotoxic doses are seen in Figure 1. The same results were seen when the data was analyzed by principal components analysis.

SUMMARY

Assessing the safety of low micron to upper nanometer scale materials and particulates has been challenging. This chapter summarized these studies by focusing on the issues raised during this research. Does the material's form and

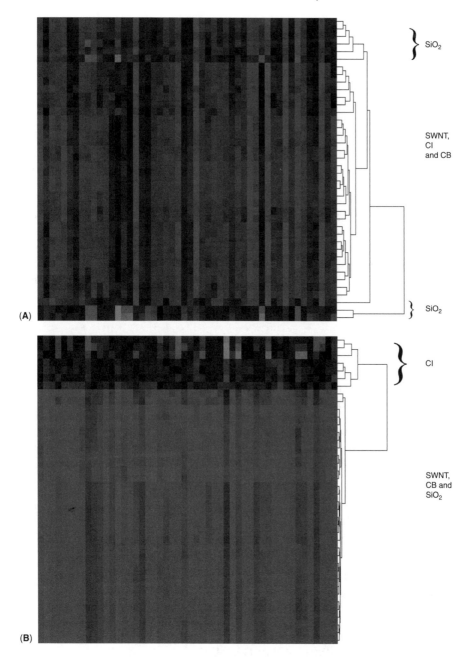

Figure 1 Gene expression profiles of single-walled nanotubes, carbonyl iron, carbon black, and silica at noncytotoxic (**A**) and cytotoxic (**B**) doses.

size, the process by which it is manufactured and prepared, the presence of any cocomponents, and whether the toxicity is due to a primary or secondary action contribute to the differences seen in standardized genotoxicity assays? The answer was yes. It was shown that all of these factors influence whether or not the material is genotoxic or not. Do these same issues pertain to low nanometer-scale materials? It may be too early to tell. Initial investigations show that some of these issues are pertinent.

The future of genetic toxicology will emphasize screening on a broader and possibly more predictive level. The focus may be on alternative tests, which are not as labor-intensive and will require less reliance on animals. Using more appropriate cell types may be emphasized. Ongoing research in embryonic cell lines may help in this regard as these cells are in the least undifferentiated state and may be artificially allowed to differentiate through specific programmatic pathways. Screening techniques, such as those methods provided by OMICs technologies, may give faster and more predictive answers. Will all of these directions help to better evaluate the newer engineered low nanometer-scale materials? Only additional focused and pertinent research will give the answer.

REFERENCES

1. Roco MC. National Nanotechnology Initiative—Past, Present, Future. In Handbook on Nanoscience, Engineering and Technology. 2nd ed. NY: Taylor and Francis, 2007.
2. Oberdorster G, Oberdorster E, Oberdorster J. Nanotoxicology: an emerging discipline evolving from studies of ultrafine particles. Environ Health Perspect 2005; 113:823–39.
3. Hoet PHM, Brueske-Hohlfeld I, Salata OV. Nanoparticles—known and unknown health risks. J Nanobiotechnol 2004; 2:12.
4. Salata OV. Applications of nanoparticles in biology and medicine. J Nanobiotechnol 2004; 2:3.
5. Jortner J, Rao CNR. Nanostructured advanced materials. Perspectives and directions. Pure Appl Chem 2002; 74:1491–506.
6. Oberdorster G. Pulmonary effects of inhaled ultrafine particles. Int Arch Occup Environ Health 2001; 74:1–8.
7. Donaldson K, Stone V, Clouter A, et al. Ultrafine particles. Occup Environ Med 2001; 58:211–6.
8. Kang YJ. New understanding in cardiotoxicity. Curr Opin Drug Discov Develop 2003; 6:110–6.
9. Delfino RJ, Sioutas C, Malik S. Potential role of ultrafine particles in associations between airborne particle mass and cardiovascular health. Environ Health Perspect 2005; 113:934–46.
10. Samet JH, Dominici F, Curriero FC, et al. Fine particulate air pollutions and mortality in 20 U.S. cities, 1987–1994. New Eng J Med 2000; 343:1742–9.
11. Dickey JH. Part VII. Air pollution: overview of sources and health effects. Dis Mon 2000; 46:566–89.

12. Antonini JM, Afshari AA, Stone S, et al. Design, construction, and characterization of a novel robotic welding fume generator and inhalation exposure system for laboratory animals. J Occup Environ Health 2006; 3:194–203.
13. Miller RW. How environmental hazards in childhood have been discovered: carcinogens, teratogens, neurotoxicants, and others. Pediatrics 2004; 113 (Suppl 4):945–51.
14. Daniel LN, Mao Y, Saffiotti U. Oxidative DNA damage by crystalline silica. Free Radic Biol Med 1993; 14:463–72.
15. Shi X, Castranova V, Halliwell B, et al. Reactive oxygen species and silica-induced carcinogenesis. J Toxicol Environ Health B Crit Rev 1998; 1:181–97.
16. Vallyathan, V, Shi X. The role of oxygen free radicals in occupational and environmental lung diseases. Environ Health Perspect 1997; 105(Suppl 1):165–77.
17. Karch J, Birringer R, Gleiter H. Ceramics ductile at low temperature. Nature 1987; 330:556–8.
18. Dey A, De S, De A, et al. Giant dielectric constant in titania nanoparticles embedded in conducting polymer matrix. J Nanosci Nanotechnol 2006; 6:1427–36.
19. Fan Z, Lu JG. Zinc oxide nanostructures: synthesis and properties. J Nanosci Nanotechnol 2005; 5:1561–73.
20. Thess A, Lee R, Nikolaev P, et al. Crystalline ropes of metallic carbon nanotubes. Science 1996; 273:483–7.
21. Ayutsede J, Gandhi M, Sugigara S, et al. Carbon nanotube reinforced *Bombyx mori* silk nanofibers by the electrospinning process. Biomacromolecules 2006; 7:208–14.
22. Durkop T, Getty SA, Cobas E, et al. Extraordinary mobility in semi-conducting carbon nanotubes. Nano Lett 2004; 4:35–9.
23. Durkop T, Cobas E, Fuhrer MS. High-mobility semiconducting nanotubes. AIP Conf Proc 2003; 685:524–7.
24. McEuen PL, Fuhrer MS, Park H. Single-walled carbon nanotube electronics. IEEE Trans Nanotechnol 2002; 1:78–85.
25. Prasher R. Predicting the thermal resistance of nanosized constrictions. Nano Lett 2005; 5:2155–9.
26. Li SD, Peng Z, Kong LX, et al. Thermal degradation kinetics and morphology of natural rubber/silica nanocomposites. J Nanosci Nanotechnol 2006; 6:541–6.
27. Zhang WX, Wang CB, Lien HL. Treatment of chlorinated organic contaminants with nanoscale bimetallic particles. Catal Today 1998; 40:387–95.
28. Chan WCW, Maxwell DJ, Gao X, et al. Luminescent quantum dots for multi-plexed biological detection and imaging. Curr Opin Biotechnol 2002; 13:40–6.
29. Alivisatos AP. Semiconductor clusters, nanocrystals and quantum dots. Science 1996; 271:933–7.
30. Jaiswal JK, Mattoussi H, Mauro JM, et al. Long-term multiple color imaging of live cells using quantum dot bioconjugates. Nat Biotechnol 2003; 21:47–51.
31. Michalet X, Pinaud FF, Bentolila LA, et al. Quantum dots for live cells, in vivo imaging, and diagnostics. Science 2005; 307:538–44.
32. Bo XZ, Tassi NG, Lee CY, et al. Pentacene-carbon nanotubes: semi-conducting assemblies for thin-film transistor applications. Appl Phys Lett 2005; 87:203510.

33. Ebron VH, Yang Z, Seyer JD, et al. Fuel-powered artificial muscles. Science 2006; 311:1580–3.

34. Collins PG, Avouris P. Nanotubes for electronics. Sci Am 2000; 283:62–9.

35. Lam CW, James JT, McCluskey R, et al. Pulmonary toxicity of single-wall carbon nanotubes in mice 7 and 90 days after intratracheal instillation. Toxicol Sci 2004; 77:126–34.

36. Warheit DB, Laurence BR, Reed KL, et al. Comparative pulmonary toxicity assessment of single wall carbon nanotubes in rats. Toxicol Sci 2004; 77:117–25.

37. Oberdorster E. Manufactured nanomaterials (fullerenes, C60) induce oxidative stress in the brain of juvenile largemouth bass. Environ Health Perspect 2004; 112:1058–62.

38. Chrisp CE, Fisher GL. Mutagenicity of airborne particles. Mutat Res 1980; 76:143–64.

39. Schins RP. Mechanisms of genotoxicity of particles and fibers. Inhal Toxicol 2002; 14:57–78.

40. Claxton LD, Matthews PP, Warren, SH. The genotoxicity of ambient outdoor air, a review: *Salmonella* mutagenicity. Mutat Res 2004; 567:347–99.

41. Borm, PJA. Toxicity and occupational health hazards of coal fly ash (CFA). A review of data and comparison to coal mine dust. Ann Occup Hyg 1997; 41:659–76.

42. Knaapen AM, Borm PJA, Albrecht C, et al. Inhaled particles and lung cancer. Part A: Mechanisms. Int J Cancer 2004; 109:799–809.

43. Cimino MC. Comparative overview of current international strategies and guidelines for genetic toxicology testing for regulatory purposes. Environ Mol Mutagen 2006; 47:362–90.

44. Hoel DG, Haseman JK, Hogan MD, et al. The impact of toxicity on carcinogenicity studies: implications for risk assessment. Carcinogenesis 1988; 9:2045–52.

45. Tennant RW, Elwell MR, Spalding JW, et al. Evidence that toxic injury is not always associated with induction of chemical carcinogenesis. Mol Carcinogen 1991; 4:420–40.

46. Yamasaki, H, Ashby, J, Bignami, M, et al. Nongenotoxic carcinogens: development of detection methods based on mechanisms: a European project. Mutat Res 1996; 353:47–63.

47. IARC Monographs on the evaluation of carcinogenic risks to humans. IARC Monograph Series, vol. 68, Silica, Some Silicates, Coal Dust and *Para*-Aramid Fibrils. Lyon, France: International Agency for Research on Cancer1997; 41:242.

48. Zhong BZ, Whong WZ, Ong TM. Detection of mineral-dust-induced DNA damage in two mammalian cell lines using the alkaline single cell gel/comet assay. Mutat Res 1997; 393:181–7.

49. Johnston CJ, Driscoll KE, Finkelstein JN, et al. Pulmonary chemokine and mutagenic responses in rats after subchronic inhalation of amorphous and crystalline silica. Toxicol Sci 2000; 56:405–13.

50. Ashikaga T, Wada M, Kobayashi H, et al. Effect of photocatalytic activity of TiO_2 on plasmid DNA. Mutat Res 2000; 466:1–7.

51. Zhang Q, Kusaka Y, Zhu X, et al. Comparative toxicity of standard nickel and ultrafine nickel in lung after intratrachael instillation. J Occup Health 2003; 45:23–30.

52. Wilson MR, Lightbody JH, Donaldson K, et al. Interactions between ultrafine particles and transition metals in vivo and in vitro. Toxicol Appl Pharmacol 2002; 184:172–9.

53. Gilmour PS, Ziesenis A, Morrison ER, et al. Pulmonary and systemic effects of short-term inhalation exposure to ultrafine carbon black particles. Toxicol Appl Pharmacol 2004; 195:35–44.

54. Donaldson K, Beswick PH, Gilmour PS. Free radical activity associated with the surface of particles: a unifying factor in determining biological activity? Toxicol Lett 1996; 88:293–8.

55. Fisher GL, Chrisp CE, Raabe, OG. Physical factors affecting the mutagenicity of fly ash from a coal-fired power plant. Science 1979; 204:879–81.

56. Johnston CJ, Finkelstein JN, Mercer P, et al. Pulmonary effects induced by ultrafine PTFE particles. Toxicol Appl Pharmacol 2000; 168:208–15.

57. Antonini JM, Lewis AB, Roberts JR, et al. Pulmonary effects of welding fumes: review of worker and experimental animal studies. Am J Ind Med 2003; 43:350–60.

58. Hedenstedt A, Jenssen D, Lidesten BM, et al. Mutagenicity of fume particles from stainless steel welding. Scand J Work Environ Health 1977; 3:203–11.

59. Maxild J, Andersen M, Kiel P. Mutagenicity of fume particles from metal arc welding on stainless steel in the *Salmonella*/microsome test. Mutat Res 1978; 56:235–43.

60. Dalal NS, Suryan MM, Vallyathan V, et al. Detection of reactive free radicals in fresh coal mine dust and their implication for pulmonary injury. Ann Occup Hyg 1989; 33:79–84.

61. Mumford JL, Lewtas J. Mutagenicity and cytotoxicity of coal fly ash from fluidized-bed and conventional combustion. J Toxicol Environ Health 1982; 10:565–86.

62. Keane MJ, Xing SG, Harrison JC, et al. Genotoxicity of diesel-exhaust particles dispersed in simulated pulmonary surfactant. Mutat Res 1991; 260: 233–8.

63. Daniel LN, Mao Y, Wang TCL, et al. DNA strand breakage, thymine glycol production, and hydroxyl radical generation induced by different samples of crystalline silica in vitro. Environ Res 1995; 71:60–73.

64. Ball JC, Straccia AM, Young WC, et al. The formation of reactive oxygen species catalyzed by neutral, aqueous extracts of NIST ambient particulate matter and diesel engine particles. J Air Waste Manag Assoc 2000; 50:1897–903.

65. Long JF, Waldman WJ, Kristovich R, et al. Comparison of ultrastructural cytotoxic effects of carbon and carbon/iron particulates on human monocyte-derived macrophages. Environ Health Perspect 2005; 113:170–4.

66. Bond JA, Johnson NF, Snipes MB, et al. DNA adduct formation in rat alveolar type II cells: cells potentially at risk for inhaled diesel exhaust. Environ Mol Mutagen 1990; 16:64–9.

67. King LC, Kohan MJ, Austin AC, et al. Evaluation of the release of mutagens from diesel particles in the presence of physiological fluids. Environ Mutagen 1981; 3:109–21.

68. Humfrey CDN, Levy LS, Faux SP. Potential carcinogenicity of foundry fumes: a comparative in vivo–in vitro study. Food Chem Toxicol 1996; 34: 1103–11.

69. Kleinjans JCS, Janssen YMW, van Agen B, et al. Genotoxicity of coal fly ash, assessed in vitro in *Salmonella typhimurium* and human lymphocytes, and in vivo in an occupationally exposed population. Mutat Res 1989; 224: 127–34.

70. Karlsson HL, Nygren J, Moller L. Genotoxicity of airborne particulate matter: the role of cell–particle interaction and of substances with adduct-forming and oxidizing capacity. Mutat Res 2004; 565:1–10.

71. Englen MD, Taylor SM, Laegreid WW, et al. The effects of different silicas on arachidonic acid metabolism in alveolar macrophages. Exp Lung Res 1990; 16:691–709.

72. Barrett EG, Johnston C, Oberdorster G, et al. Silica-induced chemokine expression in alveolar type II cells is mediated by TNF-α. Am J Physiol Lung Cell Mol Physiol 1998; 275(6 Pt 1):L1110–9.

73. Driscoll KE, Howard BW, Carter JM, et al. Alpha-quartz-induced chemokine expression by rat lung epithelial cells: effects of in vivo and in vitro particle exposure. Am J Pathol 1996; 149:1627–1637.

74. Ishihara Y, Kyono H, Kohyama N, et al. Acute biological effects of intratracheally instilled titanium dioxide whiskers compared with nonfibrous titanium dioxide and amosite in rats. Inhal Toxicol 1999; 11:131–49.

75. MacNee W, Donaldson K. Mechanism of lung injury caused by PM_{10} and ultrafine particles with special reference to COPD. Eur Respir J 2003; 21 (Suppl 40):47s–51s.

76. Moussa F, Chretien P, Dubois P, et al. The influence of C_{60} powders on cultured human leukocytes. Fullerene Sci Technol 1995; 3:333–42.

77. Baierl T, Drosselmeyer E, Seidel A, et al. Comparison of immunological effects of fullerene C_{60} and raw soot from fullerene production on alveolar macrophages and macrophage like cells *in vitro*. Exp Toxicol Pathol 1996; 48:508–11.

78. Nakajima N, Nishi C, Li FM, et al. Photo-induced cytotoxicity of water-soluble fullerene. Fullerene Sci Technol 1996; 4:1–19.

79. Tsuchiya T, Oguri I, Yamakoshi YN, et al. Novel harmful effects of [60] fullerene on mouse embryos *in vitro* and *in vivo*. FEBS Lett 1996; 393:139–45.

80. Moussa F, Chretien P, Pressac M, et al. Preliminary study of the influence of cubic C_{60} on cultured human monocytes: lack of interleukin-1β secretion. Fullerene Sci Technol 1997; 5:503–10.

81. Sakai A, Yamakoshi Y, Miyata N. Visible light irradiation of 60 fullerene causes killing and initiation of transformation of BALB/3T3 cells. Fullerene Sci Technol 1999; 7:743–56.

82. Fumelli C, Marconi A, Salvioli S, et al. Carboxyfullerenes protect human keratinocytes from ultraviolet-B-induced apoptosis. J Invest Dermatol 2000; 115:835–41.

83. Babynin EV, Nuretdinov IA, Gubskaia VP, et al. Study of mutagenic activity of fullerene and some of its derivatives using His+ reversions of *Salmonella typhimurium* as an example. Genetika 2002; 38:453–7.

84. Cusan C, Da Ros T, Spalluto G, et al. A new multi-charged C_{60} derivative: synthesis and biological properties. Eur J Org Chem 2002; 17:2928–34.

85. Rancan F, Rosan S, Boehm F, et al. Cytotoxicity and photocytotoxicity of a dendritic C_{60} mono-adduct and a malonic acid C_{60} tris-adduct on Jurkat cells. J Photochem Photobiol B 2002; 67:157–62.

86. Yang XL, Fan CH, Zhu HS. Photo-induced cytotoxicity of malonic acid [C60] fullerene derivatives and its mechanism. Toxicol In Vitro 2002; 16:41–6.
87. Mikata Y, Takagi S, Tanahashi M, et al. Detection of 1270 nm emission from singlet oxygen and photocytotoxic property of sugar-pendant (60) fullerenes. Bioorg Med Chem Lett 2003; 13:3289–92.
88. Bosi S, Feruglio L, Da Ros T, et al. Hemolytic effects of water-soluble fullerene derivatives. J Med Chem 2004; 47:6711–5.
89. Burlaka AP, Sidorik YP, Prylutska SV, et al. Catalytic system of the reactive oxygen species on the C60 fullerene basis. Exp Oncol 2004; 26:326–7.
90. Jia G, Wang H, Yan, L, et al. Cytotoxicity of carbon nanomaterials: single-wall nanotube, multi-wall nanotube and fullerene. Environ Sci Technol 2005; 39:1378–83.
91. Lyon DY, Fortner JD, Sayes CM, et al. Bacterial cell association and antimicrobial activity of a C60 water suspension. Environ Toxicol Chem 2005; 24:2757–62.
92. Sayes CM, Gobin AM, Ausman KD, et al. Nano-C60 cytotoxicity is due to lipid peroxidation. Biomaterials 2005; 26:7587–95.
93. Rancan F, Helmreich M, Molich A, et al. Fullerene-pyropheophorbide a complexes as sensitizer for photodynamic therapy: uptake and photo-induced cytotoxicity on Jurkat cells. J Photochem Photobiol B 2005; 80:1–7.
94. Fiorito S, Serafino A, Andreola F, et al. Effects of fullerenes and single-wall carbon nanotubes on murine and human macrophages. Carbon 2006; 44: 1100–5.
95. Isakovic A, Markovic Z, Todorovic-Markovic B, et al. Distinct cytotoxic mechanisms of pristine versus hydroxylated fullerene. Toxicol Sci 2006; 91:173–83.
96. Rouse JG, Yang J, Barron AR, et al. Fullerene-based amino acid nanoparticle interactions with human epidermal keratinocytes. Toxicol In Vitro 2006; 20:1313–20.
97. Xiao L, Takada H, Gan XH, et al. The water-soluble fullerene derivative 'Radical Sponge®' exerts cytoprotective action against UVA irradiation but not visible-light-catalyzed cytotoxicity in human skin keratinocytes. Bioorg Med Chem Lett 2006; 16:1590–5.
98. Yamawaki H, Iwai N. Cytotoxicity of water-soluble fullerene in vascular endothelial cells. Am J Physiol Cell Physiol 2006; 290:C1495–502.
99. Lesniak W, Bielinska AU, Sun K, et al. Silver/dendrimer nanocomposites as biomarkers: fabrication, characterization, in vitro toxicity, and intracellular detection. Nano Lett 2005; 5:2123–130.
100. Derfus A, Chan, WCW, Bhatia SN. Probing the cytotoxicity of semiconductor quantum dots. Nano Lett 2004; 4:11–8.
101. Chen F, Gerion D. Fluorescent CdSe/ZnS nanocrystal-peptide conjugates for long-term, nontoxic imaging and nuclear targeting in living cells. Nano Lett4: 1827–32.
102. Hoshino A, Hanaki KI, Suzuki K, et al. Applications of T-lymphoma labeled with fluorescent quantum dots to cell tracing markers in mouse body. Biochem Biophys Res Commun 2004a; 314:46–53.
103. Hoshino A, Fujioka K, Oku T, et al. Physicochemical properties and cellular toxicity of nanocrystal quantum dots depend on their surface modification. Nano Lett 2004b; 4:2163–9.

104. Kirchner C, Liedl T, Kudera S, et al. Cytotoxicity of colloidal CdSe and CdSe/ZnS nanoparticles. Nano Lett 2005; 5:331–8.
105. Lovric J, Bazzi HS, Cuie, Y, et al. Differences in subcellular distribution and toxicity of green and red emitting CdTe quantum dots. J Mol Med 2005; 83: 377–85.
106. Shiohara A, Hoshino A, Hanaki KI, et al. On the cytotoxicity caused by quantum dots. Microbiol Immunol 2004; 48:669–75.
107. Isobe H, Tanaka T, Maeda R, et al. Preparation, purification, characterization, and cytotoxicity assessment of water-soluble, transition-metal-free carbon nanotube aggregates. Angew Chem Int Ed Engl 2006; 45:6676–80.
108. Zhang, Q, Kusaka Y, Sato, K, et al. Differences in the extent of inflammation caused by intratracheal exposure to three ultrafine metals: role of free radicals. J Toxicol Environ Health A 1998; 53:423–38.
109. Gupta AK, Berry C, Gupta M, et al. Receptor-mediated targeting of magnetic nanoparticles using insulin as a surface ligand to prevent endocytosis. IEEE Trans Nanobiosci 2003; 2:255–61.
110. Goodman CM, McCusker CD, Yilmaz T, et al. Toxicity of gold nanoparticles functionalized with cationic and anionic side chains. Bioconj Chem 2004; 15:897–900.
111. Braydich-Stolle L, Hussain S, Schlager JJ, et al. *In vitro* cytotoxicity of nanoparticles in mammalian germline stem cells. Toxicol Sci 2005; 88:412–9.
112. Cheng FY, Su CH, Yang YS, et al. Characterization of aqueous dispersions of Fe_3O_4 nanoparticles and their biomedical applications. Biomaterials 2005; 26:729–38.
113. Gupta AK, Gupta M. Cytotoxicity suppression and cellular uptake enhancement of surface modified magnetic nanoparticles. Biomaterials 2005; 26: 1565–73.
114. Hussain SM, Hess KL, Gearhart JM, et al. In vitro toxicity of nanoparticles in BRL 3A rat liver cells. Toxicol In Vitro 2005; 19:975–83.
115. Lu ZX, Zhang ZL, Zhang MX, et al. Core/shell quantum dot-photosensitized nano-TiO_2 films: fabrication and application to the damage of cells and DNA. J Phys Chem B 2005; 109:22663–6.
116. Petri-Fink A, Chastellain, M, Juillerat-Jeanneret L, et al. Development of functionalized superparamagnetic iron oxide nanoparticles for interaction with human cancer cells. Biomaterials 2005; 26:2685–94.
117. Shukla R, Bansal V, Chaudhary M, et al. Biocompatibility of gold nanoparticles and their endocytotic fate inside the cellular compartment: a microscopic overview. Langmuir 2005; 21:10644–54.
118. Auffan M, Decome L, Rose J, et al. In vitro interactions between DMSA-coated maghemite nanoparticles and human fibroblasts: a physicochemical and cyto-genotoxical study. Environ Sci Technol 2006; 40:4367–73.
119. Dufour EK, Kumaravel T, Nohynek GJ, et al. Clastogenicity, photo-clastogenicity or pseudo-photo-clastogenicity: genotoxic effects of zinc oxide in the dark, in pre-irradiated or simultaneously irradiated Chinese hamster ovary cells. Mutat Res 2006; 607:215–24.
120. Hussain SM, Javorina AK, Schrand AM, et al. The interaction of manganese nanoparticles with PC-12 cells induces dopamine depletion. Toxicol Sci 2006; 92:456–63.

121. Qi L, Xu Z, Chen M. In vitro and in vivo suppression of hepatocellularcarcinoma growth by chitosan nanoparticles. Eur J Cancer 2007; 43:184–93.
122. Sayes CM, Wahi R, Kurian PA, et al. Correlating nanoscale titania structure with toxicity: a cytotoxicity and inflammatory response study with human dermal fibroblasts and human lung epithelial cells. Toxicol Sci 2006; 92:174–85.
123. Wang B, Feng WY, Wang TC, et al. Acute toxicity of nano- and micro-scale zinc powder in healthy adult mice. Toxicol Lett 2006; 161:115–23.
124. Warheit DB, Webb TR, Sayes CM, et al. Pulmonary instillation studies with nanoscale TiO$_2$ rods and dots in rats: toxicity is not dependent upon particle size and surface area. Toxicol Sci 2006; 91:227–36.
125. Ameller T, Marsaud V, Legrand P, et al. Pure antiestrogen RU 58668-loaded nanospheres: morphology, cell activity and toxicity studies. Eur J Pharmaceut Sci 2004; 21:361–70.
126. De S, Miller DW, Robinson DH. Effect of particle size of nanospheres and microspheres on the cellular-association and cytotoxicity of paclitaxel in 4T1 cells. Pharmaceut Res 2005; 22:766–75.
127. Park EK, Lee SB, Lee YM. Preparation and characterization of methoxy poly (ethylene glycol)/poly(ε-caprolactone) amphiphilic block copolymeric nanospheres for tumor-specific folate-mediated targeting of anticancer drugs. Biomaterials 2005; 26:1053–61.
128. Shvedova AA, Castranova V, Kisin ER, et al. Exposure to carbon nanotube material: assessment of nanotube cytotoxicity using human keratinocyte cells. J Toxicol Environ Health A 2003; 66:1909–26.
129. Kam NWS, Jessop TC, Wender PA, et al. Nanotube molecular transporters: internalization of carbon nanotube-protein conjugates into mammalian cells. J Am Chem Soc 2004; 126:6850–1.
130. Pantarotto D, Briand JP, Prato M, et al. Translocation of bioactive peptides across cell membranes by carbon nanotubes. Chem Commun (Camb) 2004a; (01):16–7.
131. Pantarotto D, Singh R, McCarthy D, et al. Functionalized carbon nanotubes for plasmid DNA gene delivery. Angew Chem Int Ed Engl 2004b; 43:5242–6.
132. Bianco A, Hoebeke J, Kostarelos K, et al. Carbon nanotubes: on the road to deliver. Curr Drug Deliv 2005a; 2:253–9.
133. Bianco A, Hoebeke J, Godefroy S, et al. Cationic carbon nanotubes bind to CpG oligodeoxynucleotides and enhance their immunostimulatory properties. J Am Chem Soc 2005b; 127:58–9.
134. Cunningham MJ, Magnuson SR, Falduto MT, et al. Gene expression profiling of nanoscale materials using a systems biology approach. Toxicol Sci 2005; 84:9.
135. Cui D, Tian F, Ozkan CS, et al. Effect of single wall carbon nanotubes on human HEK293 cells. Toxicol Lett 2005; 155:73–85.
136. Ding L, Stilwell J, Zhang T, et al. Molecular characterization of the cytotoxic mechanism of multiwall carbon nanotubes and nano-onions on human skin fibroblast. Nano Lett 2005; 5:2448–64.
137. Manna SK, Sarkar S, Barr J, et al. Single-walled carbon nanotube induces oxidative stress and activates nuclear transcription factor-kB in human keratinocytes. Nano Lett 2005; 5:1676–84.
138. Monteiro-Riviere NA, Inman AO, Wang YY, et al. Surfactant effects on carbon nanotube interactions with human keratinocytes. Nanomed: Nanotechnol Biol Med 2005a; 1:293–9.

139. Monteiro-Riviere NA, Nemanich RJ, Inman, AO, et al. Multi-walled carbon nanotube interactions with human epidermal keratinocytes. Toxicol Lett 2005b; 155:377–84.

140. Muller J, Huaux F, Moreau N, et al. Respiratory toxicity of multi-wall carbon nanotubes. Toxicol Appl Pharmacol 2005; 207:221–31.

141. Murr LE, Garza KM, Soto KF, et al. Cytotoxicity assessment of some carbon nanotubes and related carbon nanoparticle aggregates and the implications for anthropogenic carbon nanotube aggregates in the environment. Int J Environ Res Public Health 2005; 2:31–42.

142. Shvedova AA, Kisin ER, Mercer R, et al. Unusual inflammatory and fibrogenic pulmonary responses to single-walled carbon nanotubes in mice. Am J Physiol Lung Cell Mol Physiol 2005; 289:L698–708.

143. Bottini M, Bruckner S, Nika K, et al. Multi-walled carbon nanotube induce T lymphocyte apoptosis. Toxicol Lett 2006; 160:121–6.

144. Dumortier H, Lacotte S, Pastorin G, et al. Functionalized carbon nanotubes are non-cytotoxic and preserve the functionality of primary immune cells. Nano Lett 2006; 6:1522–8.

145. Magrez A, Kasas S, Salicio V, et al. Cellular toxicity of carbon-based nanomaterials. Nano Lett 2006; 6:1121–5.

146. Nimmagadda A, Thurston K, Nollert MU, et al. Chemical modification of SWNT alters in vitro cell-SWNT interactions. J Biomed Mater Res A 2006; 76:614–25.

147. Sayes CM, Liang F, Hudson JL, et al. Functionalization density dependence of single-walled carbon nanotubes cytotoxicity in vitro. Toxicol Lett 2006; 161:135–42.

148. Tian F, Cui D, Schwarz H, et al. Cytotoxicity of single-wall carbon nanotubes on human fibroblasts. Toxicol In Vitro 2006; 20:1202–12.

149. Worle-Knirsch JM, Pulskamp K, Krug, HF. Oops they did it again! Carbon nanotubes hoax scientists in viability assays. Nano Lett 2006; 6:1261–8.

150. Zanello LP, Zhao B, Hu H, et al. Bone cell proliferation on carbon nanotubes. Nano Lett 2006; 6:562–7.

151. Zhu Y, Zhao Q, Li Y, et al. The interaction and toxicity of multi-walled carbon nanotubes with *Stylonychia mytilus*. J Nanosci Nanotechnol 2006; 6:1357–64.

152. Pulskamp K, Diabate S, Krug HF. Carbon nanotubes show no sign of acute toxicity but induce intracellular reactive oxygen species in dependence on contaminants. Toxicol Lett 2007; 168:58–74.

153. Wick P, Manser P, Limbach LK, et al. The degree and kind of agglomeration affect carbon nanotube cytotoxicity. Toxicol Lett 2007; 168:121–31.

154. Zakharenko LP, Zakharov IK, Lunegov SN, et al. [Demonstration of the absence of genotoxicity of fullerene C60 using the somatic mosaic method]. Dokl Akad Naut 1994; 335:261–2.

155. Sera N, Tokiwa H, Miyata N. Mutagenicity of the fullerene C_{60}-generated singlet oxygen dependent formation of lipid peroxides. Carcinogenesis 1996; 17:2163–9.

156. Zakharenko LP, Zakharov IK, Vasiuniana EA, et al. [Determination of the genotoxicity of fullerene C60 and fullerol using the method of somatic mosaics on cells of *Drosophila melanogaster* wing and SOS-chromotest]. Genetika 1997; 33:405–9.

157. Lin AMY, Chyi, BY, Wang SD, et al. Carboxyfullerene prevents iron-induced oxidative stress in rat brain. J Neurochem 1999; 72:1634–40.

158. Kamat JP, Devasagayam TPA, Priyadarsini KI, et al. Reactive oxygen species mediated membrane damage induced by fullerene derivatives and its possible biological implications. Toxicology 2000; 155:55–61.

159. Mori T, Takada H, Ito S, et al. Preclinical studies on safety of fullerene upon acute oral administration and evaluation for no mutagenesis. Toxicology 2006; 225:48–54.

160. Xia T, Kovochich M, Brant J, et al. Comparison of the abilities of ambient and manufactured nanoparticles to induce cellular toxicity according to an oxidative stress paradigm. Nano Lett 2006; 6:1794–807.

161. Green M, Howman E. Semiconductor quantum dots and free radical induced DNA nicking. Chem Commun (Camb) 2005; (01):121–3.

162. Ye L, Su Q, Zhou XD, et al. [Genotoxicity of a new NanoHA-PA66 root filling material in vitro]. Hua Xi Kou Qiang Yi Xue Za Zhi 2004; 22:93–5.

163. Kim JS, Yoon TJ, Yu KN, et al. Toxicity and tissue distribution of magnetic nanoparticles in mice. Toxicol Sci 2006; 89:338–47.

164. Henry TB, Menn FM, Wilgus J, et al. Gene expression changes in zebrafish after exposure to aqueous C60 nanoparticles generated by different methods. Abstract presented at Overcoming Obstacles to Effective Research Design in Nanotoxicology, Boston, MA, April24–25, 2006.

165. Cunningham MJ. Genomics and proteomics: the new millennium of drug development and discovery. J Pharmacol Toxicol Meth 2000; 44:291–300.

166. Cunningham MJ, Dat DD. Microarrays-fabricating. In:Fuchs J, Podda M, eds. Encyclopedia of Diagnostic Genomics and Proteomics. New York: Marcel Dekker, 2005:819–23.

167. Cunningham MJ, Shah M. Toxicogenomics. In:Gad SC, ed. Handbook of Pharmaceutical Biotechnology. New Jersey: John Wiley & Sons, in press.

168. Sato H, Sagai M, Suzuki KT, et al. Identification, by cDNA microarray, of A-raf and proliferating cell nuclear antigen as genes induced in rat lung by exposure to diesel exhaust. Res Commun Mol Pathol Pharmacol 1999; 105: 77–89.

169. Koike E, Hirano S, Shimojo N, et al. cDNA microarray analysis of gene expression in rat alveolar macrophages in response to organic extract of diesel exhaust particles. Toxicol Sci 2002; 67:241–6.

170. Wiethoff AJ, Reed KL, Webb TR, et al. Assessing the role of neutrophil apoptosis in the resolution of particle-induced pulmonary inflammation. Inhal Toxicol 2003; 15:1231–46.

171. Wise H, Balharry D, Reynolds LJ, et al. Conventional and toxicogenomic assessment of the acute pulmonary damage induced by the instillation of Cardiff PM_{10} into the rat lung. Sci Total Environ 2006; 360:60–7.

172. Kim HJ, Ishidou E, Kitagawa E, et al. A yeast DNA microarray for the evaluation of toxicity in environmental water containing burned ash. Environ Monitor Assess 2004; 92:253–72.

173. Verheyen GR, Nuijten JM, Van Hummelen P, et al. Microarray analysis of the effect of diesel exhaust particles on in vitro cultured macrophages. Toxicol In Vitro 2004; 18:377–91.

174. Yanagisawa R, Takano H, Inoue KI, et al. Complementary DNA microarray analysis in acute lung injury induced by lipopolysaccharide and diesel exhaust particles. Exp Biol Med 2004; 229:1081–7.

175. Koike E, Hirano S, Furuyama A, et al. cDNA microarray analysis of rat alveolar epithelial cells following exposure to organic extract of diesel exhaust particles. Toxicol Appl Pharmacol 2004; 201:178–85.

176. Yamawaki H, Iwai N. Mechanisms underlying nano-sized air-pollution-mediated progression of atherosclerosis: carbon black causes cytotoxic injury/inflammation and inhibits cell growth in vascular endothelial cells. Circ J 2006; 70:129–40.

177. Ding L, Stilwell J, Zhang T, et al. Molecular characterization of the cytotoxic mechanism of multiwall carbon nanotubes and nano-onions on human skin fibroblast. Nano Lett 2005; 5:2448–64.

178. Cui D, Tian F, Ozkan CS, et al. Effect of single wall carbon nanotubes on human HEK293 cells. Toxicol Lett 2005; 155:73–85.

13

Effect of Carbon Nanotube Exposure on Keratinocyte Protein Expression

Frank A. Witzmann

Department of Cellular and Integrative Physiology, Indiana University School of Medicine, Indianapolis, Indiana, U.S.A.

Nancy A. Monteiro-Riviere

Center for Chemical Toxicology Research and Pharmacokinetics, North Carolina State University, Raleigh, North Carolina, U.S.A.

INTRODUCTION

Carbon nanotubes have been one of the most extensively used nano-materials due to their large surface areas, high electrical conductivity, and excellent strength. Carbon nanotubes are long carbon-based tubes that can be either single- or multiwalled and have the potential to act as biopersistent fibers (1). Nanotubes have aspect ratios ≥ 100, with lengths of several μm and diameters of 0.7 to 1.5 nm for single-walled nanotubes (SWNT) and 2 to 50 nm for multiwalled nanotubes (MWNT). MWNT are comparatively easy to manufacture in bulk and are finding increasingly more practical applications in a variety of areas (2–5), many with direct interaction with human tissues. The same physicochemical properties that give them broad utility may thus confer activity in biological systems. The nature of potential interactions between MWNT and cells/tissues is not known definitively, although the results of several recent studies suggest that both SWNT and MWNT exposure may have injurious cellular effects (6–12). Clearly, the rapid pace of nanoparticle commercialization and use has exceeded our understanding of potential risk (13).

While significant attention has been focused on the inspiration of airborne nanomaterials and their consequent pulmonary toxicity (14–16), another avenue for nanoparticle exposure is the skin. Shvedova et al. (17) demonstrated that unrefined SWNT may lead to dermal toxicity due to accelerated oxidative stress in keratinocytes. Quantum dots (QD) of different sizes, shapes, and surface coatings recently have been shown to penetrate intact porcine skin at an occupationally relevant dose within the span of an average-length work day (18). These results suggest that skin is surprisingly permeable to nanomaterials with diverse physicochemical properties, and thus may serve as a portal of entry for localized, and possibly systemic, exposure of humans to QD and other engineered nanoscale materials (18). Monteiro-Riviere et al. (19) documented that MWNT that were neither derivatized nor optimized for biological applications were able to localize within and initiate an irritation response in human epidermal keratinocytes (HEK), cells that constitute a potential primary route of occupational dermal exposure for manufactured nanotubes. When human skin fibroblasts were exposed to high levels of multiwall carbon nano-onions (MWNOs) and MWNT, doses that induced cell cycle arrest and increased cell death via apoptosis/necrosis (20), significant nanomaterial-specific alterations in gene expression were observed. Among the genes whose expression was altered, nanomaterials activated those involved in cellular transport, metabolism, cell cycle regulation, and stress response.

In view of these previous results and to better understand nanotube effects from a more functional standpoint, we undertook the analysis of MWNT exposure on protein expression in HEK (21). That study, described in this chapter, represents the first such proteomic analysis of nanotube exposure in an in vitro model.

METHODS

Materials

Acrylamide and immobilized pH gradient (IPG) strips were purchased from BioRad Inc. (Richmond, California, U.S.A.). Other ultrapure electrophoretic reagents were obtained from BioRad, Sigma (St. Louis, Missouri, U.S.A.), or BDH (Poole, U.K.). Sequence grade trypsin was obtained from Promega (Madison, Wisconsin, U.S.A.). Ammonium bicarbonate was purchased from Mallinckrodt Chemicals (Paris, Kentucky, U.S.A.). Proteomics grade formic acid, iodoethanol, and triethylphosphine were obtained from Sigma (St. Louis, Missouri, U.S.A.). Acetonitrile and hydrochloric acid solution $N/10$ were obtained from Fisher Scientific (Fair Lawn, New Jersey, U.S.A.). All other chemicals used were of the highest grade obtainable. Fully characterized MWNT were manufactured using a microwave plasma-enhanced chemical vapor deposition system, as described previously (19).

Cell Culture and MWNT Exposure

Cryopreserved HEK (approximately 260 K cells/vial) were purchased from Cambrex BioScience (Walkerville, Maryland, U.S.) and plated onto three 75-cm^2 culture flasks, each containing 15 mL of serum-free keratinocyte growth media (KGM-2; from HEK basal media supplemented with 0.1 ng/mL human epidermal growth factor, 5 mg/mL insulin, 0.4% bovine pituitary extract, 0.1% hydrocortisone, 0.1% transferrin, 0.1% epinephrine, and 50 mg/mL gentamicin/50 ng/mL amphotericin-B). The culture flasks were maintained in a humidified incubator at 37°C with a 95% O_2/5% CO_2 atmosphere. After reaching approximately 60% confluency, the HEK were passed into eight 75-cm^2 culture flasks and grown in 15 mL of KGM-2. HEK were harvested and plated in six-well culture plates (9.6 cm^2) in 2 mL of media at a concentration of approximately 96,000 cells per well.

Upon reaching 80% HEK confluency, each six-well plate was exposed to MWNT in KGM-2, as well as media alone, served as the controls. Immediately prior to treating the cells, nanotubes were added to the KGM-2 to provide a 0.4 mg/mL stock solution. The solution was thoroughly sonicated to disperse the structures and 2 mL added to each well. The HEK medium was harvested at 24 and 48 h posttreatment (six wells/plate/time point), and stored at −80°C until assayed. Cells destined for proteomic analysis remained adherent to wells from which medium was removed, frozen, and stored at −80°C.

Cytokine Assay

We assayed human cytokines IL-1β, IL-6, IL-8, IL-10, and TNF-α using the Bio-Plex™ Suspension Array System (Bio-Rad Laboratories, Hercules, California, U.S.). In this assay system, duplicate 50 μL samples of media were added to filter wells in a 96-well plate containing antibody-conjugated beads and incubated in the dark with agitation for 30 min. In this experiment, the wells were rinsed and incubated for 30 min with 25 μL of the biotinylated detection antibody. The beads were incubated for 10 min with streptavidin–phycoerythrin after the initial wash, were washed again, and then resuspended in 125 μL of the assay buffer. The samples were then quantified on a Bio-Plex Array Reader using multiplexing to simultaneously assay all 5 cytokines within the 50 μL culture medium sample. The contents of each well were analyzed using Bioplex Manager™ v4.0 and the cytokine data were statistically compared using ANOVA (SAS 6.12 for Windows; SAS Institute, Cary, North Carolina, U.S.).

Sample Preparation

Following cell culture and treatment, HEKs were solubilized directly in well (in situ) (22) by adding 550 μL of lysis buffer containing 9 M urea, 4% Igepal

CA-630 ([octylphenoxy] polyethoxyethanol), 1% DTT, and 2% carrier ampholytes (pH 8–10.5) directly to the frozen cells adhering to the bottom of each well. The culture plates were then placed in a 37°C incubator for 1 h with intermittent manual agitation. After 1 h, the entire volume was removed from each well and placed in 2 mL Eppendorf tubes. Each sample was then sonicated with a Fisher Sonic Dismembranator using 3×2 s bursts. Sonication was carried out every 15 min for 1 h after which the fully solubilized samples were transferred to a cryotube for storage at −80°C until thawed for proteomic analysis. Protein concentration was determined using amido black 10B (23), an approach that enables the sensitive and accurate assay of solubilized proteins to be performed without interference from lysis buffer constituents.

Two-Dimensional Electrophoresis and Image Analysis

500 µg protein were loaded onto IPG strips (24 cm, nonlinear pH 3–10) using overnight, passive rehydration at room temperature. Isoelectric focusing was then performed simultaneously on all 20 IPG strips randomly assigned to two Protean IEF Cells (BioRad) (10 strips/instrument), by a program of progressively increasing voltage (150 V for 2 h, 300 V for 4 h, 1500 V for 1 h, 5000 V for 5 h, 7000 V for 6 h, and 10,000 V for 3 h) for a total of 100,000 V h. A computer-controlled gradient casting system was used to prepare second-dimension SDS gradient slab gels ($20 \times 25 \times 0.15$ cm) in which the acrylamide concentration varied linearly from 11% to 17% T. First-dimension IPG strips were loaded directly onto the slab gels following equilibration for 10 min in Equilibration Buffer I and 10 min in Equilibration Buffer II (Equilibration Buffer I: 6 M urea, 2% SDS, 0.375 M Tris–HCl pH 8.8, 20% glycerol, 130 mM DTT; Equilibration Buffer II: 6 M urea, 2% SDS, 0.375 M Tris–HCl pH 8.8, 20% glycerol, 135 mM iodoacetamide). All of the 20 second-dimension polyacrylamide slab gels were run in parallel at 8°C for 18 h at 160 V and subsequently fixed and stained using a colloidal Coomassie Blue G-250 procedure (24) for 96 h. After complete staining, gels were washed several times with water and scanned at 95.3 µm/pixel resolution using a GS-800 Calibrated Imaging Densitometer (Bio-Rad, Hercules, California, U.S.).

The gel images were analyzed using PDQuest™ software (Bio-Rad, v.7.1) in which background was subtracted and protein spot density peaks detected and counted. A reference pattern was constructed and each of the 20 gels in the matchset was matched to the reference gel. Numerous proteins that were uniformly expressed in all patterns were used as landmarks to facilitate rapid gel matching. Individual protein quantities were expressed as parts-per-million (ppm) of the total integrated optical density, after normalization against total image density enabling accurate comparisons of individual protein spot abundance. The raw quantitative data for each protein spot was exported to Excel for statistical analysis and group comparisons using an unpaired, two-tailed Student's *t*-test.

Peptide Mass Fingerprinting

Protein spots were excised manually from the gels and processed automatically using the multifunctional MultiProbe II Station robot (PerkinElmer). The protein spots were destained, reduced with dithiothreitol, alkylated with iodoacetamide, and tryptically digested using Promega sequence grade, modified trypsin in preparation for matrix-assisted laser desorption ionization mass spectrometry (MALDI-TOF MS) of the resulting peptides. The tryptic peptides were eluted and manually spotted on the sample target along with α-cyano-4-hydroxycinnamic acid matrix. The target was then analyzed directly using the prOTOF™ 2000 MALDI Orthogonal Time of Flight Mass Spectrometer (PerkinElmer/SCIEX, Concord ON) using TOF Works™ software for automated batch database searches of the NCBIR protein sequence database. Accuracy of monoisotopic peptide mass measurements ranged between 5 and 15 ppm, resulting in high confidence protein identifications. Alternatively, some peptide mass spectra were submitted for online interrogation of the ProFound™ Peptide Mass Database. Protein identity was deemed acceptably robust, though not necessarily conclusive, when the TOF Works expectation probability was < .01 or the Profound™ Z-score exceeded 1.30, corresponding to the 90th percentile.

To give meaning to differential protein expression and enable accurate interpretation, the altered proteins were categorized according to three ontological aspects: cell component, cell process, and physiological function using the Generic Gene Ontology (GO) (25) Term Mapper (http://go.princeton.edu/cgi-bin/GOTermMapper).

RESULTS

Comparative levels of IL-8, IL-1β, IL-6, and TNF-α measured in the culture media from control and MWNT-exposed HEK are illustrated in Figure 1. Treatment of HEK with 0.4 mg/mL of MWNT resulted in a significant ($p < .05$) increase in IL-8 at both the 24 and 48 h time points as compared to controls. IL-1β concentrations showed a significant ($p < .05$) increase only at 48 h. Il-6 release was actually lower than the controls. TNF-α levels were extremely low (< 0.01 pg/mL), an observation that likely reflects the detection of background noise rather than an actual quantity.

In Figure 2, we illustrate a raw gel image from PDQuest 2D gel analysis software representative of all images in the experiment. This gel

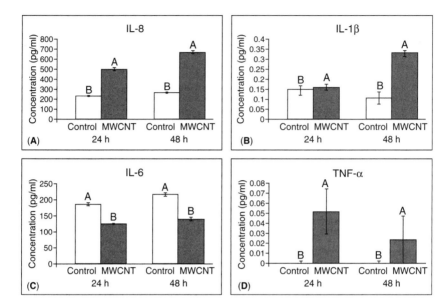

Figure 1 (A) Mean IL-8 concentrations (±SEM). Histogram with different letters (A,B) denote mean values that are statistically different at $p < .05$. (B) Mean IL-β concentrations (±SEM). Histogram with different letters (A,B) denote mean values that are statistically different at $p < .05$. (C) Mean IL-6 concentrations (±SEM). Histogram with different letters (A,B) denote mean values that are statistically different at $p < .05$. (D) Mean TNF-α concentrations (±SEM). Histogram with different letters (A,B) denote mean values that are statistically different at $p < .05$. *Abbreviation*: MWCNT, multi-walled carbon nanotube.

pattern illustrates the ~1750 protein spots resolved and detected in each of the various HEK samples studied. To determine expression differences resulting from MWNT exposure and the effect of culture duration, spot quantities (determined as described in the methods section) of all matched proteins were compared in the following manner: 24 h Control versus 24 MWNT; 48 h Control versus 48 h MWNT; and 24 h Control versus 48 h Control. As a result of these group comparisons, we determined that 152 proteins were significantly ($p < .01$) differentially expressed. These proteins, along with other notable proteins, were thus cut from the gel, subjected to peptide mass fingerprinting. 117 were positively identified, are illustrated by spot number (SSP) in Figure 2, and listed accordingly in Table 1.

As a result of 24 h of MWNT exposure, the expression of 36 HEK proteins was altered while 48 h of MWNT exposure altered 106 protein spots. When we compared the proteins in untreated, 24 and 48 h control groups, the abundance of 48 protein spots were significantly different ($p < .01$). These results, along with the relative direction (up or down) of differential expression, are presented in Table 2.

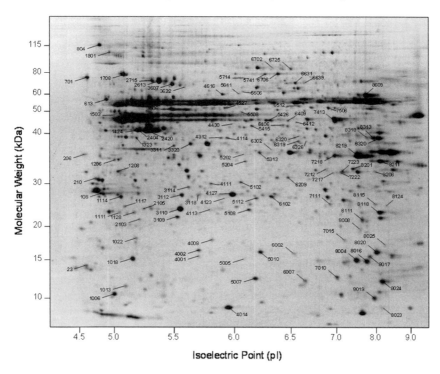

Figure 2   Large-format 2D gel $(20 \times 25 \times 0.15\,\text{cm}$; stained with colloidal CBB) image of whole HEK lysate. Numbered protein spots are those altered by MWNT exposure and identified by mass spectrometry. Quantitative differences in protein staining intensity were analyzed statistically and are listed in Table 1 along with protein identifiers. Molecular weight and p*I* calibrations are estimates based on the calculated MW and p*I* of protein spots identified in the pattern. *Abbreviation*: HEK, human epidermal keratinocytes; MW, _____; MWNT, multiwalled nanotube.

DISCUSSION

To assess the potential dermal toxicity of MWNT, HEK were exposed at a level and duration previously shown to cause an inflammatory response (19). Decreased cell viability under such conditions have been described before (19), and the elevated levels of the proinflammatory cytokines IL-8, and IL-1β observed here (Fig. 1) indicate that MWNT exposure initiates an inflammatory response at 0.4 mg/mL dose in HEK. Transmission electron micrographs (TEMs) have previously verified that MWNT are capable of entering into HEK in the absence of a vehicle or surfactant (19). The presence of IL-8, IL-6, and IL-1β coincide with reports of dermal irritation in humans (26–29). Normal HEKs respond rapidly to injury by activating molecules that are capable of promptly signaling a need for tissue repair (30). The observed TNF-α levels were extremely low, but TNF-α and IL-1β

(*text continues on p. 214*)

Table 1 Proteins Identified from Human Epidermal Keratinocyte (HEK) Lysates Separated by 2DE—Effect of MWCNT Exposure

Spot #	Protein ID	24 h fold change	48 h fold change	p*I*	kDa	SwissProt ID	SwissProt accession
23	Thiopurine S-methyltransferase	—	−2.6	4.6	13.3	TPMT_HUMAN	P51580
108	Protein kinase C inhibitor protein-1; phospholipase A2; 14-3-3 zeta	+1.3	+2.6	4.7	27.9	1433Z_HUMAN	P63104
117	Keratin 17	+6.5	+50.8	5.0	47.9	K1C17_HUMAN	Q04695
206	NF-kappaB inhibitor beta	—	−1.5	4.7	35.9	IKBB_HUMAN	Q15653
210	Tropomyosin 3	—	−1.7	4.7	32.9	TPM3_HUMAN	P06753
613	Prolyl 4-hydroxylase, beta subunit; protein disulfide isomerase	—	+1.6	4.8	57.5	PDIA1_HUMAN	P07237
701	Calreticulin precursor (calregulin)	—	+1.7	4.3	48.1	CRTC_HUMAN	P27797
804	Serine/threonine kinase 31 isoform a	—	+1.5	5.0	116.7	Q6PCD3_HUMAN	Q6PCD3
1006	Ubiquitin activating enzyme E1	—	−1.4	4.5	5.1	UBE1L_HUMAN	P41226
1013	MHC class II antigen	—	−1.7	5.1	10.8	Q9GIL6_HUMAN	Q9GIL6
1018	Hypothetical protein FLJ20972	—	−1.5	5.3	16.1	Q9H7F6_HUMAN	Q9H7F6
1022	Myosin light chain kinase, smooth muscle and non-muscle isozymes	—	−1.5	4.2	17.2	MYLK_HUMAN	Q15746

				pI	MW		
1107	Keratin 14	+24.7	+99.6	5.1	51.4	K1C14_HUMAN	P02533
1111	Atrial/embryonic alkali myosin light chain		+1.7	5.0	21.7	MYL4_HUMAN	P12829
1114	Keratin 18	—	-1.3	4.9	33.8	K1C18_HUMAN	P05783
1117	Rab11-family interacting protein 4	—	-1.7	5.2	35.1	RFIP4_HUMAN	Q86YS3
1128	Transmembrane gamma-carboxyglutamic acid protein 3 precursor	—	-1.7	5.8	26.0	TMG3_HUMAN	Q9BZD7
1206	Cell growth regulator with RING finger domain 1 (CGR19)	—	+1.4	5.1	39.1	CGRF1_HUMAN	Q99675
1208	GNB3 protein (transducin beta)	—	+1.7	6.0	32.6	Q96B71_HUMAN	Q96B71
1323	Tubulin-specific chaperone C	—	-1.5	5.3	40.4	TBCC_HUMAN	Q15814
1424	Actin, cytoplasmic 1 (beta)	+1.6	+1.2*	5.6	41.4	ACTB_HUMAN	P60709
1503	Keratin, type I cytoskeletal 16	-1.9	—	5.0	52.3	K1C16_HUMAN	P08779
1708	BiP protein; 78 kDa glucose-regulated protein	+1.6	+2.3	5.2	73.5	GRP78_HUMAN	P11021
1801	Endoplasmin; heat shock protein gp96 precursor	—	+2.9	4.8	92.7	ENPL_HUMAN	P14625
2103	Visinin-like protein 3; calcium-binding protein BDR-1	—	-1.6	5.2	22.4	HPCL1_HUMAN	P37235

(Continued)

Table 1 Proteins Identified from Human Epidermal Keratinocyte (HEK) Lysates Separated by 2DE—Effect of MWCNT Exposure (*Continued*)

Spot #	Protein ID	24 h fold change	48 h fold change	p*I*	kDa	SwissProt ID	SwissProt accession
2105	MHC alpha chain	—	−1.6	5.3	21.3	1A11_HUMAN	P13746
2404	Actin, gamma	+1.9	+4.2	5.3	42.0	ACTG_HUMAN	P63261
2420	Actin, beta	—	+1.9	5.3	42.1	ACTB_HUMAN	P60709
2613	Heat shock cognate protein,71-kDa; hsc70	—	+1.3	5.4	70.9	HSP7C_HUMAN	P11142
2715	Heat shock cognate protein,71-kDa; hsc70	—	+1.6	5.4	70.9	HSP7C_HUMAN	P11142
3109	UMP-CMP kinase (cytidylate kinase) (deoxycytidylate kinase)	—	−1.5	5.4	22.4	KCY_HUMAN	P30085
3110	Glutathione S-transferase, Pi class	—	−1.3	5.4	23.3	GSTP1_HUMAN	P09211
3112	Heat-shock protein beta-1; heat shock 27kDa protein 1	+1.3	+1.6	6.0	23.1	HSPB1_HUMAN	P04792
3114	Similar to 3'(2'), 5'-bisphosphate nucleotidase 1	—	−1.4	5.5	36.1	BPNT1_HUMAN	O95861
3118	Heat shock 27kDa protein 1	+1.6	+1.3*	6.0	22.8	Q96EI7_HUMAN	Q96EI7
3311	Keratin, type I cytoskeletal 9	+1.5	+2.3	5.2	63.4	K1C9_HUMAN	P35527
3320	Annexin A4 (Annexin IV) (Lipocortin IV) (Endonexin I) (Chromobindin 4)	—	+1.3	5.8	36.1	ANXA4_HUMAN	P09525

Spot	Protein			pI	MW	Name	Accession
3506	Keratin 7; cytokeratin 7	–	+1.8	5.4	51.5	K2C7_HUMAN	P08729
3607	Heat shock 70k Da protein 1B; heat shock 70kD protein 1B	–	+4.5	5.5	70.3	HSP71_HUMAN	P08107
3622	Keratin, type I cytoskeletal 9	-2.4	–	5.2	63.4	K1C9_HUMAN	P35527
4001	T-cell receptor beta	–	-2.2	5.3	15.3	TVB2_HUMAN	P04435
4002	Copper-zinc Superoxide Dismutase	–	-1.6	5.7	15.9	SODC_HUMAN	P00441
4008	Keratin-like protein – (fragment)	–	-1.8	5.5	28.5	KRHB1_HUMAN	Q14533
4014	Immunoglobulin lambda light chain variable region	–	-1.2	5.6	11.4	Q96SB0_HUMAN	Q96SB0
4111	TOLLIP protein; Toll-interacting protein	–	-1.2	5.7	30.5	TOLIP_HUMAN	Q9H0E2
4113	GDP dissociation inhibitor 2	+4.7	+1.9	5.7	21.6	Q8TB95_HUMAN	Q8TB95
4123	GRB2 growth factor receptor-bound protein 2; ash protein (see SOS1)	Undetect.	Undetect.	5.9	25.2	GRB2_HUMAN	P62993
4127	Heat shock 27kDa protein 1	+1.2	-1.4	6.0	23.1	Q6F147_HUMAN	Q6F147
4312	RAB3A interacting protein-like 1	–	-1.3	6.7	36.1	Q9P1Q8_HUMAN	Q9P1Q8
4314	Calpain 3 isoform d; calpain, large polypeptide L3; calpain p94	–	-1.4	6.6	36.1	CAN3_HUMAN	P20807

(Continued)

Table 1 Proteins Identified from Human Epidermal Keratinocyte (HEK) Lysates Separated by 2DE—Effect of MWCNT Exposure (*Continued*)

Spot #	Protein ID	24 h fold change	48 h fold change	p*I*	kDa	SwissProt ID	SwissProt accession
4430	Annexin A4; annexin IV; lipocortin IV; endonexin I	−4.5	—	5.6	37.2	ANXA4_HUMAN	P09525
4527	Keratin, type II cuticular Hb5	−1.5	−2.7	6.3	57.2	KRHB5_HUMAN	P78386
4616	T-complex protein 1, alpha subunit	−1.7	—	5.8	62.5	TCPA_HUMAN	P17987
5005	Chain A, dynamin (pleckstrin homology domain) (fragment)	−1.6	−2.1	5.9	14.8	DYN1_HUMAN	Q05193
5007	Leucocyte antigen HLA-DRB5 (fragment)	—	−1.1	5.9	10.9	Q9MY54_HUMAN	Q9MY54
5010	Heme-binding protein	—	−2.1	5.7	21.2	Q9Y5Z5_HUMAN	Q9Y5Z5
5102	Ketohexokinase, isoform a	—	−1.2	5.6	33.1	Q53G56_HUMAN	Q53G56
5108	Ras-related protein Rab-23 (HSPC137)	—	−1.7	6.2	26.9	RAB23_HUMAN	Q9ULC3
5112	Manganese superoxide dismutase	−1.4	−1.9	6.9	22.2	SODM_HUMAN	P04179
5202	3-Hydroxyanthranilate 3,4-dioxygenase	+3.3	+1.8	5.6	33.2	3HAO_HUMAN	P46952
5204	WDFY3 protein	—	−1.3	5.8	32.4	Q96D33_HUMAN	Q96D33
5313	Annexin I (charge variant)	—	+1.2	7.9	35.3	ANXA1_HUMAN	P04083
5415	proliferation-associated protein 2G4 (Cell cycle protein p38-2G4)	—	−1.8	6.1	44.1	PA2G4_HUMAN	Q9UQ80

Spot	Protein			pI	MW	Name	Accession
5426	Flotillin	−3.6	−1.5	7.1	48.8	FLOT1_HUMAN	O75955
5508	Galactosyltransferase-associated protein kinase p58/GTA	−1.4	−1.7	5.6	51.1	CD2L1_HUMAN	P21127
5606	Aspartate-ammonia ligase (Asparagine synthetase)	−2.1	−1.4	6.4	66.6	ASNS_HUMAN	P08243
5611	Hop, stress-induced-phosphoprotein 1 (Hsp70/Hsp90-organizing protein)	−1.8	—	6.4	65.9	STIP1_HUMAN	P31948
5714	Annexin VI isoform 2; calcium-binding protein p68; annexin VI (p68)	−4.1	—	5.6	75.6	ANXA6_HUMAN	P08133
5741	Moesin	—	+2.3	6.1	70.5	MOES_HUMAN	P26038
6002	Kinesin light chain 1P	—	−2.9	6.8	15.8	KLC1_HUMAN	Q07866
6007	Sos1 (Son of sevenless protein homolog 1; pleckstrin homology domain)	—	−1.7	6.5	15.0	SOS1_HUMAN	Q07889
6102	Peroxiredoxin 6; antioxidant protein 2;	—	−1.3	6.0	25.1	PRDX6_HUMAN	P30041
6209	Purine nucleoside phosphorylase	—	−1.4	6.5	32.4	PNPH_HUMAN	P00491
6302	Type II hair keratin 5	−1.6	−1.6	6.3	58.3	KRHB5_HUMAN	P78386
6319	Sulfatase modifying factor 1 (formylglycine-generating enzyme)	—	−1.2	6.2	41.1	SUMF1_HUMAN	Q8NBK3
6320	YWHAZ protein (unique 14-3-3 zeta/delta)	+1.8	+1.8	7.0	35.6	1433Z_HUMAN	P63104

(Continued)

Table 1 Proteins Identified from Human Epidermal Keratinocyte (HEK) Lysates Separated by 2DE—Effect of MWCNT Exposure (*Continued*)

Spot #	Protein ID	24 h fold change	48 h fold change	p*I*	kDa	SwissProt ID	SwissProt accession
6326	N-acetylneuraminic acid phosphate synthase; sialic acid synthase	−2.2	—	6.3	40.8	SIAS_HUMAN	Q9NR45
6406	ARP1 actin-related protein 1 (centractin)	−1.5	—	6.2	42.7	ACTZ_HUMAN	P61163
6409	Squamous cell carcinoma antigen 1	—	—	6.3	44.6	SCCA1_HUMAN	P29508
6412	Flotillin (variant, cleavage?)	Undetect.	Undetect.	7.1	48.8	FLOT1_HUMAN	O75955
6512	Similar to Keratin, type I cytoskeletal 18 (Cytokeratin 18) (K18) (CK 18)	—	−1.5	6.9	46.4	K1C18_HUMAN	P05783
6631	Actin-interacting protein 1; (Aip1)	−1.5	—	6.2	68.5	WDR1_HUMAN	O75083
6639	Actin-interacting protein 1; (Aip1) (charge variant)	−2.3	—	6.2	68.5	WDR1_HUMAN	O75083
6702	Exocyst complex component 7	+11.3	+8.8	6.4	83.0	EXOC7_HUMAN	Q9UPT5
6706	Moesin	—	+2.4	6.1	67.9	MOES_HUMAN	P26038
6725	Transferrin	+3.0	+2.2	6.9	79.3	TRFE_HUMAN	P02787
7010	Galectin-7	—	−1.9	7.0	15.0	LEG7_HUMAN	P47929

				pI	MW		
7015	Interleukin 18 binding protein isoform D precursor	—	−1.6	9.2	17.5	Q9NZA9_HUMAN	Q9NZA9
7111	Endoplasmic reticulum protein 29 precursor; ERp28	+2.8	−2.9	6.8	29.0	ERP29_HUMAN	P30040
7212	Voltage-dependent anion channel 2; VDAC2 protein	+1.6	—	6.8	31.8	Q9BWK8_HUMAN	Q9BWK8
7217	Inorganic pyrophosphatase 2, mitochondrial (Precursor)]	+1.5	—	7.1	38.5	IPYR2_HUMAN	Q9H2U2
7218	Annexin A2; annexin II; annexin II (lipocortin II)	+1.8	+1.8	7.7	38.8	ANXA2_HUMAN	P07355
7222	ATP sulfurylase/APS kinase isoform SK2 (Fragment)	+1.5	—	8.5	30.3	Q9UIR2_HUMAN	Q9UIR2
7223	Transcription factor mammalian MafA	—	+1.4	7.5	37.1	Q8NHW3_HUMAN	Q8NHW3
7413	Phosphopyruvate hydratase beta (beta enolase)	—	−1.3	7.1	47.3	ENOB_HUMAN	P13929
7506	P58 galactosyltransferase-associated protein kinase	—	−1.5	9.7	49.6	CD2L1_HUMAN	P21127
8004	Cyclophilin	—	−1.4	7.9	18.1	Q71V99_HUMAN	Q71V99
8008	Cyclophilin (variant MW)	+5.5	+5.8	8.1	18.1	PPIA_HUMAN	P62937

(Continued)

Table 1 Proteins Identified from Human Epidermal Keratinocyte (HEK) Lysates Separated by 2DE—Effect of MWCNT Exposure (*Continued*)

Spot #	Protein ID	24 h fold change	48 h fold change	p*I*	kDa	SwissProt ID	SwissProt accession
8016	Profilin I	—	−3.1	8.7	15.1	PROF1_HUMAN	P07737
8017	Profilin I	−9.8	−6.8	8.7	15.1	PROF1_HUMAN	P07737
8019	GTP binding protein Rab1a (fragment)	—	−2.7	9.1	10.0	Q96RD8_HUMAN	Q96RD8
8020	Cofilin 1	−2.2	−2.6	8.5	18.7	COF1_HUMAN	P23528
8023	Heat shock 10kDa protein 1 (chaperonin 10)	Undetect.	Undetect.	8.9	11.4	CH10_HUMAN	P61604
8024	Profilin I	Undetect.	Undetect.	8.1	12.2	PROF1_HUMAN	P07737
8025	Actin related protein 2/3 complex subunit 4 (ARP2/3)	Undetect.	Undetect.	8.8	19.8	ARPC4_HUMAN	P59998
8111	phosphatidy-lethanolamine-binding protein	—	−2.3	7.5	21.0	PEBP_HUMAN	P30086
8115	proteasome beta 1 subunit	−2.6	−2.2	8.7	27.2	PSB1_HUMAN	P20618

ID	Protein						
8118	peroxiredoxin 1; natural killer-enhancing factor A	Undetect.	Undetect.	8.7	22.3	PRDX1_HUMAN	Q06830
8124	peroxiredoxin 1; natural killer-enhancing factor A	Undetect.	Undetect.	8.7	23.1	PRDX1_HUMAN	Q06830
8201	Voltage-dependent anion channel 2	+1.2	–	7.7	33.0	Q9BWK8_HUMAN	Q9BWK8
8208	Ras-related protein, RASD1, DEXRAS1	Undetect.	-2.2	9.5	32.0	RASD1_HUMAN	Q9Y272
8211	Lactate dehydrogenase M Chain	–	-2.6	8.7	36.8	LDHA_HUMAN	P00338
8219	Annexin A2	–	+1.8	7.7	38.8	Q8TBV2_HUMAN	Q8TBV2
8313	Aldolase A	Undetect.	Undetect.	8.8	39.7	ALDOA_HUMAN	P04075
8318	Pseudouridine synthase 1 (dyskerin)	–	-1.7	8.4	41.4	TRUA_HUMAN	Q9Y606
8320	Aldolase A	Undetect.	Undetect.	8.8	39.7	ALDOA_HUMAN	P04075
8609	Pyruvate kinase M2-type	-1.5	–	8.4	58.5	KPYM_HUMAN	P14618

Abbreviation: MWCNT, multiwalled carbon nanotube.

are two of the most common initiators of keratinocyte activation (26,30). In response to injury or irritation, keratinocytes release TNF-α and IL-1β, which stimulate IL-8 in a time-dependent manner (19,31–34). IL-8 is not present in normal skin, but can play a significant role in dermal injuries and inflammatory skin diseases (35). IL-6 is a major proinflammatory mediator that is produced by keratinocytes in response to skin irritants, contact allergens, viruses, UV irradiation, and thermal damage so the decrease in IL-6 shows that MWNT probably modulates a different mechanism. Detectable levels of IL-1β show that the HEK triggered an activation state in response to the MWNT and then initiated the proinflammatory response indicated by the IL-8 increase. Many of these responses are associated with several related functional changes in the HEK as indicated by significant alterations in protein expression.

A previous investigation of the effect of prolonged monolayer cell culture in hepatocytes (36) showed significant temporal, postplating differences in gene expression. Similar effects have been observed in keratinocytes during differentiation in culture (37). When we compared protein expression in untreated (control) HEK cultured for 24 and 48 h, we found that 48 proteins were differentially expressed, the majority (67%) of which increased in abundance after 48 h (Table 2). Two of these proteins, hsp27 and profilin 1, were found to be altered in all conditions experimental conditions, including nanotube exposure. Hsp27 levels are known to increase during the late phase of the keratinocyte differentiation (38), most likely as a marker of endogenous stress conditions that may arise when extensive changes in the intracellular protein organization occur, such as during differentiation, dedifferentiation, and perhaps MWNT invasion. Like hsp27, many of the other proteins altered by culture duration alone are related to protein folding and binding activities, and responses to the stress of cell growth (e.g., cyclophilin, galectin-7, cytidylate kinase, GSTP1-1, SOD, and heme-binding protein).

When protein expression in MWNT exposed cells is compared to culture duration-matched controls, a very different picture emerges. At 24 h of exposure, 36 proteins underwent altered expression, nearly two-thirds of which were significant decreases in abundance. In similar fashion (70% decrease in abundance) and to a significantly greater extent, at 48 h of MWNT exposure 106 proteins were differentially expressed. As is the case in discovery-based proteomic investigations such as this, numerous proteins were found to be altered by nanotube exposure and subsequently were identified, yet their impact on the keratinocyte specifically, and the skin more generally, remains difficult to define. To better understand the meaning of the protein alterations observed and to assess their toxicologic relevance, we have categorized the proteins listed in Table 2 according to various ontological characteristics and, in view of changes occurring in the expression of many of these proteins in the course of 24 and 48 h of cell

Table 2 Differentially Expressed Proteins — Nanotube-Exposed Keratinocytes

Comparison	Proteins altered $p < .01$	# ↑	# ↓	% ↑	% ↓
Control 24 h vs. MWCNT 24 h	36	13	23	36	64
Control 48 h vs. MWCNT 48 h	106	33	73	31	69
Control 24 h vs. Control 48 h	48	32	16	66	34

Abbreviation: MWCNT, multiwalled carbon nanotube.

culture, MWNT toxicity will therefore be discussed accordingly. The results of GO TermMapper categorization of the proteins altered by MWNT exposure are illustrated in Table 3.

For instance, two proteins normally upregulated during differentiation, cell cycle-related proliferation-associated protein 2G4 p38 (39) and the peroxiredoxins (40) were decreased by MWNT exposure. Proliferating/differentiating HEK normally display unique regulation of protein expression (41) where, for example, keratin 5 is downregulated in quiescent HEK, as it is here in response to nanotube exposure. This is also consistent with the observed decrease in IL-6 expression (Fig. 1). The keratins K6, K16, and K17 (two of which declined or were fragmented here) are also known to be prominently expressed in stratified epithelia featuring hyperproliferation or abnormal differentiation, including psoriasis and cancer (42). Whether HEK have stopped growing or have started dying in response to MWNT exposure, both or either suggested by a significant decrease in viability observed under exposure conditions identical to those here (19) is debatable, as is the potential mode of cell death.

While the classic apoptotic marker proteins are absent from the results, several apoptosis-related proteins were clustered by the Gene Ontology search. Galectin-7 is a protein with the potential to mediate corneal epithelial cell migration and re-epithelialization of wounds (43) and its overexpression is known to be proapoptotic during cell injury in for instance UV-irradiation (44). Its apparent downregulation here is consistent with nonapoptotic mechanisms. This is consistent with the TEM observations seen in HEK-treated with 0.4 mg/mL of MWNT that did not observe any apoptotic cells (19). In a recent study, fullerene exposure in vitro changed the morphology of vascular endothelial cells in a dose-dependent manner (45). The maximal fullerene dose caused cytotoxic injury, cell death, and inhibited cell growth. Cell death seemed to be caused by activation of ubiquitin–autophagic death pathways. The nature and direction of protein alterations listed in the various categories in Table 3 suggest that in addition to stress and inflammation, cellular MWNT invasion may interfere with normal HEK growth, development and proliferation, though not via apoptosis.

Table 3 Functional Classes of Differentially Expressed Proteins Determined by Gene Ontology Database Mining

Apoptosis
Annexin I (charge variant)↑
Cyclophilin ↓ (charge variant ↑)
Galectin-7 ↓
Proteasome beta 1 subunit ↓
Voltage-dependent anion channel 2
  (& charge variant) ↑

Cytoskeleton
Actin, beta ↑
Actin, gamma ↑
ARP1 ↓
ARP 2/3 complex
  subunit 4 ↓
Cofilin ↓
Dynamin ↓
GDP dissociation inhibitor ↑
Keratin 5 ↓
Keratin 7 ↑
Keratin 9 ↑
keratin 14 (fragment) ↑↑
Keratin 16 ↓
Keratin 17 (fragment) ↑↑
Keratin 18 ↓
Keratin HB5 ↓
Kinesin light chain 1 ↓
MHC class II antigen ↓
Moesin ↑ (charge variant ↓↑)
Profilin 1 ↓
Tropomyosin 3 ↓
Tubulin-specific chaperone C ↓

Membrane Trafficking/Exocytosis
Annexin A2 ↑
Annexin I ↑
Annexin IV ↑
Annexin VI ↓
Dynamin ↓
Exocyst complex
  component 7 ↑
Flotillin ↓
Kinesin light chain 1 ↓
Moesin ↑ (charge variant ↓↑)
  Profilin 1 ↓

Tox/Detox
GSTP1↓
Peroxiredoxin 1 ↓ (charge Δ)
Peroxiredoxin 6 ↓
Superoxide dismutase (Mn) ↓
Thiopurine methyltransferase ↓

Signaling (pathways)
14-3-3 protein zeta/delta (two types ↓↑)
Atrial/embryonic alkali light chain ↑
DexRas 1 ↓
Galactosyltransferase-associated protein
  kinase ↓
GRB2 ↓
IL-18 binding protein ↑
MLCK, nonmuscle ↓
Moesin ↑ (charge variant ↓↑)
NF*K*B inhibitor beta ↓
Serine/threonine kinase 31 isoform a ↑
Transducin beta ↑
Transmembrane gamma-carboxyglutamic
  acid protein 3 precursor ↓
Protein Degradation
Calpain 3 ↓
Ubiquitin activating enzyme E1 ↓

Growth/Differentiation
Cell cycle protein P38 2G4 homolog ↓
Cell growth regulator ↑
Galactosyltransferase-associated
  protein kinase ↓
Galectin-7 ↓
p58 galactosyltransferase-associated
  protein kinase ↓
Phosphatidylethanolamine binding
  protein ↓
Sialic acid synthase ↓
Transcription factor
  mammalian MafA ↑
UMP-CMP kinase (cytidylate kinase) ↓

(Continued)

Table 3   Functional Classes of Differentially Expressed Proteins Determined by Gene Ontology Database Mining (*Continued*)

Rab1A ↓	**Stress Proteins/Chaperones**
Rab3A interacting protein ↓	Calreticulin ↑
Rab11 interacting protein 4 ↓	Cyclophilin ↑ ↓ (variants)
Rab23 ↓	erp29 ↑ ↓
	grp78 ↑
Metabolism	grp94 ↑
3-Hydroxyanthranilate	HOP (hsp70/hsp90
3,4-dioxygenase ↑	organizing protein) ↓
Aldolase A ↓ (charge variant ↑)	hsc70 ↑
ATP sulfurylase/APS kinase ↑	hsp10 (mito) ↓
Enolase, beta ↓	hsp27 ↑ (all charge forms)
Ketohexokinase ↓	hsp70 ↑
LDH ↓	Protein disulfide isomerase ↑
Pseudouridine synthase 1 (dyskerin) ↓	T-complex protein 1α ↓
Purine nucleoside phosphorylase ↑	
Pyrophosphatase 2 ↑	
Pyruvate kinase ↓	
Sulfatase modifying factor 1	
(formylglycine-generating enzyme) ↓	

Perhaps the most striking of the functional categories that are listed in Table 3 and are populated by differentially expressed proteins are these three related groups: signaling, cytoskeleton, and membrane trafficking proteins. Recent evidence suggests that the Golgi apparatus, in addition to its function in protein secretion, may be the site of signaling events important for diverse cellular processes (46–48), acting as a signaling platform in the regulation of downstream events. The Golgi apparatus responds to extracellular signals by reorienting in cells at experimental wound edges through migration and polarization processes. This involves a complex series of signaling events coordinated with reorientation of the microtubule cytoskeleton and changes in actin dynamics involving the Arp2/3 complex, particularly in endocytotic processes (49). It is also possible that membrane traffic and signaling via the Golgi apparatus are integral components of this process. We have observed altered expression in a number of proteins associated with just such processes, and they provide clues to the possible mechanism of MWNT toxicity in HEK.

For example, the expression of four unique annexins, I, A2, IV, and VI was altered by nanotube exposure. Only annexin VI was upregulated by exposure. Annexins are a class of Ca^{++}-regulated proteins linked to many membrane-related events, such as the regulated organization of membrane domains and/or membrane–cytoskeleton linkages, certain exocytotic and

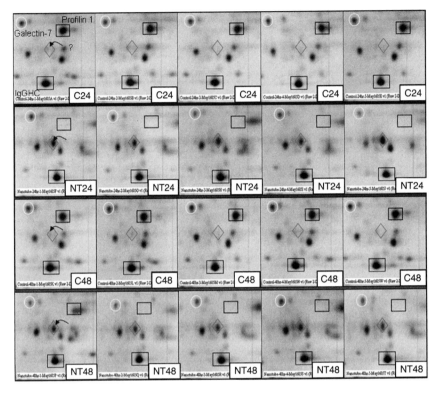

Figure 3 Gel pattern sections ($n = 5$ per group) representing each of the HEK samples studied and illustrating the expression of proteins identified as profilin 1, galectin-7, and IgGHC and one unidentified protein, labeled "?" These frames document the huge decrease in profilin, the moderate increase in galectin-7, the uniform expression of IgGHC, and what appears to be a charge shift in the unidentified protein. Fold-changes for altered proteins appear in Table 1. *Abbreviation*: HEK, human epidermal keratinocytes.

endocytotic transport steps and the regulation of ion fluxes across membranes (50). Annexin A2 in particular is associated with F-actin in scaffolding functions related to endocytic vesicle internalization, multi-vesicular endosomes formation, receptor cycling, and lipid raft formation. Perhaps its downregulation is somehow related to the decrease observed in flotillin, a lipid raft marker. Annexin 1 is associated with inward vesicle budding and multivesicular endosomes formation, VI is involved in membrane actin/myosin interactions, and IVs function remains unclear. Their collective alterations, while difficult to interpret, strongly suggest altered vesicular trafficking mechanisms. A decline in the four Rab (Rab23 and Rab1a) or Rab-associated proteins (Rab11-family interacting protein 4,

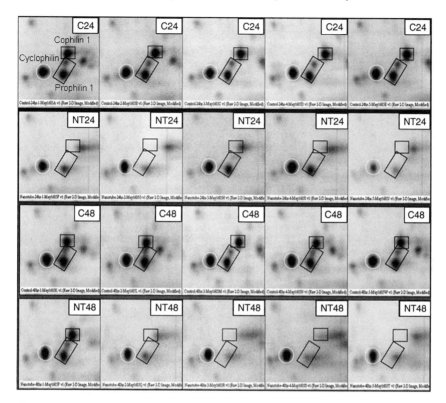

Figure 4 Gel pattern sections ($n = 5$ per group) representing each of the HEK samples studied and illustrating the expression of proteins identified as profilin 1, cophilin 1, and cyclophilin. These frames document the huge decrease in profilin 1 and cophilin 1, and the minor but insignificant decrease in cyclophilin. Fold-changes for altered proteins appear in Table 1. *Abbreviation*: HEK, human epidermal keratinocytes.

RAB11-FIP4) detected in this study also points toward impaired actin-driven, clathrin-independent, and Rab GTPase-related endocytosis (51).

With respect to the actin cytoskeleton, spot numbers 6631 and 6639 were both identified as actin-interacting protein 1 (Aip1), the former likely a negatively charged variant (posttranslationally modified) and both were decreased at 24 h of exposure. Other apparently downregulated proteins include Arp1 (actin-related protein 1) (52), which is involved in microtubule-based vesicle trafficking and mitosis (e.g., centractin) (53) and other cytoskeleton-associated chaperones (54) like TCP-1 identified here. In contrast, exocyst complex component 7 was the most upregulated protein of those identified, and was unaffected by culture alone. The exocyst complex associates with microtubules to mediate vesicle targeting and

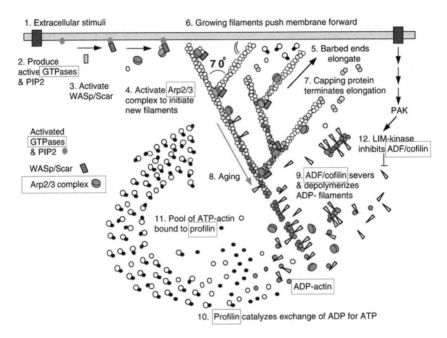

Figure 5 This diagram models the putative participation of the Arp2/3 proteins (and other actin-related proteins the expression for which was altered by MWNT in the present study) and activated Rho family GTPases in regulation of actin filament assembly at the leading edge of motile cells. *Source*: Ref. 54a.

neurite outgrowth in neurons (55) and may also play a role in modulating microtubule dynamics by inhibiting tubulin polymerization (56). Indirect evidence of impaired vesicular trafficking, particularly exocytosis, is provided by increased intracellular transferrin levels. Transferrin associates with specific cell surface receptors to be internalized and delivered to the endocytic pathway. Unlike many other ligands, transferrin (devoid of its iron cargo) remains bound to its receptor and is recycled back to the cell surface, where it can be released for further rounds of iron delivery (57). Accumulation of intracellular transferrin might be the result of a failure to complete its recycling due to impaired exocytotic mechanisms.

Related evidence of altered actin dynamics is provided through increased expression of GDP dissociation inhibitor as overexpression of GDI proteins leads to disruption of the actin cytoskeleton, rounding up of the cells, and loss of stress fibers and focal contact sites (58). Likewise, proteins such as tropomyosin, which stabilizes the actin polymer, and profilin and Arp2/3 were all downregulated by MWNT exposure. Profilin and Arp2/3, along with Aip1 mentioned above all participate in enhancing actin filament disassembly in the presence of actin-depolymerizing factor

(ADF)/cofilin (59), the latter decreased by MWNT exposure as well. The differential expression of these proteins is illustrated in Figures 3 and 4. Interestingly, both beta and gamma actin monomers displayed increased abundance after exposure. This may be explained by an alteration in the soluble, nonpolymerized pool of these proteins and enhanced recovery for detection by 2DE. The role of actin-related proteins ARP, AIP, cofilin, profiling, and potential GTPase-related proteins in actin polymerization and depolymerization are illustrated in Figure 5.

Altogether, the alterations in protein expression observed after 24 and 48 h of HEK culture in the presence of MWNT, at a level that results in both irritation and decreased cell viability, are evidence of the injurious nature of this nanoparticle. If one hypothesizes that the responses observed here might also occur in vivo, epidermal MWNT exposure creates the potential for chronic inflammation and injury which, in turn, may contribute to the development or progression of disease states in the skin.

REFERENCES

1. Nel A, et al. Toxic potential of materials at the nanolevel. Science 2006; 311: 622–7.
2. Xiong X, et al. Enhanced separation of purine and pyrimidine bases using carboxylic multiwalled carbon nanotubes as additive in capillary zone electrophoresis. Electrophoresis, 2006.
3. Chen S, et al. Amperometric third-generation hydrogen peroxide biosensor based on the immobilization of hemoglobin on multiwall carbon nanotubes and gold colloidal nanoparticles. Biosens Bioelectron, 2006.
4. Marrs B, et al. Augmentation of acrylic bone cement with multiwall carbon nanotubes. J Biomed Mater Res A 2006; 77:269–76.
5. Firkowska I, et al. Highly ordered MWNT-based matrixes: topography at the nanoscale conceived for tissue engineering. Langmuir 2006; 22:5427–34.
6. Bottini M, et al. Multi-walled carbon nanotubes induce T lymphocyte apoptosis. Toxicol Lett 2006; 160:121–6.
7. Soto KF, et al. Comparative in vitro cytotoxicity assessment of some manufactured nanoparticulate materials characterized by transmission electron microscopy. J Nanoparticle Res 2005; 7:145–69.
8. Muller J, et al. Respiratory toxicity of multi-wall carbon nanotubes. Toxicol Appl Pharmacol 2005; 207:221–31.
9. Jia G, et al. Cytotoxicity of carbon nanomaterials: single-wall nanotube, multi-wall nanotube, and fullerene. Environ Sci Technol 2005; 39:1378–83.
10. Warheit DB, et al. Comparative pulmonary toxicity assessment of single-wall carbon nanotubes in rats. Toxicol Sci 2004; 77:117–25.
11. Lam CW, et al. Pulmonary toxicity of single-wall carbon nanotubes in mice 7 and 90 days after intratracheal instillation. Toxicol Sci 2004; 77:126–34.
12. Magrez A, et al. Cellular toxicity of carbon-based nanomaterials. Nano Lett 2006; 6:1121–5.

13. Service RF. Nanotechnology: calls rise for more research on toxicology of nanomaterials. Science 2005; 310:1609–.

14. Kipen HM, Laskin DL. Smaller is not always better: nanotechnology yields nanotoxicology. Am J Physiol Lung Cell Mol Physiol 2005; 289:L696–7.

15. Tsuji JS, et al. Research strategies for safety evaluation of nanomaterials. Part IV. Risk assessment of nanoparticles. Toxicol Sci 2006; 89:42–50.

16. Carrero-Sanchez JC, et al. Biocompatibility and toxicological studies of carbon nanotubes doped with nitrogen. 2006.

17. Shvedova AA, et al. Exposure to carbon nanotube material: assessment of nanotube cytotoxicity using human keratinocyte cells. J Toxicol Environ Health A 2003; 66:1909–26.

18. Ryman-Rasmussen JP, Riviere JE, Monteiro-Riviere NA. Penetration of intact skin by quantum dots with diverse physicochemical properties. Toxicol Sci 2006; 91:159–65.

19. Monteiro-Riviere NA, et al. Multi-walled carbon nanotube interactions with human epidermal keratinocytes. Toxicol Lett 2005; 155:377–84.

20. Ding L, et al. Molecular characterization of the cytotoxic mechanism of multiwall carbon nanotubes and nano-onions on human skin fibroblast. Nano Lett 2005; 5:2448–64.

21. Witzmann F, Monteiro-Riviere NA. Multi-walled carbon nanotube exposure alters protein expression in human keratinocytes. Nanomed: Nanotechnol Biol Med 2006; 2:158–68.

22. Witzmann FA, et al. Proteomic evaluation of cell preparation methods in primary hepatocyte cell culture. Electrophoresis 2002; 23:2223–32.

23. Kaplan RS, Pedersen PL. Determination of microgram quantities of protein in the presence of milligram levels of lipid with amido black 10B. Anal Biochem 1985; 150:97–104.

24. Candiano G, et al. Blue silver: a very sensitive colloidal Coomassie G-250 staining for proteome analysis. Electrophoresis 2004; 25:1327–33.

25. Gene Ontology C. The Gene Ontology (GO) database and informatics resource. Nucl Acids Res 2004; 32:D258–61.

26. Barker JN, et al. Keratinocytes as initiators of inflammation. Lancet 1991; 337:211–4.

27. Corsini E, Galli CL. Cytokines and irritant contact dermatitis. Toxicol Lett 1998; 102–103:277–82.

28. Grone A. Keratinocytes and cytokines. Vet Immunol Immunopathol 2002; 88: 1–12.

29. Nickoloff BJ. The cytokine network in psoriasis. Arch Dermatol 1991; 127: 871–84.

30. Freedberg IM, et al. Keratins and the keratinocyte activation cycle. J Invest Dermatol 2001; 116:633–40.

31. Allen DG, Riviere JE, Monteiro-Riviere NA. Identification of early biomarkers of inflammation produced by keratinocytes exposed to jet fuels jet A, JP-8, and JP-8(100). J Biochem Mol Toxicol 2000; 14:231–7.

32. Allen DG, Riviere JE, Monteiro-Riviere NA. Analysis of interleukin-8 release from normal human epidermal keratinocytes exposed to aliphatic hydrocarbons: delivery of hydrocarbons to cell cultures via complexation with alpha-cyclodextrin. Toxicol In Vitro 2001; 15:663–9.

33. Chou CC, Riviere JE, Monteiro-Riviere NA. The cytotoxicity of jet fuel aromatic hydrocarbons and dose-related interleukin-8 release from human epidermal keratinocytes. Arch Toxicol 2003; 77:384–91.

34. Monteiro-Riviere NA, Baynes RE, Riviere JE. Pyridostigmine bromide modulates topical irritant-induced cytokine release from human epidermal keratinocytes and isolated perfused porcine skin. Toxicology 2003; 183:15–28.

35. Chabot-Fletcher M, et al. Interleukin-8 production is regulated by protein kinase C in human keratinocytes. J Invest Dermatol 1994; 103:509–15.

36. Baker TK, et al. Temporal gene expression analysis of monolayer cultured rat hepatocytes. Chem Res Toxicol 2001; 14:1218–31.

37. Steele BK, Meyers C, Ozbun MA. Variable expression of some "housekeeping" genes during human keratinocyte differentiation. Anal Biochem 2002; 307:341–47.

38. Arrigo A.-P, Ducasse C. Expression of the anti-apoptotic protein Hsp27 during both the keratinocyte differentiation and dedifferentiation of HaCat cells: expression linked to changes in intracellular protein organization? Exp Gerontol 2002; 37:1247–55.

39. Radomski N, Jost E. Molecular cloning of a murine cDNA encoding a novel protein, p38-2G4, which varies with the cell cycle. Exp Cell Res 1995; 220: 434–45.

40. Yun SJ, et al. Peroxiredoxin I and II are up-regulated during differentiation of epidermal keratinocytes. Arch Dermatol Res 2005; 296:555–9.

41. Olsen E, Rasmussen HH, Celis JE. Identification of proteins that are abnormally regulated in differentiated cultured human keratinocytes. Electrophoresis 1995; 16:2241–8.

42. Paladini RD, Coulombe PA. Directed expression of keratin 16 to the progenitor basal cells of transgenic mouse skin delays skin maturation. J Cell Biol 1998; 142:1035–51.

43. Cao Z, et al. Galectin-7 as a potential mediator of corneal epithelial cell migration. Arch Ophthalmol 2003; 121:82–6.

44. Bernerd F, Sarasin A, Magnaldo T. Galectin-7 overexpression is associated with the apoptotic process in UVB-induced sunburn keratinocytes. PNAS 1999; 96:11329–34.

45. Yamawaki H, Iwai N. Cytotoxicity of water soluble fullerene in vascular endothelial cells. Am J Physiol Cell Physiol 2006; 290:C1495–502.

46. Ferri KF, Kroemer G. Organelle-specific initiation of cell death pathways. Nat Cell Biol 2001; 3:E255–63.

47. Bivona TG, Philips MR. Ras pathway signaling on endomembranes. Curr Opin Cell Biol 2003; 15:136–42.

48. Rios RM, Bornens M. The Golgi apparatus at the cell centre. Curr Opin Cell Biol 2003; 15:60–6.

49. Schafer DA. Coupling actin dynamics and membrane dynamics during endocytosis. Curr Opin Cell Biol 2002; 14:76–81.

50. Gerke V, Creutz CE, Moss SE. Annexins: linking Ca^{2+} signalling to membrane dynamics. Nat Rev Mol Cell Biol 2005; 6:449–61.

51. Weigert R, et al. Rab22a regulates the recycling of membrane proteins internalized independently of clathrin. Mol Biol Cell 2004; 15:3758–70.

52. Muller J, et al. Sequence and comparative genomic analysis of actin-related proteins. Mol Biol Cell 2005; 16:5736–48.
53. Clark SW, Meyer DI. Centractin is an actin homologue associated with the centrosome. Nature 1992; 359:246–50.
54. Liang P, MacRae TH. Molecular chaperones and the cytoskeleton. J Cell Sci 1997; 110:1431–40.
54a. Reprinted with permission from Pollard et al., Ann Rev Biophys Biomol Struct 2000; 29:545–576
55. Vega IE, Hsu S.-C. The exocyst complex associates with microtubules to mediate vesicle targeting and neurite outgrowth. J Neurosci 2001; 21:3839–48.
56. Wang S, et al. The mammalian exocyst, a complex required for exocytosis, inhibits tubulin polymerization. J Biol Chem 2004; 279:35958–66.
57. Ciechanover A, et al. Kinetics of internalization and recycling of transferrin and the transferrin receptor in a human hepatoma cell line. Effect of lysosomotropic agents. J Biol Chem 1983; 258:9681–9.
58. Leffers H, et al. Identification of two human Rho GDP dissociation inhibitor proteins whose overexpression leads to disruption of the actin cytoskeleton. Exp Cell Res 1993; 209:165–74.
59. Balcer HI, et al. Coordinated regulation of actin filament turnover by a high-molecular-weight Srv2/CAP complex, cofilin, profilin, and Aip1. Curr Biol 2003; 13:2159–69.

14

Critical Issues in the Evaluation of Possible Adverse Pulmonary Effects Resulting from Airborne Nanoparticles

Anna A. Shvedova, Tina Sager, Ashley R. Murray, Elena Kisin,
Dale W. Porter, Stephen S. Leonard, Diane Schwegler-Berry,
Victor A. Robinson, and Vincent Castranova
*National Institute for Occupational Safety and Health, Morgantown,
West Virginia, U.S.A.*

INTRODUCTION

Nanotechnology is the manipulation of matter on a near-atomic scale to produce new structures, materials, and devices. Engineered nanoparticles are defined as having at least one dimension <100 nm. Because of their small size, nanoparticles have a high particle surface area/mass and exhibit physicochemical properties that differ dramatically from fine-sized particles of the same composition. These unique properties are being exploited for a number of applications, including integrated sensors, semiconductors, structural materials, drug delivery systems, medical imaging, sunscreens, cosmetics, and coatings (1). Therefore, nanotechnology has the ability to transform many industries from manufacturing to medicine. By 2015, the National Science Foundation estimates that nanotechnology will have a $1 trillion impact on the global economy and employ 2 million workers, 1 million of which may be in the United States.

Since nanoparticles are engineered to exhibit unique physicochemical properties, it would be reasonable to expect that these nanoparticles would interact with biological systems in ways that may be dramatically different from fine-sized particles of the same composition. The Royal Society and

Royal Academy of Engineering recognized the challenge of predicting whether exposure to nanoparticles would be a health concern, which routes of entry should be avoided, and which nanoparticle exposures should be controlled (2).

If nanoparticles become airborne during production or use, the effects of pulmonary exposure require evaluation. Thus, far little information is available concerning airborne levels of nanoparticles in the nanotechnology industry. Maynard et al. (3) reported that respirable airborne dust levels in laboratory settings producing single-walled carbon nanotubes (SWCNT) by either a high-pressure carbon monoxide (HiPCO) or laser ablation process were generally low, $53 \, \mu g/m^3$. However, peaks were noted during certain handling processes. In addition, laboratory studies indicate that airborne levels of SWCNT can be increased significantly by agitation, i.e., using a vortex shaker or a fluidized bed generator. Therefore, airborne levels in nanotechnology workplaces would depend on the energetics of the processes involved during production and use as well as the presence of control systems.

Given that aerosolization of nanoparticles is possible, adverse respiratory effects are a concern. This chapter will review some properties of nanoparticles, which are critical issues for investigation of pulmonary toxicology. These issues include: deposition, interstitialization, translocation, role of surface area, and role of oxidant stress in the pulmonary toxicity of nanoparticles.

Deposition

For a given particle, pulmonary response is dependent on the fraction of inhaled particles, which remain deposited in the lung. Deposition fraction is dependent on the aerodynamic diameter of the particle (4–6). Deposition models predict that deposition of coarse (>2.5 µm) and fine (0.1–2.5 µm) particles is governed by the processes of sedimentation and impaction. In the case of nanoparticles (<100 nm), particle mass and momentum are extremely small; thus, sedimentation and impaction are not significant factors in pulmonary deposition. Rather, nanoparticles behave like gas molecules, moving randomly by Brownian motion. Such movement would result in the random contact of nanoparticles with the epithelial and/or fluid lining the lung. Models predict that the deposition of nanoparticles in both the tracheobronchial and pulmonary regions of the lung can far exceed that of fine or coarse particles (4–6). In addition, as nanoparticles become smaller than 10 nm, nasal deposition by diffusional mechanisms becomes very high.

Experimental data are available supporting the high deposition of inhaled nanoparticles in the lung. Kreyling et al. (7) exposed rats ventilated via an endotracheal tube by inhalation to radioactive iridium particles (^{192}Ir) with a primary particle size of either 15 or 80 nm. They reported thoracic deposition fraction (deposited in the tracheobronchial plus the pulmonary regions) to be 49% and 28% for the 15 or 80 nm nanoparticles, respectively. Daigle et al. (8) conducted a deposition study in humans upon inhalation of 8.7 or 26 nm carbon particles. They reported that deposition fraction for the respiratory tract was 66% and 80% for 8.7 or 26 nm particles, respectively, at rest. Deposition fraction increased significantly to 83% or 94%, respectively, upon exercise.

In conclusion, both deposition models and experimental results indicate that a high fraction of inhaled nanosized particles can deposit in airways of the conducting and respiratory zones of the lungs. This deposition of nanosized particles is much higher than lung burdens expected after inhalation of equivalent amounts of coarse or fine particles. These relatively high lung burdens are an area of concern when considering the potential pulmonary toxicity of a nanoparticle.

INTERSTITIALIZATION

Since a relatively high percentage of inhaled nanosized particles are likely to deposit on the alveolar surfaces, an issue is whether nanosized particles are effectively phagocytized and cleared by alveolar macrophages or whether a significant number of particles enter the alveolar interstitium where they may cause interstitial damage, inflammation, and/or fibrosis. Results from Kreyling and Scheuch (9) indicate that upon pulmonary exposure fine particles are more effectively phagocytized and cleared by alveolar macrophages than nanosized particles. The fact that a fraction of nanosized particles may avoid phagocytosis results in a greater interstitial burden of nanosized TiO_2 than with an equivalent mass exposure of fine-sized TiO_2 (10). A careful investigation of the interstitialization of fine versus nanosized particles was reported by Oberdorster et al. (11). In this study, rats were exposed to nanosized (20 nm) or fine (250 nm) particles by inhalation for 12 weeks at respective concentrations that resulted in a similar mass deposition of the two particle types. The amount of nanosized TiO_2 in the alveolar interstitium and lymph nodes significantly exceeded the amount of fine TiO_2 in these sites at all time points studied over a 1-year postexposure period. At 1-year postexposure, 44% of deposited nanosized TiO_2 had migrated to the interstitium compared to 13% for fine TiO_2.

In a recent investigation, Roberts et al. (12) exposed rats by intratracheal instillation to fluorescently labeled quantum dots (30–50 nm) and monitored the deposition and fate of these nanoparticles from 2 h to 5 days postexposure. At 2 h postexposure, some quantum dots were located in the alveolar airspaces and on the alveolar epithelial surface, while other quantum dots had already been phagocytized by alveolar macrophages.

At 24 h postexposure, most quantum dots were found within alveolar macrophages. However, a small fraction of deposited quantum dots had avoided phagocytosis and could be found in the alveolar interstitium after 24 h. It appears that the fraction of deposited nanoparticles that are phagocytized can vary greatly with particle type. Unlike quantum dots, which were avidly phagocytized by alveolar macrophages both in vitro and in vivo (12), SWCNT appear to be poorly phagocytized by macrophages in culture (13). Mercer et al. (14) evaluated phagocytosis and interstitialization of aspired SWCNT, which had been labeled with colloidal gold nanoparticles. Only a small fraction of deposited gold-labeled SWCNT was engulfed by alveolar macrophages, while most of the SWCNT were rapidly incorporated into the alveolar interstitium. In contrast, aspiration of gold nanoparticles resulted in avid phagocytosis by alveolar macrophages with only a few gold particles in the interstitium.

In conclusion, not only are nanoparticles highly deposited in the alveoli, but particle number/mass is so great that some nanoparticles escape phagocytosis by alveolar macrophages and can enter the alveolar interstitium. The recognition of nanoparticles by alveolar macrophages is dependent on particle type, i.e., quantum dots and nanogold particles are rapidly phagocytized by alveolar macrophages while SWCNT are not. Therefore, a large fraction of deposited SWCNT rapidly migrates to the alveolar interstium. This high interstitial deposition of SWCNT after aspiration has been associated with diffuse interstitial fibrosis of rapid onset, which progresses over 60 days postexposure (13).

TRANSLOCATION

If a large fraction of inhaled nanoparticles can deposit in the alveoli and a significant number of these nanoparticles can escape phagocytosis and enter the alveolar interstitium, an issue is whether nanoparticles within the alveolar walls can enter pulmonary capillaries and translocate to systemic sites. A study by Oberdorster et al. (15) involving whole body inhalation of ^{13}C nanoparticles (20–24 nm) in rats indicated that substantial numbers of ^{13}C nanoparticles were found in the liver within 18 h postexposure. Relatively rapid translocation of nanoparticles from the lung to the blood was also reported in hamsters after inhalation of nanosized carbon labeled with technetium (16). Similarly, Stone and Godleski (17) reported migration of nanosized particles in the liver and heart following inhalation exposure. In contrast to the reports above, Kreyling et al. (7) investigated translocation of ^{192}Ir (15 or 80 nm) and reported than 1% of these nanoparticles given by inhalation via an endotracheal tube were found in the liver between 6 h and 2 days postexposure. Kreyling and colleagues (7) explained these disparate results by suggesting that the Oberdoster et al. (15) study involved whole body exposure. Therefore, oral exposure during grooming and absorption of particles via the gastrointestinal tract was possible. They also argued that the technetium label may have dissociated from the carbon nanoparticles and entered the blood.

In conclusion, nanoparticles can enter the alveolar interstitium. Once in the interstitium they can migrate into pulmonary capillaries and translocate to systemic sites. At present, the rate of this translocation is a matter of debate and requires further investigation. Investigations are currently in progress at the National Institute for Occupational Safety and Health to quantify the extent of translocation of gold-labeled SWCNT or metal oxide nanoparticles following pulmonary exposure by monitoring the metal content of systemic organs by neutron activation analysis. If nanoparticles translocate from the lungs to systemic organs, then the possible adverse effects of inhalation of nanoparticles on the function of these organs requires investigation. Indeed, there is evidence that aspiration of SWCNT can cause oxidant stress in cardiac and aortic tissue and augment plaque formation in an atherosclerotic susceptible mouse model (18–20).

ROLE OF SURFACE AREA IN TOXICITY

Nanoparticles are characterized by a high surface area per mass. A current hypothesis is that particulate surface area and available surface-active sites play an important role in the biological activity of a particle. Support for this hypothesis can be provided from a simple experiment to evaluate the cytotoxicity of crystalline silica particles of different diameters on human alveolar type II epithelial cell line (A549) in culture (Fig. 1). In this experiment, surface area of SiO_2 (<2 µm) was 5.90 ± 0.03 m^2/g while SiO_2 (<10 µm) was 1.75 ± 0.03 m^2/g, as measured by gas absorption (BET analysis). When exposure dose was on an equivalent mass basis (µg/mL), the smaller silica particles with the greater surface area were 1.9-fold more cytotoxic than the larger silica particles at 70 µg/mL (Fig. 1A). However, when dose was normalized to equivalent particle surface area/cell surface area, there was no difference in the toxicity of the two sizes of silica (Fig. 1B). Similar results were reported for exposure of a human alveolar type II epithelial cell line (A549) to fine or ultrafine TiO_2 and stimulation of message for IL-8. When exposure dose was normalized to equivalent particle surface area, both fine and ultrafine TiO_2 were equipotent in induction of mRNA for this chemokine (21). This dependence of biological activity on particle surface area has also been demonstrated in vivo (22). In this study, rats were exposed to fine (250 nm) or ultrafine (20 nm) TiO_2 particles by intratracheal instillation and pulmonary inflammation determined by the number of polymorphonuclear (PMN) leukocytes harvested by bronchoalveolar lavage

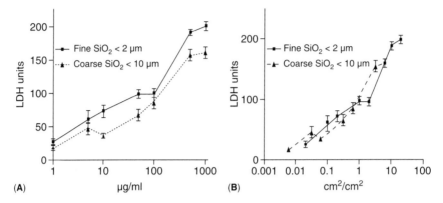

Figure 1 Size dependence of silica cytotoxicity. Human alveolar type II epithelial cells (A549; 1.5×10^5 cells/mL/well) were exposed to various concentrations of crystalline silica of two particle sizes ($<2\,\mu m$; surface area $= 5.9\ m^2/g$ or $<10\,\mu m$, surface area $= 1.75\ m^2/g$). Cytotoxicity was measured as the leakage of lactate dehydrogenase (LDH) into the medium. (**A**) Response versus dose on an equivalent mass/mL basis. (**B**) Response versus dose on an equivalent particle surface area/cell surface area basis. Data are means ± SE of three experiments.

(BAL) at 24 h postexposure. On an equivalent mass basis, ultrafine TiO_2 was more inflammogenic than fine TiO_2 (1.9-fold more potent at $500\,\mu g/rat$). However, when Oberdorster (22) normalized exposure dose to equivalent surface area, the inflammatory potency of ultrafine and fine TiO_2 was similar. A similar relationship between particle surface area and inflammatory potential or depression of particle clearance was reported after inhalation exposure to fine versus ultrafine TiO_2 (11).

Nanoparticles have a tendency to agglomerate into μm-sized particles when suspended in saline. If particle surface area is critical to pulmonary response, would the presence of agglomerates affect the biological responses of cells or the lung to in vitro or in vivo (intratracheal instillation or pharyngeal aspiration) exposure to suspensions of nanoparticles? As shown in Figure 2A, suspension of ultrafine carbon black (Printex 90, Degussa Corporation, Parsippany, New Jersey, U.S.; 14 nm primary particle diameter) in phosphate-buffered saline (PBS) resulted in μm-sized agglomerates even after sonication. Since inhaled nanoparticles would come in contact with alveolar lining fluid, we hypothesized that one could collect diluted alveolar lining fluid by a single BAL of rat lungs and use this BAL fluid to suspend nanoparticles (23,24). Suspension of ultrafine carbon black in acellular BAL fluid resulted in a much improved dispersion of ultrafine carbon black with many structures in the submicrometer size (Fig. 2B). Better dispersion of nanoparticle suspensions had a dramatic effect on the biological activity of ultrafine carbon black in rat lungs 24 h after intratracheal instillation. Pulmonary exposure to ultrafine carbon black

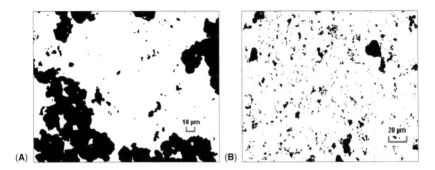

Figure 2 Dispersion of ultrafine carbon black. Ultrafine carbon black (Printex 90, 14 nm) was suspended in media and briefly sonicated (5 individual pulses) then viewed under a light microscope at ×40. (**A**) Suspension in PBS showing μm-sized agglomerates. (**B**) Suspension in bronchoalveolar lavage fluid, i.e., diluted lung lining fluid, showing substantially improved dispersion. *Abbreviation*: PBS, phosphate-buffered saline.

suspended in PBS caused a dose-dependent inflammatory response (PMN infiltration) 24 h postexposure (Fig. 3A). However, ultrafine carbon black suspended in BAL fluid was significantly more potent at doses ranging from 0.047 to 1.5 mg/rat. Maximum inflammation at 1.5 mg/rat was twofold greater for nanoparticles suspended in BAL fluid with an equivalent level of inflammation seen at a 16-fold lower dose of the well-dispersed carbon black compared to the nanoparticles suspended in PBS. Likewise, exposure of rat lungs to ultrafine carbon black suspended in PBS caused dose-dependent lung damage as indicated by elevated lactate dehydrogenase (LDH) activity in the BAL fluid (Fig. 3B). However, particles dispersed in BAL fluid were more cytotoxic at all exposure doses. Maximum cytotoxicity was 1.7-fold greater in the BAL fluid-dispersed nanoparticles with an equivalent level of toxicity seen at a 16-fold lower dose.

Improved dispersion of nanoparticles also alters the character as well as the magnitude of pulmonary response. Pharyngeal aspiration of SWCNT to mice resulted in granulomatous lesions at deposition sites of large agglomerates and interstitial fibrosis at sites containing more dispersed SWCNT structures (13). Mercer et al. (14) reported that when efforts are made to improve the dispersion of SWCNT the mean diameter of SWCNT agglomerates can be significantly decreased. In contrast to the initial study by Shvedova et al. (13), pharyngeal aspiration of mice with dispersed SWCNT did not result in granulomas while the potency in initiating diffuse interstitial fibrosis increased by at least fourfold (14).

In conclusion, there is support for the hypothesis that the high surface area of nanoparticles plays a significant role in their bioactivity. Evidence also exists that efforts to improve the dispersion of nanoparticles and decrease the size of agglomerates delivered to in vitro or in vivo test systems

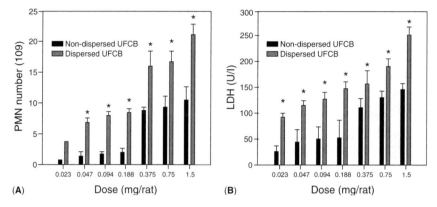

Figure 3 Pulmonary response to exposure to ultrafine carbon black. Rats were exposed to ultrafine carbon black by intratracheal instillation. (**A**) Inflammation was monitored by BAL PMN counts 24 h postexposure. (**B**) Toxicity was monitored by BAL LDH activity 24 h postexposure. Values are means ± SE of 5 experiments. * indicates that particles dispersed in BAL fluid produce a significantly greater pulmonary response than particles suspended in PBS. *Abbreviations*: BAL, bronchoalveolar lavage; LDH, lactate dehydrogenase; PBS, phosphate-buffered saline; PMN, polymorphonuclear.

increases the magnitude of response, and in the case of SWCNT alters the site and character of the pulmonary response. Therefore, efforts should be made to increase the dispersion of nanoparticles in the delivery vehicle for in vitro and in vivo exposure. Sager et al. (23,24) demonstrated the effectiveness of BAL fluid in dispersing nanoparticles and have reported that a mixture of disaturated phosphatidylcholine (DSPC) and protein, at levels found in BAL fluid, was also effective.

ROLE OF OXIDANT STRESS IN TOXICITY

Nel et al. (25), in a recent review of nanotoxicology, noted that oxidant generation by nanoparticles and resultant oxidant stress to cells is the "best developed paradigm for nanoparticle toxicity." Shvedova et al. (26) conducted a study on the effects of exposure of human bronchial epithelial cells (BEAS-2B) to unpurified SWCNT containing 30% iron by mass. Unpurified SWCNT-generated oxidant species in a cell-free system and hydroxyl (OH) radical in the presence of BEAS-2B cells, which served as a source of H_2O_2 to induce a Fenton reaction. Unpurified SWCNT were cytotoxic to BEAS-2B cells and addition of the iron chelator, deferoxamine, reversed both radical generation and cytotoxicity. The radical generation by unpurified SWCNT was associated with depletion of cell antioxidants and enhancement of lipid peroxidation in BEAS-2B cells, indicating that oxidant stress had occurred.

To further evaluate the hypothesis that oxidant generation and resultant oxidant stress were predictors of cytotoxicity, BEAS-2B cells were exposed to three types of engineered carbon nanoparticles, i.e., fullerenes, SWCNT produced by the HiPCO process, and SWCNT, i.e., LM-90, produced by the laser ablation method. The HiPCO SWCNT sample contained 30% iron by mass, while the LM-90 sample contained 20% nickel by mass. In these studies, the carbon nanoparticles were suspended in PBS and dispersed by sonication prior to use. Figure 4 shows TEM micrographs of HiPCO SWCNT (A), fullerenes (B), and LM-90 (C) in suspension. HiPCO SWCNT structures were loose networks of nanotubes with iron nanoparticles (arrows) bound to the nanotubes. LM-90 structure also appeared to be loose networks of nanotubes in suspension with nickel nanoparticles (arrows) bound to the nanotubes. Fullerenes formed agglomerates of widely variable diameters in suspension. Suspension of the carbon nanoparticles in PBS containing 1 mM H_2O_2 and 100 mM DMPO as a spin trap resulted in the generation of 'OH radical measured by electron spin resonance (ESR) spectroscopy. From the peak heights, the

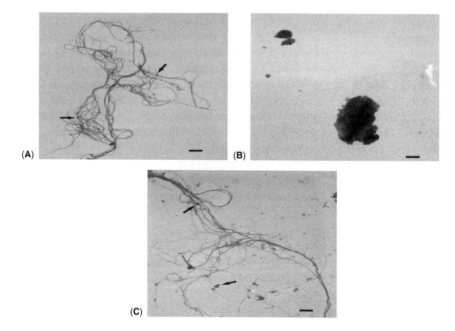

(A)

(B)

(C)

Figure 4 Structure of carbon nanoparticles in suspension. Particles were added to distilled H_2O and sonicated. Morphology of HiPCO SWCNT (**A**), fullerenes (**B**), or LM-90 (**C**) under TEM. Arrows indicate adherent iron (**A**) or nickel (**C**) nanoparticles identified by EDX. Scale bars are 200 nm. *Abbreviations*: EDX, HiPCO SWCNT, high-pressure carbon monoxide single-walled carbon nanotubes; TEM, transmission electron micrograph.

potency sequence for ˙OH generation was fullerenes >LM-90 > HiPCO SWCNT (Table 1). Exposure of BEAS-2B cells to these carbon nanoparticles ($8.5\,\mu g/cm^2$) caused oxidant stress, measured as a decline in cellular levels of glutathione (GSH). The potency sequence was HiPCO SWCNT $\approx$ LM-90 > fullerenes (Table 1). Exposure of BEAS-2B cells to these carbon nanoparticles ($8.5\,\mu g/cm^2$) caused a significant decrease in cell viability. The potency sequence was HiPCO SWCNT > fullerenes > LM-90 (Table 1).

In summary, the data indicate that carbon nanoparticles can generate reactive oxygen species, which results in oxidant stress and cytotoxicity. However, the relationship among these events is not simple in that radical generation of three types of carbon nanoparticles did not directly predict the degree of oxidant stress and these events did not directly predict the degree of cytotoxicity (Table 1). Therefore, other characteristics, such as agglomerate size or density of the agglomerates, may also contribute to bioactivity, interaction with the cell membrane, and/or uptake into the cells.

CONCLUSION

Concern that inhalation of engineered nanoparticles may have adverse pulmonary effects arises from the fact that, compared to coarse or fine particles, nanoparticles exhibit a high deposition in the conducting and respiratory zones of the lung. Once deposited, some nanoparticles may escape clearance by alveolar macrophages and enter the alveolar interstitium. There is some evidence that nanoparticles can migrate from the alveolar interstitium to the pulmonary capillary blood and translocate to systemic organs. Thus, systemic toxicity after pulmonary exposure is also an issue for further research. At present, two of the most promising mechanisms for the toxicity of nanoparticles involve their high surface area and the ability to generate reactive species and cause oxidant injury. Research is needed to determine whether these mechanisms are universally

Table 1   Effect of Different Nanoparticles on Viability, Glutathione Levels, and Oxidant Generation in BEAS-2B Cells ($8.50\,\mu g/cm^2$; 18 h)

Particle	Viability % of control	GSH % of control	˙OH generation average peak height
Fullerenes	$88.43 \pm 1.42^{a,b}$	91.02 ± 1.63^a	$116 \pm 6.821^{b,c}$
LM-90	93.664 ± 0.625^a	$71.35 \pm 0.84^{a,d}$	68.0 ± 7.0^c
SWCNT	$84.232 \pm 1.166^{a,b,d}$	$68.75 \pm 1.60^{a,d}$	42.50 ± 2.754

Note: Values are means $\pm$ SE of 3 experiments.
[a] $p < .05$ versus control.
[b] $p < .05$ versus LM-90.
[c] $p < .05$ versus control.
[d] $p < .05$ versus SWCNT.

predictive of cytotoxicity and pulmonary response. Clearly the effects of agglomeration, particle shape, particle coatings or surface groups, particle charge, etc. on bioactivity are issues requiring further investigation.

REFERENCES

1. Roco MC. Science and technology integration for increased human potential and societal outcomes. Ann N Y Acad Sci 2004; 1013:1–6.
2. Royal Society and Royal Academy of Engineering. Nanoscience and Nanotechnologies. London: Royal Society and Royal Academy of Engineering (accessed 2004 at http://www.nanotec.org.uk/FinalReport.htm).
3. Maynard AD, Baron PA, Foley M, et al. Exposure to carbon nanotube material: aerosol release during the handling of unrefined single-walled carbon nanotube material. J Toxicol Environ Health Part A 2004; 67:87–107.
4. International Commission on Radiological Protection. Human Respiratory Tract Model for Radiological Protection. Oxford: Elsevier Science, 1994. ICRP Publication 66, Ann ICRP 24(4).
5. Jarvis NS, Birchall A, James AC, et al. LUDEP 2.0 personal computer program for calculating internal doses using the ICRP publication 66 respiratory tract model. NRPB-SR287. Oxon, UK: National Radiological Protection Board, 1996.
6. International Commission on Radiological Protection. Supporting guidance 3, guide for the practical application of the ICRP human respiratory tract model. Ann ICRP 2002; 32:1–2.
7. Kreyling WG, Semmler M, Erbe F, et al. Minute translocation of inhaled ultrafine insoluble iridium particles from lung epithelium to extrapulmonary tissues. J Toxicol Environ Health Part A 2002; 65:1513–30.
8. Daigle CC, Chalupa DC, Gibb FR, et al. Ultrafine particle deposition in humans during rest and exercise. Inhal Toxicol 2003; 15:839–52.
9. Kreyling WC, Scheuch G. Clearance of particles deposited in the lungs. In: Gehr P, Heyder J, eds. Particle Lung Interaction. New York: Marcel Dekker, 2000:323–76.
10. Ferin J, Oberdorster G, Soderholm SC, et al. The rate of dose delivery affects pulmonary interstitialization of particles in rat. Ann Occup Hyg 1994; 38: 289–93.
11. Oberdorster G, Ferin J, Lehnert BE. Correlation between particle size, in vivo particle persistence and lung injury. Environ Health Perspect 1994; 102 (Suppl 15):173–9.
12. Roberts JR, Mercer RR, Young S-H, et al. Inflammation and fate of quantum dots following pulmonary treatment of rats. The Toxicol 2007; 96(1):A1112.
13. Shvedova AA, Kisin ER, Mercer R, et al. Unusual inflammatory and fibrogenic pulmonary responses to single-walled carbon nanotubes in mice. Am J Physiol: Lung Cell Mol Physiol 2005; 289:L698–708.
14. Mercer RR, Scabilloni JF, Wang L, et al. Dispersion significantly enhances the pulmonary toxicity of single-walled carbon nanotubes. The Toxicol 2007; 96(1):A1115.

15. Oberdorster G, Sharp Z, Atudorei V, et al. Extrapulmonary translocation of ultrafine carbon particles following whole-body inhalation exposure of rats. J Toxicol Environ Health Part A 2002; 65:1531–43.

16. Nemmar A, Vanbilloen H, Hoylaerts MF, et al. Passage of intratracheally instilled ultrafine particles from the lungs into systemic circulation in hamster. Am J Respir Crit Care Med 2002; 165:1671–2.

17. Stone PH, Godlesk JJ. First steps toward understanding the pathophysiologic link between air pollution and cardiac mortality. Am Heart J 1999; 138:804–7.

18. Li Z, Salmen R, Hulderman T, et al. Pulmonary exposure to carbon nanotubes induces vascular toxicity. The Toxicol 2005; 84:A1045.

19. Li Z, Salmen R, Hulderman T, et al. Pulmonary carbon nanotube exposure and oxidative status in vascular system. Free Radic Biol Med 2004; 37:S142.

20. Li Z, Chapman R, Hulderman T, et al. Relationship of pulmonary exposure to multiple doses of single wall carbon nanotubes and atherosclerosis in APOE–/– mouse model. The Toxicol 2006; 90:A1555.

21. Faux SP, Tran CL, Miller BG, et al. In vitro determinants of particulate toxicity: the dose metric for poorly soluble dusts. HSE Research Report 154, 2003.

22. Oberdorster G. Pulmonary effects of inhaled ultrafine particles. Int Arch Occup Environ Health 2001; 74:1–8.

23. Sager T, Robinson V, Porter D, et al. An improved method to prepare suspensions of nanoparticles for treatment of lung cells in culture or in vivo exposure by pharyngeal aspiration or intratracheal instillation. The Toxicol 2007; 6(1):A1120.

24. Sager TM, Porter DW, Robinson VA, et al. Improved method to disperse nanoparticles for in vitro and in vivo investigation of toxicity. Nanotoxicology 2007.

25. Nel A, Xia T, Madler L, et al. Toxic potential of materials at the nanolevel. Science 2006; 311:622–7.

26. Shvedova AA, Kisin E, Murray A, et al. Exposure of human bronchial epithelial cells to carbon nanotubes caused oxidative stress and cytotoxicity. Proceedings of the Society of Free Radical Research Meeting—European Section, Ioannina, Greece, June 26–29, 2003, 2004, 91–103.

15

Carbon Nanotube Exposure and Risk for Cardiovascular Effects

Petia P. Simeonova, Aaron Erdely, and Zheng Li

Tissue Injury Team, Toxicology and Molecular Biology Branch, Health Effects Laboratory Division, National Institute for Occupational Safety and Health, Morgantown, West Virginia, U.S.A.

INTRODUCTION

Engineered nanosized particles are new materials of emerging technological importance in different industries (1,2). The U.S. National Science Foundation estimated that millions of workers would be needed to support nanotechnology industries worldwide within 15 years. One direction of the nanomaterial industries is developing new carbon nanomaterials. Carbon atoms can be arranged into diverse geometries, forming a number of stable nanostructures. For example, a graphene sheet is rolled up, usually using a metal catalyst, to form a long single-walled carbon nanotube (SWCNT) with a diameter of ~1 nm. Bare carbon atoms can also be organized into spherical structures as fullerenes ("buckyballs"). The most stable and readily available fullerene is C_{60} having an average diameter of 0.72 nm. In addition to these single layer structures, large nanotubes and fullerenes can also be synthesized forming multiwalled nanotubes (MWNT) or onion-like clusters, respectively (3). Fullerenes, because of their strong electronegativity, can be combined with metals and other molecules to form metallofullerenes.

From the carbon nanomaterials, SWCNT recently elicited a great deal of interest due to their unique electronic and mechanical properties. SWCNT can be metallic or semiconducting thus offering amazing possibilities to create a broad spectrum of nanoelectronic devices as well as composite materials with extraordinary features (4,5). Global revenues from CNT in 2006 are estimated at—US \$230 million, which provides potential for workplace and general exposure (6). Concerns have been raised over occupational SWCNT exposure because adverse effects related to lung deposition have been found in the first animal studies.

Nanotechnologies will influence significantly our life but they also pose important toxicological questions that are related to the unique nature of materials and processes at the nanometer scale. Human contact with nanomaterials can be related to targeted exposure through therapeutics and cosmetics or untargeted exposure through occupational and environmental contamination. The most attractive features of nanomaterials including their small size, large surface area, and reactivity might also be the main factors for their toxicity. In this regard, nanomaterials, specifically nanoparticles, hypothetically can induce not only damage at the penetration site but can lead to unexpected distant responses, involving the immune system, cardiovascular system, liver, kidney, and brain, as a result of their reactivity and/or translocation through the body. The exposure may induce or modify the progression of existing pathophysiological conditions including cardiovascular diseases. Our research efforts are currently directed to evaluate the cardiovascular effects, including vascular inflammation, blood cell coagulation status, atherosclerosis, as well as the related molecular mechanisms associated with respiratory exposure to different types of nanosized materials using animal and cellular models.

SWCNT TOXICITY STUDIES

Several studies evaluated the potential pulmonary toxicity of SWCNTs (7–9). All three studies demonstrated that SWCNT induce pulmonary toxicity, which is different than this induced by graphite. SWCNTs accumulate as agglomerates in the lung, followed by granuloma formation and fibrotic reaction. Inflammatory responses as a result of SWCNT lung deposition are reported in some of these studies (7,9).

The unique physical characteristics (shape, size, surface area) and the metal impurities of the SWCNT as well as the pulmonary toxicity are major predictors for potential cardiovascular injury. The generation of reactive oxygen species in the lung, may result in release of mediators into the circulation leading to impaired endothelial as well as blood cell homeostasis (coagulation activation). Furthermore, SWCNTs may penetrate into the circulatory system and induce direct vascular toxicity. All stages of atherosclerosis can be modified by oxidative stress and inflammation. In addition to the well-established cardiovascular risk factors, such as high cholesterol levels, diabetes mellitus, and hypertension, many nontraditional risk factors, including concomitant infections, systemic autoimmune diseases, and chemical exposure, have been suggested to influence atherosclerotic process through these mechanisms and precipitate disease complications (10–12). In this respect, epidemiological and experimental studies have recently found a positive association between particulate matter in air pollution and adverse cardiovascular outcomes (13–16). The potential of SWCNT respiratory exposure to induce systemic effects related to cardiovascular diseases was evaluated in several model systems summarized below.

SWCNT CARDIOVASCULAR EFFECTS

In Vitro Data Related to Oxidative Potential

Oxidative modification of low-density lipoprotein (LDL) particles is a dominant hypothesis of atherogenesis (17–19). Oxidized LDL particles are readily taken by macrophage scavenger receptors, leading to "foam cell" formation (macrophage loading with lipids), an obligatory step in atheroma development. Bioactive lipids derived from LDL oxidation can also modulate intracellular signal transduction and expression of genes coding inflammatory mediators and adhesion molecules (20–22). Consistent with the "LDL oxidative-modification hypothesis" of atherosclerosis, free transition metal ions, such as copper and iron, have been shown to stimulate the lipoprotein oxidation by vascular cells in vitro (23). We tested whether SWCNTs induce oxidation of human plasma LDL, measured as malondialdehyde (MDA) formation, in presence of human aortic endo-thelial cells (HAECs). As demonstrated in Figure 1, unpurified SWCNTs dose-dependently while purified SWCNTs only in the highest tested concentration-induced LDL oxidation. This demonstrated that at least in vitro metal impurities of SWCNTs augment LDL oxidation.

In Vivo Data Related to Oxidative Effects

The vessel wall is normally composed of an endothelial cell lining on a medial layer of vascular-smooth muscle cells and enwrapped by an adventitial layer of connective tissue. The endothelial cells provide the transduction of signals in the microenvironment between the blood and vessel wall, and they orchestrate the homeostatic balance of the vessels by production of mediators regulating vascular tone, coagulation status, cell death, and inflammatory cell trafficking. The disruption or activation of endothelial cells leads to series of events including vasoconstriction, increased adhesion molecule expression resulting in leukocyte adhesion and inflammatory cell infiltration and platelet-thrombus formation (10,23). Endothelial cell dysfunction is associated with an alteration of the cellular oxidative state. We applied several approaches to screen for

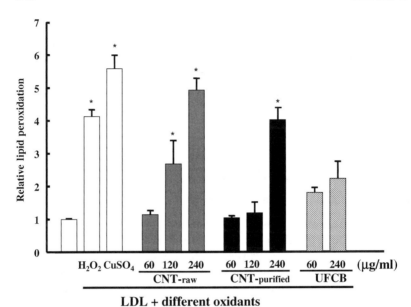

Figure 1 Evaluation of LDL oxidation in HAECs. The cells were cultured in serum-free medium containing 200 mg/mL LDL for 3 h. CuSO₄ (20 μM), H₂O₂ (250 μM) used as positive controls or the tested compounds including SWCNTs unpurified, SWCNT purified, ultrafine carbon black (UFCB) were simultaneously added. The oxidation state of LDL was assayed by the determination of MDA formation and the results presented as a fold increases from the control (LDL). Each value represents the mean ± of four cultures. *p < .001. *Abbreviations*: HAEC, human aortic endothelial cell; LOL, low-density lipoprotein; MDA, malondialdehyde; SWCNT, single-walled carbon nanotube.

systemic oxidative effects of SWCNT pulmonary exposure (24). First, the activation of HO-1 gene expression, a biomarker of oxidative stress (25), was evaluated using Ho1-luc reporter mice; second, mitochondrial homeostasis, a sensitive marker of oxidative insults (26), was evaluated by measuring mitochondrial DNA damage, protein oxidation, and glutathione levels in C57BL/6 mice. Based on these assays we demonstrated that exposure to purified SWCNT in doses ranging between 10 and 40 μg/mouse by single intrapharyngeal instillation induces cardiovascular-oxidative modifications including mitochondrial perturbations. Mitochondria have been reported to be highly susceptible to oxidative stress, mediated by metabolic defects and environmental insults (26,27) and mitochondrial dysfunction is emerging as an important pathophysiological factor in a number of cardiovascular diseases including atherosclerosis (26,28).

ATHEROMA FORMATION

Since there is a strong link between oxidation and atherosclerosis, the effect of SWCNT on atherosclerosis progression was evaluated in ApoE–/– transgenic mice, a widely used model of human atherosclerosis. Recently, we characterized the application of this experimental model for studying the role of metals in atherosclerosis (29). Interestingly, the findings supported the epidemiological data linking arsenic exposure and atherosclerosis. To evaluate SWCNT effects on atherosclerosis progression, ApoE–/– mice were exposed by pharyngeal aspiration to SWCNT (20 µg/mouse) via multiple exposures (once every other week for 8 weeks). Although SWCNT exposure did not alter lipid profiles, ApoE–/– mice had exacerbated plaque development in the aorta and brachiocephalic arteries (24). The histopathology, including granulomas resulting from agglomerated SWCNT, fibrotic tissue in the granulomas and along the small SWCNT-depositions (more dispersed material), in the lung of the ApoE–/– mice were similar to previously described pulmonary alterations in C57BL/6 mice exposed to a single dose of SWCNT (9).

CONCLUSION/HYPOTHESIS

Overall, these initial studies demonstrate that respiratory exposure to high concentrations, mostly agglomerated, SWCNTs provokes not only pulmonary toxicity but vascular effects related to mitochondrial oxidative modifications and accelerated atheroma formation. Pulmonary exposure to SWCNT may induce cardiovascular effects either directly or indirectly through mitochondrial oxidative perturbations, which can result in altered vessel homeostasis (Fig. 2).

It is possible that individual SWCNTs can translocate from the lung into the systemic circulation causing direct cardiovascular endothelial damage. It has been reported that nanoparticles treated with albumin and/or surfactant proteins cross the alveolocapillary barrier to gain access to the systemic circulation (30,31). The proximity between epithelial type I and endothelial cell caveolar membrane structures might play a role in the particle translocation mechanisms (32). Since the SWCNT are not well recognized and cleared by lung macrophages (9,33), nanotubes, dispersed or disintegrated from the agglomerates, may persist in the alveolar space, which will facilitate their access into the systemic circulation. Behavior and fate of SWCNTs have been addressed only in several pharmacokinetic studies evaluating the body distribution of the material after injection for the purposes of biomedical application development (34,35). These studies applied water-soluble SWCNTs (functionalized in the first two or covered with an artificial surfactant in the last reference) and did not find acute toxicity or adverse reactions. The SWCNTs have been traced by linking

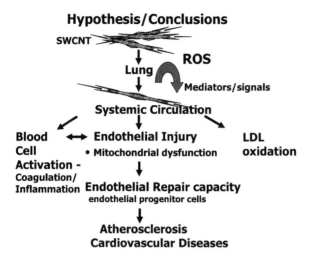

Figure 2 Diagram of possible mechanisms of cardiovascular effects related to SWCNT respiratory exposure. *Abbreviations*: LOL, low-density lipoprotein; ROS, reactive oxygen species; SWCNT, single-walled carbon nanotube.

them covalently or noncovalently to external fluorophores or chelated radioisotopes (34). Cherukuri et al. (35) applied near-infrared fluorescence technique to monitor SWCNT with sensitivity high enough to detect a single intracellular nanotube. This method might find an application for evaluation of SWCNT distribution in the experimental settings simulating occupational paradigm of exposure and to provide insights the partition of single tubes from the lung into the systemic circulation.

Indirect processes are also possible to play a role in the cardiovascular effects induced by SWCNT exposure. Increased circulating cytokine levels (e.g., IL-6, IL-8, IL-1β, GM-CSF) have been found in humans with pulmonary inflammation due to chronic obstructive pulmonary disease (COPD), asbestos, zinc oxide, particulate matter exposure, and endotoxin (36–38). Although SWCNT exposure was associated with atherosclerosis acceleration, significant differences in the plasma levels of IL-6, IL-10, MCP-1, TNF-α, and IFN-γ were not observed although more acute effects cannot be ruled out (24). If unpurified SWCNTs are deposited in the lung, chronic inflammation in the lung as well as systemic circulation might be triggered. In addition to low inflammation, recently it has been suggested that inefficient metabolism in blood vessels as a result of ischemic events can cause vascular diseases through mitochondrial dysfunction (39). Mediators, released from the lung into the systemic circulation or ischemic events, associated with altered pulmonary function seen after SWCNT exposure, may lead to vascular-oxidative modifications.

A third hypothesis for SWCNT exposure-mediated cardiovascular effects is through platelet activation in the lung circulation. The pulmonary circulation is considered a site for platelet maturation (40,41) and recently, it has been demonstrated that SWCNT can directly stimulate platelet aggregation in vitro (42). Furthermore, transforming growth factor β 1 (TGFβ1), which is involved in platelet activation (43), was found to be significantly increased in the lung of SWCNT-treated mice (9) and the time course of its increase paralleled the occurrence of cardiovascular mitochondrial dysfunction.

In addition to induction of endothelial dysfunction, SWCNT exposure directly or indirectly may affect the bone marrow capacity to provide endothelial progenitor cells (EPCs) for endothelium repair mechanisms (44,45). The number of circulating EPCs has been shown to correlate negatively with several established cardiovascular risk factors such as aging, chronic hypercholesterolemia, increased plasma C-reactive protein levels (46,47). Although the mechanisms of EPC depletion are not understood, it is speculated that inflammation/oxidative stress may directly influence the mobilization/properties of EPCs and/or lead to the exhaustion of their bone marrow pool.

Most recently, studies have shown that circulating peripheral blood cells, which come into contact with all tissue and contribute to homeostasis, are valuable sources of information on the state of health or disease in the body. For example, human coronary artery disease as well as cancer has been approached using blood cell transcripts (48). Blood gene expression studies can provide evaluation of many genes and the analysis of these data can reveal clusters of biomarker genes that signify a healthy or diseased state, or to predict exposure-related outcomes. This information can help in prediction of nanoparticle exposure-related cardiovascular outcomes.

Studies in progress, involving labeled SWCNT as well as detailed analysis of the role of lung platelet activation, bone marrow EPCs, and blood cell gene transcripts will provide more insight the mechanisms of the cardiovascular perturbations in SWCNT-treated animals. The current studies demonstrate that evaluation for systemic effects in parallel with pulmonary toxicity studies provides more complete toxicological information, which will help in predicting the risk and development of safety regulations for the nanomaterial production and use.

DISCLAIMER

The findings and conclusions in this report are those of the author(s) and do not necessarily represent the views of the National Institute for Occupational Safety and Health.

ABBREVIATIONS

BCA   brachiocephalic artery
HO-1   heme oxygenase-1
IFN-γ interferon γ
IL-6   interleukin 6
IL-12   interleukin 12
LDL   low-density lipoprotein
MCP-1   monocyte chemoattractant protein 1
MDA   malondialdehyde
MtDNA   mitochondrial DNA
SWCNT   single-walled carbon nanotubes
TNF-α tumor necrosis factor α
VCAM-1   vascular cell adhesion molecule 1
UfCB   ultrafine carbon black

REFERENCES

1. Colvin VL. The potential environmental impact of engineered nanomaterials. Nat Biotechnol 2003; 21:1166–70.
2. Hood E. Nanotechnology: looking as we leap. Environ Health Perspect 2004; 112:A740–9.
3. Park KH, Chhowalla M, Iqbal Z, et al. Single-walled carbon nanotubes are a new class of ion channel blockers. J Biol Chem 2003; 278:50212–6.
4. Sinnott SB, Andrews R. Carbon nanotubes: synthesis, properties, and applications. Crit Rev Solid State Mater Sci 2001; 26:145–249.
5. Subramoney S. Novel nanocarbons—structure, properties, and potential applications. Adv Mater 1998; 10:1157–71.
6. Donaldson K, Aitken R, Tran L, et al. Carbon nanotubes: a review of their properties in relation to pulmonary toxicology and workplace safety. Toxicol Sci 2006; 92:5–22.
7. Lam CW, James JT, McCluskey R, et al. Pulmonary toxicity of single-wall carbon nanotubes in mice 7 and 90 days after intratracheal instillation. Toxicol Sci 2004; 77:126–34.
8. Warheit DB, Laurence BR, Reed KL, et al. Comparative pulmonary toxicity assessment of single-wall carbon nanotubes in rats. Toxicol Sci 2004; 77:117–25.
9. Shvedova AA, Kisin ER, Mercer R, et al. Unusual inflammatory and fibrogenic pulmonary responses to single-walled carbon nanotubes in mice. Am J Physiol Lung Cell Mol Physiol 2005; 289:L698–708.
10. Libby P. Coronary artery injury and the biology of atherosclerosis: inflammation, thrombosis, and stabilization. Am J Cardiol 2000; 86:3J–8.
11. Ross R. Atherosclerosis is an inflammatory disease. Am Heart J 1999; 138: S419–20.
12. Simeonova PP, Luster MI. Arsenic and atherosclerosis. Toxicol Appl Pharmacol 2004; 198:444–9.

13. Brook RD, Franklin B, Cascio W, et al. Air pollution and cardiovascular disease: a statement for healthcare professionals from the Expert Panel on Population and Prevention Science of the American Heart Association. Circulation 2004; 109:2655–71.

14. Kunzli N, Jerrett M, Mack WJ, et al. Ambient air pollution and atherosclerosis in Los Angeles. Environ Health Perspect 2005; 113:201–6.

15. Peters A, Von KS, Heier M, et al. Exposure to traffic and the onset of myocardial infarction. N Engl J Med 2004; 351:1721–30.

16. Pope CA III, Burnett RT, Thurston GD, et al. Cardiovascular mortality and long-term exposure to particulate air pollution: epidemiological evidence of general pathophysiological pathways of disease. Circulation 2004; 109:71–7.

17. Steinberg D, Parthasarathy S, Carew TE, et al. Beyond cholesterol. Modifications of low-density lipoprotein that increase its atherogenicity. N Engl J Med 1989; 320:915–24.

18. Daugherty A, Roselaar SE. Lipoprotein oxidation as a mediator of atherogenesis: insights from pharmacological studies. Cardiovasc Res 1995; 29: 297–311.

19. Mertens A, Holvoet P. Oxidized LDL and HDL: antagonists in atherothrombosis. FASEB J 2001; 15:2073–84.

20. Kita T, Kume N, Minami M, et al. Role of oxidized LDL in atherosclerosis. Ann N Y Acad Sci 2001; 947:199–205; discussion 205–196.

21. Chen K, Thomas SR, Keaney JF. Beyond LDL oxidation: ROS in vascular signal transduction. Free Radic Biol Med 2003; 35:117–32.

22. Harrison D, Griendling KK, Landmesser U, et al. Role of oxidative stress in atherosclerosis. Am J Cardiol 2003; 91:7A–11.

23. Cai H, Harrison DG. Endothelial dysfunction in cardiovascular diseases: the role of oxidant stress. Circ Res 2000; 87:840–4.

24. Li Z, Hulderman T, Salmen R, et al. Cardiovascular effects of pulmonary exposure to single-wall carbon nanotubes. Environ Health Perspect 2006; 115(3):377–382.

25. Prawan A, Kundu JK, Surh AJ. Molecular basis of heme oxygenase-1 induction: implications for chemoprevention and chemoprotection. Antioxid Redox Signal 2005; 7:1688–703.

26. Ballinger SW. Mitochondrial dysfunction in cardiovascular disease. Free Radic Biol Med 2005; 38:1278–95.

27. Madamanchi NR, Vendrov A, Runge MS. Oxidative stress and vascular disease. Arterioscler Thromb Vasc Biol 2005; 25:29–38.

28. Binkova B, Strejc P, Boubelik O, et al. DNA adducts and human atherosclerotic lesions. Int J Hyg Environ Health 2001; 204:49–54.

29. Simeonova PP, Hulderman T, Harki D, et al. Arsenic exposure accelerates atherogenesis in apolipoprotein E(–/–) mice. Environ Health Perspect 2003; 111:1744–8.

30. Kato T, Yashiro T, Murata Y, et al. Evidence that exogenous substances can be phagocytized by alveolar epithelial cells and transported into blood capillaries. Cell Tissue Res 2003; 311:47–51.

31. Oberdörster G, Oberdörster E, Oberdörster J. Nanotoxicology: an emerging discipline evolving from studies of ultrafine particles. Environ Health Perspect 2005; 113:823–39.

32. Heckel K, Kiefmann R, Dorger M, Stoeckelhuber M, Goetz AE. Colloidal gold particles as a new in vivo marker of early acute lung injury. Am J Physiol Lung Cell Mol Physiol 2004; 287:L867–78.

33. Kagan VE, Tyurina YY, Tyurin VA, et al. Direct and indirect effects of single walled carbon nanotubes on RAW 264.7 macrophages: role of iron. Toxicol Lett 2006; 165:88–100.

34. Singh R, Pantarotto D, Lacerda L, et al. Tissue biodistribution and blood clearance rates of intravenously administered carbon nanotube radiotracers. PNAS 2006; 103:3357–62.

35. Cherukuri P, Gannon CJ, Leeuw TK, et al. Mammalian pharmacokinetics of carbon nanotubes using intrinsic near-infrared fluorescence. PNAS 2006; 103:18882–6.

36. Agusti AG, Noguera A, Sauleda J, et al. Systemic effects of chronic obstructive pulmonary disease. Eur Respir J 2003; 21:347–60.

37. van Eeden SF, Tan WC, Suwa T, et al. Cytokines involved in the systemic inflammatory response induced by exposure to particulate matter air pollutants (PM(10)). Am J Respir Crit Care Med 2001; 164:826–30.

38. Copeland S, Warren HS, Lowry SF, et al. Acute inflammatory response to endotoxin in mice and humans. Clin Diagn Lab Immunol 2005; 12:60–7.

39. Bernal-Mizrachi C, Gates AC, Weng S, et al. Vascular respiratory uncoupling increases blood pressure and atherosclerosis. Nature 2005; 435:502–6.

40. Martin JF, Slater DN, Trowbridge EA. Abnormal intrapulmonary platelet production: a possible cause of vascular and lung disease. Lancet 1983; 1:793–6.

41. O'Sullivan BP, Michelson AD. The inflammatory role of platelets in cystic fibrosis. Am J Respir Crit Care Med 2006; 173:483–90.

42. Radomski A, Jurasz P, Onso-Escolano D, et al. Nanoparticle-induced platelet aggregation and vascular thrombosis. Br J Pharmacol 2005; 146:882–93.

43. Hoying JB, Yin M, Diebold R, et al. Transforming growth factor beta1 enhances platelet aggregation through a non-transcriptional effect on the fibrinogen receptor. J Biol Chem 1999; 274:31008–13.

44. Hill JM, Zalos G, Halcox JP, et al. Circulating endothelial progenitor cells, vascular function, and cardiovascular risk. N Engl J Med 2003; 348:593–600.

45. Khakoo AY, Finkel T. Endothelial progenitor cells. Annu Rev Med 2005; 56: 79–101.

46. Rauscher FM, Goldschmidt-Clermont PJ, Davis BH, et al. Aging, progenitor cell exhaustion, and atherosclerosis. Circulation 2003; 108:457–63.

47. Verma S, et al. C-reactive protein attenuates endothelial progenitor cell survival, differentiation, and function: further evidence of a mechanistic link between C-reactive protein and cardiovascular disease. Circulation 2004; 109(17):2058–67.

48. Gibbons GH, Liew CC, Goodarzi MO, et al. Genetic markers: progress and potential for cardiovascular disease. Circulation 2004; 109(25 Suppl 1): IV47–58.

16

Hemostatic and Thrombotic Effects of Particulate Exposure: Assessing the Mechanisms

Peter H.M. Hoet

Unit of Lung Toxicology,
Laboratorium of Pneumology, K.U. Leuven, Leuven, Belgium

Abderrahim Nemmar

Department of Physiology, College of
Medicine & Health, Sultan Qaboos University, Al-Khod, Sultanate of Oman

Benoit Nemery

Unit of Lung Toxicology, Laboratorium of Pneumology, K.U. Leuven,
Leuven, Belgium

Marc Hoylaerts

Center for Molecular and Vascular Biology, K.U. Leuven, Leuven, Belgium

INTRODUCTION

This chapter provides an overview of the most important findings concerning cardiopulmonary effects of (inhaled) particle matter (PM). In the second part the focus is on techniques successfully used in studies on the mechanisms of particle-induced atherothrombosis.

AIR POLLUTION—NANOPARTICLES AND CARDIOPULMONARY EFFECTS

Background

It has been known for many years that episodes of air pollution could be responsible for increases in morbidity and mortality (1). Several epidemiological studies have reported associations between urban air pollution and cardiopulmonary morbidity and mortality (reviewed by Brunekreef and Holgate (2) and Pope and Dockery (3)). Most studies reporting the health effects of inhaled particulate matter concentrate on the short-term (acute) changes in exposure. It has been shown that acute increases in outdoor air pollution are associated with increases in daily deaths and hospitalizations for cardiovascular conditions, including acute myocardial infarction. These data suggest that peak exposures *trigger* clinical manifestations of cardiorespiratory disease. Besides the acute effect studies, a limited number of long-term exposure studies have demonstrated an association between chronic exposure to urban air pollution and an increased risk of cardiovascular mortality and morbidity. This observation suggests that chronic exposure to particulate matter influences the *progression* of atherosclerosis.

During the past decades, a large body of epidemiological studies linking particulate air pollution and increased cardiovascular morbidity and mortality have been reported (2,3). Numerous time-series studies, including our recent analysis of data from Flanders (4), have shown associations between short-term increases in particulate matter with a diameter equal to or lower than 10 μm (PM_{10}) and daily mortality, even at relatively low concentrations of air pollutants (5–7). These epidemiological observations have indicated that particulate air pollution not only exerts respiratory effects, but also increases cardiovascular morbidity and mortality (8). In fact, more people die from cardiovascular than from pulmonary diseases during episodes of urban air pollution (9). A growing number of epidemiological and clinical studies support the concept that components of the cardiovascular system are affected by particulate air pollutants (10,11). Thus, increases in PM have been associated with increased plasma viscosity (12), changes in blood parameters such as fibrinogen levels or red blood cell counts (13), arterial vasoconstriction (14), increased heart rate (15), elevated systolic blood pressure (16), and decreased heart rate variability (11). These effects can be responsible for pathophysiological changes in cardiac function, such as reported in PM-related exacerbations in patients with ischemic heart disease (17), cardiac arrhythmias (18), and congestive heart failure (19).

Studies on the effects of long-term (chronic) exposure to air pollution are less numerous. The Harvard Six Cities Studies (20) was the first longitudinal study to document an adverse effect of chronic exposure to urban air pollution on mortality. Later, Pope et al. (21) concluded that for every $10\,\mu g/m^3$ increase in fine particles ($PM_{2.5}$), mortality increased by 6% annually and cardiopulmonary mortality by 9%. Larger risks of (fatal and nonfatal) cardiovascular events were found in a recently published study of more than 65,000 postmenopausal women followed up for 6 years (22). Künzli et al. (23) studied the association between long-term exposure to

$PM_{2.5}$ and carotid intima-media thickness in subjects living in different areas of Los Angeles. Those living in the areas with the highest annual mean concentrations of ambient $PM_{2.5}$ had an increased intima-media thickness.

An important feature of the epidemiological associations between air pollution and morbidity or mortality is that the acute adverse effects appear to be most marked in people with preexisting compromised cardiovascular function. This increased risk is particularly apparent in at-risk populations such as those with underlying cardiovascular disease or risk factors such as high cholesterol level, diabetes mellitus, hypertension, previous myocardial infarction, atherosclerosis, and heart failure (23–29).

This aspect has only recently started to be investigated experimentally. It has been shown that spontaneously hypertensive rats exhibited greater pulmonary vascular leakage and oxidative stress than healthy normotensive rats after inhalation of residual oil fly ash particles (30). With respect to atherosclerosis, two studies have assessed, in Watanabe heritable hyperlipidemic rabbits, naturally developing atherosclerotic plaques, the possibility that the increased levels of circulating inflammatory mediators induced by PM cause progression and instability of atherosclerosis (31,32). These studies showed that 4 weeks of exposure of these animals to ambient particles induced a local inflammatory response in the lung, a systemic inflammatory response including stimulation of the bone marrow, and caused progression of atherosclerosis in both the aorta and coronary arteries (31,32). More recently, Sun et al. have shown, in an $apoE^{-/-}$ mouse model, that long-term exposure to relevant concentrations of $PM_{2.5}$ altered vasomotor tone, induced vascular inflammation, and potentiated atherosclerosis (33).

The epidemiological and clinical studies have mainly investigated the link between PM_{10} or $PM_{2.5}$ and cardiovascular morbidity and mortality, but recent evidence (essentially from experimental studies) suggests that the ultrafine fraction of these particles (UFPs) shows more toxicity. These particles are formed by condensation of hot vapor from combustion sources or can be produced as nanoparticles. It has been generally accepted that most of the particles of this size are relatively short-lived and grow into larger particles, but they may remain suspended for up to several weeks in the air. Such very small particles have a high chance of deposition in the gas-exchanging (alveolar) part of the lung, and in addition, they have a larger surface area than larger sized particles, thus having a higher potential for interactions with biological targets and causing a greater inflammatory response (34–36). A large part of UFPs in the environment are emitted from combustion engines (e.g., diesel-powered engines) and other high-temperature processes in the form of fractal-like aggregates composed of solid nanoparticles (37). It has been established that more than 100,000 particles per cm^3 may be found in the vicinity of a busy road (38). Many concepts derived from studies of the toxicity of ultrafine particles in air pollution have given rise to concerns about the hazards of engineered nanoparticles (39–41).

Although recent advances have been made to try and understand the extrapulmonary effects of particulate pollution, we are still far away from a complete experimental verification—biological plausibility—of the cardiovascular effects of current levels of particle pollutants. Moreover, solid experimental data are also needed to improve the risk assessment process that should lead, together with good epidemiological data, to scientifically valid standards for the protection of public health.

Proposed Mechanisms

One line of investigation is that inhaled particles may affect the autonomic nervous system, and thus cause perturbations in heart rhythm (11,42). Two other, complementary, hypotheses have been proposed to explain the cardiovascular effects of PM. The first hypothesis is based on the occurrence of pulmonary inflammation, leading to the release of mediators, which may influence platelets, coagulation, or other cardiovascular endpoints (13,43). The second hypothesis is that some particles translocate from the lungs into the systemic circulation and thus, directly or indirectly, influence haemostasis or cardiovascular integrity. In studies investigating the latter two hypotheses, several methods, normally used in the clinical environment, have examined platelet activation and blood clotting in blood of laboratory animals (44).

Effect of Particles on Thrombogenesis

Thrombogenesis has been used as a relevant cardiovascular endpoint to study the effects of particulate matter. Nemmar et al. (45–48) used a hamster model in which a local endothelial lesion is produced by a photochemical reaction (produced by light activation of Rose Bengal) in a peripheral vessel, and hence a (venous or arterial) thrombus is formed, which can be followed online and quantitated by image analysis (49). The developed thrombi are platelet-rich, and they resemble clinical thrombi, as shown by electron microscopic analysis (50). Thus, by combining transillumination and photochemical vessel wall injury, it has become possible to link the degree of vessel wall injury with the intensity of thrombosis that develops as a consequence of endothelial cell injury.

Commercially available polystyrene particles of 60 nm diameter were used in these studies as a model of UFPs (45). These offered the advantage of being well-characterized and chemically relatively inert, and it was possible to investigate the effects of surface modification by comparing particles with neutral, negative or positive surface charges. Intravenous injection of such ultrafine particles affected haemostasis, dependent on the surface properties of the particles. Thus, positively charged (amine-modified) particles led to a marked increase in prothrombotic tendency resulting, at least in part, from platelet activation (45), as demonstrated by platelet aggregation in vitro and strongly increased the adenosine diphosphate (ADP)-triggered aggregation in a dose-dependent manner. In subsequent experiments using i.t. administration, a neutrophil influx in the lung was found and similar effects on thrombosis were obtained 1 h after the instillation of ultrafine positively charged polystyrene particles (60 nm) (46). Larger particulates (400-nm positive particles) also caused pulmonary inflammation, but they did not enhance in vivo thrombosis at all after intratracheal instillation, within 1 h. These findings indicate that the enhanced thrombotic complications at 1 h cannot be solely explained by pulmonary inflammation but that a direct passage of UFPs and activation of circulating platelets probably contributes to the observed extrapulmonary peripheral thrombotic effects.

Subsequently, Silva et al. (51) assessed, in a rat model of ear vein thrombosis, the effect of intravenous and intratracheal administration of amine- and carboxylate-modified polystyrene of similar diameter, resulting in comparable effects. Similarly, Khandoga et al. (52) observed that intra-arterial injection of ultrafine carbon particles led to prothrombotic changes in mice. Using the same hamster model Nemmar et al. (47) showed that diesel exhaust particles (DEP), given intratracheally, caused a dose-dependent enhancement of peripheral venous and arterial thrombosis within an hour after their deposition in the lungs.

Ex vivo, i.e., in blood samples collected from hamsters i.t. instilled with DEP, platelet activation was apparent 30 min after instillation as measured with the platelet function analyzer (PFA-100). The addition of DEP to hamster blood in vitro caused platelet activation within 5 min with as little as 0.5 µg of DEP/mL (47), indicating a central role for platelets in particulate-dependent thrombogenesis.

Histamine levels have been correlated with the onset of myocardial infarction (53–55), but the evidence linking exposure to DEP and release of histamine is not straightforward. Thus, an increase in mast cell numbers in the submucosa and elevated BAL histamine levels were observed, in humans, 6 h after exposure to DEP (56). DEP have also been demonstrated to directly degranulate mast cells and to increase histamine levels and symptom severity in humans (57,58). Our laboratory measured histamine, both in the respiratory tract and in the peripheral circulation, at different time points (1, 6, and 24 h) after i.t. instillation of DEP, and investigated pulmonary inflammation and vascular thrombosis following pretreatment with a histamine receptor-1 blocking agent (diphenhydramine). Pretreatment with diphenhydramine attenuated both pulmonary inflammation and the prothrombotic effect at 6 and 24 h, but at 1 h only pulmonary inflammation was diminished whereas platelet activation and the enhancement of thrombosis were not affected (59). In another study it was shown, 24 h after DEP exposure, that pretreatment with dexamethasone or with cromoglycate blocked the DEP-induced pulmonary inflammation, prothrombotic events and histamine release in BAL and plasma. This possibly means that the systemic inflammatory and prothrombotic effects observed 24 h after DEP administration are secondary to lung inflammation, and that they can be prevented by mast cell stabilization (60). No increased level of plasma von Willebrand factor (vWF), which is a marker of endothelial activation, after DEP administration was found (60,61). This apparent absence of endothelial effects may have been due to the short-term nature (max. 24h) of the experimental protocol in these studies.

Conclusions

From the large pool of data it can be suggested that the relationship between inhaled particles and cardiovascular morbidity and mortality is causal. Unfortunately, the biologic plausibility behind these associations has not yet been fully revealed (8). Currently, three different research lines are being followed to explain the epidemiological observations (41,44). Two hypotheses are, generally spoken, based on particle-induced changes in hemostasis or cardiovascular integrity. In exploring these changes, the use of sophisticated techniques, describing the effect of coagulation factors, platelets activity and/or general hemostasis, is needed. A few of these techniques are described in the following section.

ASSESSING THE ATHEROTHROMBOTIC EFFECTS

Atherothrombosis and the Role of Platelets

Platelets (primary haemostasis) and the coagulation cascade (secondary haemostasis) both play a central role in atherothrombosis, and therefore are good targets in the study of the effects of inhaled particles on hemostasis (see reviews (8,44,62)). The whole process of atherothrombosis is complex; below a brief description is given, highlighting only the most important steps— stages (63,64).

Platelet Adhesion

In nonhemostatic (normal) conditions, platelets are at rest and flow through blood vessels without interacting with any other cells or each other. Upon vessel damage, platelets adhere within seconds to the subendothelium. The most important factors inducing this adhesion are the constituents of the exposed subendothelium: collagen, vWF, fibronectin, laminin, and thrombospondin, of which collagen and vWF are the most important ones, interacting with $\alpha_2\beta$, GPVI, and the GPIb membrane complex, respectively.

Platelet Activation, Promotion of Coagulation and Aggregation

The adherent platelet changes its shape and this is accompanied by biochemical changes. Finally the hemispherical-shaped platelet—with a large surface area—is strongly anchored to the artery wall. This process is known as platelet activation and is reversible during the early phase.

The activated platelets synthesise and release platelet-activating substances such as ADP, serotonin, and thromboxane A2 in association with enhanced surface expression of $\alpha_{IIb}\beta_3$. Circulating agonists such as thromboxane A2, ADP, α-thrombin and epinephrine, bind to adherent and freshly recruited platelets and synergistically induce their activation. Thus, platelet activation is amplified by several feedback pathways.

Another important level of regulation in hemostasis is the coagulation cascade, resulting from the stepwise activation of coagulation factors, and formation of insoluble fibrin, stabilizing the growing thrombus via cross-links between adjacent platelets.

The coagulation cascade initiates when tissue factor (TF), e.g., at damaged vessel walls, is exposed to circulating factor VII and/or VIIa. A complex is formed with the activated factor VII (TF-FVIIa). This event, in turn, initiates the activation of factor IX and factor X. Factor VII plays a central role in this cascade and can be activated by thrombin, activated factor XI, plasmin, factor XII, and activated factor X. Thrombin (formed from prothrombin) plays a role in stabilizing the hemostatic plug by converting fibrinogen to fibrin, and is involved in the activation of coagulation cofactors VIII and V (see Fig. 1).

The activation of the different factors involved in the coagulation cascade occurs in close relationship with the activated surface of the platelets exposing negatively charged phospholipids. Platelet aggregation occurs when the activated $\alpha_{IIb}\beta_3$ receptors bind to various adhesion proteins, including soluble fibrinogen. In the final blood clot, platelets also interact with the strong network of fibrin formed by the coagulation cascade.

Assessing Vascular Damage and Thrombus Formation In Vivo

Techniques to induce and to monitor thrombosis at the vessel wall have been described by Kawasaki et al. (65), Rosen et al. (66), and Kurz et al. (67).

Rose Bengal Technique

The technique of Kawasaki et al. (65) was slightly modified by Nemmar et al. (45) to assess the effects of PM on the formation of venous or arterial

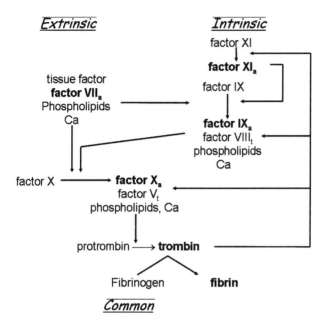

Figure 1 Simplified schematic overview of the coagulation cascade and fibrin formation. Activated factors are presented in bold, subscript "a" indicates activated, subscript "t" indicates platelet bound.

thrombi. Hamsters are anesthetized and placed supine on a heating pad (37°C) and a venous catheter is inserted in the right jugular vein. Distal from this side, the right femoral vein (or artery—depending on the setup of the experiment) is uncovered. In order to irradiate and to follow the thrombus formation, a transilluminator with optic fibers located only 5 mm above the vessel is mounted on the micromanipulator. After the intravenous administration of Rose Bengal (20 mg/kg), via the jugular vein, the segment of the femoral vessel is irradiated with green light (540 nm) for 1.5 or 2 min for artery and vein injury induction, respectively. The thrombus can be monitored using a surgical microscope at × 40 magnification. The change over time in light transmission through the blood vessel (clots are white and allow more light to pass compared to blood) at the site of the trauma is recorded using a microscope-attached camera. Every 10 s an image is record-ed over a period of 40 min. Finally image analysis is used to quantitate thrombus intensity, with light intensity plotted against time, often expressed in arbitrary units as the total area under the curve (68).

Animals can be dosed at several time-points before Rose Bengal admin-istration, allowing to study time-dependent changes. The model can also be used in mice, in which case the carotid artery rather than the femoral artery is studied.

Laser-Induced Injury

Another model to inflict vascular damage and consequent thrombus formation has been described by Rosen et al. (66). Vascular injury was induced using an argon-ion laser. The laser was focused on the target site using a low-intensity light then an injury was induced with a short- but high-intensity light. After laser exposure, an image of the injury was generated by backlighting the injured vessel. In order to allow quantification, the images were recorded, digitized, and analyzed. This method has the advantage of being noninvasive, thus reducing the handling and preparation of the vessel. Multiple injuries can be induced and recorded in a single animal over a longer time period, which allows follow-up and a reduction of animal numbers. The destruction of the vessel wall with the laser is probably accompanied by heat-induced destruction of subendothelial factors at the site of the injury, which can affect outcome of the assay.

Originally the technique was developed in mice but it was used by Silva et al. (51) using rats, illuminating ear veins or arteries. The ear of an anesthetized rat was placed on a glass table of an inverted microscope and the blood vessels and flow could be visualized with a digital camera. A 2-mm green laser beam (532 nm) was introduced to the optical system. To facilitate focusing without damage, a filter was placed between the laser and the microscope objective. Light intensity was measured with an optical power meter. A thrombus should occur normally within 30 s after exposure to green laser. Silva et al. (51) compared the model with and without Rose Bengal and found that the thrombus-inducing time (TIT) after exposure to damaging laser light is longer compared to TIT in the presence of Rose Bengal.

Ferric Chloride Technique

This technique has been described for several laboratory animals, including mouse, rat, and rabbit (67,69,70), and is based on the iron-mediated oxidative tissue damage at the vessel wall initiating thrombus formation. The carotid artery (or vein) of the anesthetized animals is exposed. The blood flow in the vessel is measured with a Doppler flow probe. Thrombosis is induced by applying two pieces of filter paper saturated with ferric chloride to each side of the vessel in contact with the adventitial surface of the vessel for 3 min. The carotid blood flow reduction is a measure of thrombus formation. Until now this technique has not been used in studies investigating particulate-related effects, but is now generally accepted as a standard technique to study thrombosis upon vascular damage.

This technique, together with the Rose Bengal techniques, has, in comparison to the laser technique, the disadvantage of being invasive, and does not allow for assessing effects at different time points in one animal. In comparison to the Rose Bengal technique, ferric chloride only induces local damage, at the site of exposure, for a short period of time without dosing a circulating toxic compound.

Preanalytical Factors Influencing the Reliability for Assessing Platelet Activity and Thrombus Formation In Vitro

In this paragraph, a few points will be addressed to illustrate the importance of applying correct and standardized blood sampling procedures prior to testing platelet activity in vitro.

Damaged blood cells release hemoglobin, intracellular components, and thromboplastic substances. Slight hemolysis in blood samples (as low as 0.9%) already affects the reliability of routine coagulation testing. An increase in prothrombin time (PT) and a decrease in activated partial thromboplastin time (aPTT) and fibrinogen can be observed. Mathematical models exist to correct for a certain amount of hemolysis, but these corrections do not take into account the large interindividual variability. Therefore, it is advised to quantify the free hemoglobin and collect new samples if necessary (71).

Since shear stress is an important trigger for the activation of platelets, the needle bore size can influence significantly platelet activity assessment. For chemical analysis of blood, needles of 23 G are used, while for testing platelet activation, blood is drawn traditionally with ordinary straight needles with bore size of 21 G (or larger) (72). Recently this has been challenged by Lippi et al. (2005) (73) who used a "butterfly" device (also 21 G) successfully for routine coagulation testing. A factor influencing the quality of a blood sample, which is difficult to study in an unprejudiced way, is the experience of the person drawing blood from the patient or volunteer.

Blood collected for platelet activity measurements is in most instances drawn into containers (tubes) with sodium citrate. Specific measurements of platelet activity such as platelet microparticles (PMP), submicroscopic membrane vesicles released by platelets during activation, require specific sampling and sample treatment. The numbers of PMP collected into citrate-theophylline-adenosine-dipyridamole (CTAD) tubes seemed more stable with time compared to samples collected into sodium citrate tubes. The PMP assay is regarded as a useful marker of in vivo platelet activation, and it was also observed that the PMP assay is well correlated with (beta)-thromboglobulin levels. Caution must be taken with delayed measurement because artifactual platelet activation can occur during storage; therefore, it is necessary to evaluate samples within 2 or 3 h (74).

In view of the difficulties and uncertainty that can arise from poor blood samples it is imperative to verify the quality of the samples and to reject all samples of poor quality because these will increase the variability and/or will lead to false conclusions.

Platelet Aggregometry

Principle

Platelet aggregation is one of the oldest and most widely used methods for assaying platelet function.

A sample of citrated blood is collected from the patient and centrifuged to prepare platelet-rich plasma (PRP) ($200g$ for 10 min or $1000g$ for 2 min). At this point, care must be taken not to introduce artifacts (red blood cell lysis, too high shear stress, insufficient use of citrate) (75). The platelet-poor plasma (PPP) is also separated from the sample and serves as an autologous control.

Both PRP and PPP are placed in cuvettes at 37°C and stirred with a magnetic stirrer in an aggregometer to monitor the aggregation. Various platelet-activating agonists such as ADP, collagen, thrombin, or epinephrine are added to the sample of PRP to initiate platelet aggregation. As platelets are activated, they start forming aggregates, decreasing the turbidity of the sample (larger groups of platelets—aggregates—allow more light transmission). A light beam passes through the sample and the amount of light passing through is a measure of aggregation.

Platelet adhesion needs to be studied under flow conditions to mimic the physiological situation. Platelet accumulation is the result of platelet adhesion and platelet detachment. Detachment may vary depending on the adhesive protein to which platelets stick and on the shear rate used for the study. It was found that attachment is in the first place determined by the shear rate, followed by the time platelets are allowed to settle, then by the nature of the surface, and finally by the degree of spreading. These parameters have to be controlled relatively strictly (76).

Platelet aggregation can also be measured in whole blood. In this case it is not the light transmission that is measured but impedance. Alternatively, the number of nonaggregated platelets is counted and used as a parameter to calculate the degree of platelet aggregation (75,77,78).

In the experimental laboratory, the assays for measuring platelet activation due to nanomaterials will need some changes compared to routine measurements. For instance, in a experiment in which the thrombotic or prothrombotic effect of specific nanomaterials is examined, the experimenter can adapt the agonist concentrations added to the sample, in order to preactivate platelets without irreversible aggregation (44,45).

It is impossible to discuss dissimilarities between species in details within the scope of this chapter, care must be taken that all settings of the aggregometer are cor-rectly adapted to the species used (79). For instance hematological values (platelet number, white blood cell numbers, etc.) as well as the size of platelets vary largely between species. Also, distinctive differences are found in the activation of platelets in the presence of specific agonists, e.g., rat platelets lack the PAF receptor, which makes these platelets nonresponsive to this agonist (78).

Another important remark is that aggregation values between samples can simply differ because of abnormally low or high numbers of platelets in one of the samples. These abnormal counts can result from pretreatment of the animals or due to clotting, reducing the circulating platelets, before sampling. Therefore, it is important to report platelet numbers together with aggregation values (77).

Platelet Activation

Bleeding Time
Probably the most logical and presumably the most simple way to evaluate hemostasis is measuring the bleeding time after a standardized incision. This assay was developed almost 100 years ago and is known as the bleeding time (80).

Unfortunately, the bleeding time proved not to be a very good measure for platelet disorders because severe inhibition (80%) of platelet function is necessary to cause significant prolongation of the bleeding time. Despite this questionable sensitivity, the large variation between individuals, and the fact that the test is not suitable for serial testing, the test is still widely used.

In the laboratory the mouse tail bleeding time has been used frequently. Anesthetized mice are placed on a 37°C heating pad. About 2 to 4 mm from the tip of mouse tail, where the tail is approximately 1 mm in diameter, an amputation is made. The tail is placed in a tube filled with 37°C saline solution and the bleeding time is recorded. This technique has proven its value provided the environmental and individual variability is well controlled (mice from one strain with the same age, diet, etc.), but reliable measurements need large experimental groups and this may pose ethical problems.

Platelet Function Analyzer
A good alternative for the bleeding time measurement is the PFA-100 (Dade-Behring) (81) that assesses the closure time of an artificial wound, which is a quantitative measure of primary (platelet-related) hemostasis at high shear stress. In this system membranes precoated with collagen/ epinephrine or collagen/ADP, mimicking vessel wall damage, are used to stimulate platelet aggregation. A small sample of citrated blood (0.8 mL) is placed in a specific disposable cartridge. Briefly, the sample is warmed to 37°C, and is drawn (under vacuum) through a capillary (200 μm) to a punctured (150 μm diameter) nitrocellulose membrane coated with collagen/ epinephrine (CEPI) or collagen/ADP (CADP). This procedure is fully automated. In response to the shear stress ($5000–6000 \, s^{-1}$) and the agonists, platelets will aggregate and block blood flow through the punctured

membrane. The time to occlude the membrane is the closure time. The normal value for human blood is about 100 s (82).

The use of the PFA-100 with blood of experimental animals is possible but because of the blood volume needed for the test it is not advised to run the PFA-100 for small animals such as mice. One of the advantages of this system is that not only the activity or the activation of platelets can be measured in blood from treated animals/persons, but that test materials can be added to blood samples in vitro in order to measure the direct effect of the test compound on the platelet activity. If relatively large blood samples are available, the experimenter can run several experiments in one sample, thus reducing the individual differences.

For nanotoxicology research, an experimenter may try to evaluate the (pro)thrombotic effect, which is equivalent to a shortening of the closure time (83). In these instance it is sometimes useful to prolong the closure time in control samples in order to have a larger window of time in which activation can be measured. This can be obtained by using higher concentrations of sodium citrate, e.g., 12.9 mM compared to the classic 10.9 mM (84).

Coagulation Cascade

PT and partial thromboplastin time (PTT) are both tests that measure the time for blood to clot following recalcification, and are routinely used in the clinical laboratory to monitor for clotting and bleeding disorders.

The PT measures the presence and activity of prothrombin (or factor II) and four other blood clotting factors (factors I, V, VII, and X) of what is "classically" referred to as the extrinsic and common pathway.

The PTT and the aPTT evaluate the efficacy of both the intrinsic and the common coagulation pathways. These tests detect deficiencies of factors VIII, IX, XI, and XII.

In the experimental laboratory, and specifically in view of the (pro) thrombotic effect of inhaled nanomaterials, these tests have been used to detect both the shortening or prolongation of the control (normal) time. Changes can be linked to:

1. Reduced (or increased) concentrations of blood clotting factors and/or a decrease in activity of any of the factors.
2. The presence of a substance that impedes the activity of any of the factors.

Since several of these factors are released from liver or kidney, changes can be an indication of impairment of liver or kidney.

Nemmar et al. (45) used these techniques in their acute studies but could not detect significant changes, which is not surprising because PT and

PTT vary among individuals and therefore such a study would have required enough power to show significant shortening of the time. In a recent epidemiologic study, however, it has been shown that the PT but not the aPTT was shorter with higher ambient air concentrations of PM_{10}, CO, and NO_2 (85), suggestive of coagulation factor changes by air pollutants.

In experimental studies it is probably more convenient to measure changes in concentration of some key factors in the coagulation cascade. The most plausible candidates are TF and factor VIIa.

CONCLUSIONS AND REMARKS

There is evidence that inhaled particles can increase the risk of cardiovascular diseases (as reviewed by Oberdörster et al. [41] and Nemmar et al. [44]).

To uncover the biologic plausibility of these effects, more mechanistic studies have to be performed. Techniques exist to study the atherothrombotic consequence, but care must be taken to adapt these techniques for the specific experimental conditions. In models, using laboratory animals, the differences in thrombogenesis between animal and human must be taken into account.

It should be repeated that the collection of high-quality blood samples is a prerequisite to study blood clotting. Poor sampling will lead to incorrect conclusions.

For the study of complex systems such as hemostasis and thrombogenesis, it is highly advisable to conduct such studies in close collaboration with an expert in the field of coagulation and vascular biology.

REFERENCES

1. Nemery B, Hoet PH, Nemmar A. The Meuse Valley fog of 1930: an air pollution disaster. Lancet 2001; 357:704–8.
2. Brunekreef B, Holgate ST. Air pollution and health. Lancet 2002; 360: 1233–42.
3. Pope CA III, Dockery DW. Health effects of fine particulate air pollution: lines that connect. J Air Waste Manag Assoc 2006; 56:709–42.
4. Nawrot TS, Torfs R, Fierens F, et al. Stronger associations between daily mortality and fine particulate air pollution in summer than in winter: evidence from a heavily polluted region in western Europe. J Epidemiol Commun Health 2007; 61:146–9.
5. Schwartz J. Air pollution and daily mortality: a review and meta analysis. Environ Res 1994; 64:36–52.
6. Wordley J, Walters S, Ayres JG. Short term variations in hospital admissions and mortality and particulate air pollution. Occup Environ Med 1997; 54: 108–16.

7. Samet JM, Dominici F, Curriero FC, et al. Fine particulate air pollution and mortality in 20 U.S. cities, 1987–1994. N Engl J Med 2000; 343: 1742–9.

8. Brook RD, Franklin B, Cascio W, et al. Air pollution and cardiovascular disease—a statement for healthcare professionals from the expert panel on population and prevention science of the American Heart Association. Circulation 2004; 109:2655–71.

9. Pope CA III, Verrier RL, Lovett EG, et al. Heart rate variability associated with particulate air pollution. Am Heart J 1999; 138(5 Pt 1):890–9.

10. Liao D, Creason J, Shy C, et al. Daily variation of particulate air pollution and poor cardiac autonomic control in the elderly. Environ Health Perspect 1999; 107:521–5.

11. Gold DR, Litonjua A, Schwartz J, et al. Ambient pollution and heart rate variability. Circulation 2000; 101:1267–73.

12. Peters A, Doring A, Wichmann HE, et al. Increased plasma viscosity during an air pollution episode: a link to mortality? Lancet 1997; 349:1582–7.

13. Seaton A, Soutar A, Crawford V, et al. Particulate air pollution and the blood. Thorax 1999; 54:1027–32.

14. Brook RD, Brook JR, Urch B, et al. Inhalation of fine particulate air pollution and ozone causes acute arterial vasoconstriction in healthy adults. Circulation 2002; 105:1534–6.

15. Peters A, Perz S, Doring A, et al. Increases in heart rate during an air pollution episode. Am J Epidemiol 1999; 150:1094–8.

16. Urch B, Silverman F, Corey P, et al. Acute blood pressure responses in healthy adults during controlled air pollution exposures. Environ Health Perspect 2005; 113:1052–5.

17. Schwartz J, Morris R. Air pollution and hospital admissions for cardiovascular disease in Detroit, Michigan. Am J Epidemiol 1995; 142:23–35.

18. Rich DQ, Schwartz J, Mittleman MA, et al. Association of short-term ambient air pollution concentrations and ventricular arrhythmias. Am J Epidemiol 2005; 161:1123–32.

19. Wellenius GA, Bateson TF, Mittleman MA, et al. Particulate air pollution and the rate of hospitalization for congestive heart failure among Medicare beneficiaries in Pittsburgh, Pennsylvania. Am J Epidemiol 2005; 161:1030–6.

20. Dockery DW, Pope CA III, Xu X, et al. An association between air pollution and mortality in six U.S. cities. N Engl J Med 1993; 329:1753–9.

21. Pope CA III, Burnett RT, Thun MJ, et al. Lung cancer, cardiopulmonary mortality, and long-term exposure to fine particulate air pollution. JAMA 2002; 287:1132–41.

22. Miller KA, Siscovick DS, Sheppard L, et al. Long-term exposure to air pollution and incidence of cardiovascular events in women. N Engl J Med 2007; 356:447–58.

23. Kunzli N, Jerrett M, Mack WJ, et al. Ambient air pollution and atherosclerosis in Los Angeles. Environ Health Perspect 2005; 113:201–6.

24. O'Neill MS, Veves A, Zanobetti A, et al. Diabetes enhances vulnerability to particulate air pollution—associated impairment in vascular reactivity and endothelial function. Circulation 2005; 111:2913–20.

25. Bateson TF, Schwartz J. Who is sensitive to the effects of particulate air pollution on mortality? A case-crossover analysis of effect modifiers. Epidemiology 2004; 15:143–9.

26. Pope CA, Burnett RT, Thurston GD, et al. Cardiovascular mortality and long-term exposure to particulate air pollution—epidemiological evidence of general pathophysiological pathways of disease. Circulation 2004; 109:71–7.

27. Peters A, Dockery DW, Muller JE, et al. Increased particulate air pollution and the triggering of myocardial infarction. Circulation 2001; 103:2810–5.

28. Peters A, von Klot S, Heier M, et al. Exposure to traffic and the onset of myocardial infarction. N Engl J Med 2004; 351:1721–30.

29. Ruckerl R, Ibald-Mulli A, Koenig W, et al. Air pollution and markers of inflammation and coagulation in patients with coronary heart disease. Am J Respir Crit Care Med 2006; 173:432–41.

30. Kodavanti UP, Schladweiler MC, Ledbetter AD, et al. The spontaneously hypertensive rat as a model of human cardiovascular disease: evidence of exacerbated cardiopulmonary injury and oxidative stress from inhaled emission particulate matter. Toxicol Appl Pharmacol 2000; 164:250–63.

31. Suwa T, Hogg JC, Quinlan KB, et al. Particulate air pollution induces progression of atherosclerosis. J Am Coll Cardiol 2002; 39:935–42.

32. Goto Y, Hogg JC, Shih CH, et al. Exposure to ambient particles accelerates monocyte release from bone marrow in atherosclerotic rabbits. Am J Physiol Lung Cell Mol Physiol 2004; 287:L79–85.

33. Sun Q, Wang A, Jin X, et al. Long-term air pollution exposure and acceleration of atherosclerosis and vascular inflammation in an animal model. JAMA 2005; 294:3003–10.

34. Oberdorster G, Ferin J, Lehnert BE. Correlation between particle-size, in-vivo particle persistence, and lung injury. Environ Health Perspect 1994; 102:173–9.

35. Nemmar A, Delaunois A, Nemery B, et al. Inflammatory effect of intratracheal instillation of ultrafine particles in the rabbit: role of C-fiber and mast cells. Toxicol Appl Pharmacol 1999; 160:250–61.

36. Xia T, Kovochich M, Brant J, et al. Comparison of the abilities of ambient and manufactured nanoparticles to induce cellular toxicity according to an oxidative stress paradigm. Nano Lett 2006; 6:1794–807.

37. Xiong C, Friedlander SK. Morphological properties of atmospheric aerosol aggregates. Proc Natl Acad Sci USA 2001; 98:11851–6.

38. Shi JP, Mark D, Harrison RM. Characterization of particles from a current technology heavy-duty diesel engine. Environ Sci Technol 2000; 34:748–55.

39. Oberdorster G. Pulmonary effects of inhaled ultrafine particles. Int Arch Occup Environ Health 2001; 74:1–8.

40. Hoet PH, Bruske-Hohlfeld I, Salata OV. Nanoparticles—known and unknown health risks. J Nanobiotechnol 2004; 2:12.

41. Oberdorster G, Oberdorster E, Oberdorster J. Nanotoxicology: an emerging discipline evolving from studies of ultrafine particles. Environ Health Perspect 2005; 113:823–39.

42. Riediker M, Cascio WE, Griggs TR, et al. Particulate matter exposure in cars is associated with cardiovascular effects in healthy young men. Am J Respir Crit Care Med 2004; 169:934–40.

43. Seaton A, MacNee W, Donaldson K, et al. Particulate air pollution and acute health effects. Lancet 1995; 345:176–8.
44. Nemmar A, Hoylaerts MF, Hoet PH, et al. Possible mechanisms of the cardiovascular effects of inhaled particles: systemic translocation and prothrombotic effects. Toxicol Lett 2004; 149:243–53.
45. Nemmar A, Hoylaerts MF, Hoet PHM, et al. Ultrafine particles affect experimental thrombosis in an *in vivo* hamster model. Am J Respir Crit Care Med 2002; 166:998–1004.
46. Nemmar A, Hoylaerts M, Hoet PH, et al. Size effect of intratracheally instilled ultrafine particles on pulmonary inflammation and vascular thrombosis. Toxicol Appl Pharmacol 2003; 186:38–45.
47. Nemmar A, Hoet PH, Dinsdale D, et al. Diesel exhaust particles in lung acutely enhance experimental peripheral thrombosis. Circulation 2003; 107:1202–8.
48. Nemmar A, Nemery B, Hoet PHM, et al. Pulmonary inflammation and thrombogenicity caused by diesel particles in hamsters—role of histamine. Am J Respir Crit Care Med 2003; 168:1366–72.
49. Kawasaki T, Kaida T, Arnout J, et al. A new animal model of thrombophilia confirms that high plasma factor VIII levels are thrombogenic. Thromb Haemost 1999; 81:306–11.
50. Matsuno H, Uematsu T, Umemura K, et al. Effects of vapiprost, a novel thromboxane receptor antagonist, on thrombus formation and vascular patency after thrombolysis by tissue-type plasminogen activator. Br J Pharmacol 1992; 106:533–8.
51. Silva VM, Corson N, Elder A, et al. The rat ear vein model for investigating in vivo thrombogenicity of ultrafine particles (UFP). Toxicol Sci 2005; 85:983–9.
52. Khandoga A, Stampfl A, Takenaka S, et al. Ultrafine particles exert prothrombotic but not inflammatory effects on the hepatic microcirculation in healthy mice in vivo. Circulation 2004; 109:1320–5.
53. Zaca F, Benassi MS, Ghinelli M, et al. Myocardial infarction and histamine release. Agents Actions 1986; 18:258–61.
54. Clejan S, Japa S, Clemetson C. Blood histamine is associated with coronary artery disease, cardiac events and severity of inflammation and atherosclerosis. J Cell Mol Med 2002; 6:583–92.
55. Laine P, Kaartinen M, Penttila A, et al. Association between myocardial infarction and the mast cells in the adventitia of the infarct-related coronary artery. Circulation 1999; 99:361–9.
56. Salvi S, Blomberg A, Rudell B, et al. Acute inflammatory responses in the airways and peripheral blood after short-term exposure to diesel exhaust in healthy human volunteers. Am J Respir Crit Care Med 1999; 159:702–9.
57. Devouassoux G, Saxon A, Metcalfe DD, et al. Chemical constituents of diesel exhaust particles induce IL-4 production and histamine release by human basophils. J Allergy Clin Immunol 2002; 109:847–53.
58. Diaz-Sanchez D, Penichet-Garcia M, Saxon A. Diesel exhaust particles directly induce activated mast cells to degranulate and increase histamine levels and symptom severity. J Allergy Clin Immunol 2000; 106:1140–6.

59. Nemmar A, Hoylaerts MF, Hoet PH, et al. Role of histamine in thrombus formation and pulmonary inflammation induced by diesel exhaust particles. Am J Respir Crit Care Med 2003; 167:A107.

60. Nemmar A, Hoet PHM, Vermylen J, et al. Pharmacological stabilization of mast cells abrogates late thrombotic events induced by diesel exhaust particles in hamsters. Circulation 2004; 110:1670–7.

61. Gilmour PS, Ziesenis A, Morrison ER, et al. Pulmonary and systemic effects of short-term inhalation exposure to ultrafine carbon black particles. Toxicol Appl Pharmacol 2004; 195:35–44.

62. Napoli C, De Nigris F, Pignalosa O, et al. In vivo veritas: thrombosis mechanisms in animal models. Scand J Clin Lab Invest 2006; 66:407–27.

63. Jurk K, Kehrel BE. Platelets: physiology and biochemistry. Semin Thromb Hemost 2005; 31:381–92.

64. Vorchheimer DA, Becker R. Platelets in atherothrombosis. Mayo Clin Proc 2006; 81:59–68.

65. Kawasaki T, Kaida T, Arnout J, et al. A new animal model of thrombophilia confirms that high plasma factor VIII levels are thrombogenic. Thromb Haemost 1999; 81:306–11.

66. Rosen ED, Raymond S, Zollman A, et al. Laser-induced noninvasive vascular injury models in mice generate platelet- and coagulation-dependent thrombi. Am J Pathol 2001; 158:1613–22.

67. Kurz KD, Main BW, Sandusky GE. Rat model of arterial thrombosis induced by ferric chloride. Thromb Res 1990; 60:269–80.

68. Stockmans F, Stassen JM, Vermylen J, et al. A technique to investigate mural thrombus formation in small arteries and veins. I. Comparative morphometric and histological analysis. Ann Plast Surg 1997; 38:56–62.

69. Wang X, Xu L. An optimized murine model of ferric chloride-induced arterial thrombosis for thrombosis research. Thromb Res 2005; 115:95–100.

70. Konstantinides S, Schafer K, Thinnes T, et al. Plasminogen activator inhibitor-1 and its cofactor vitronectin stabilize arterial thrombi after vascular injury in mice. Circulation 2001; 103:576–83.

71. Lippi G, Montagnana M, Salvagno GL, et al. Interference of blood cell lysis on routine coagulation testing. Arch Pathol Lab Med 2006; 130:181–4.

72. Lippi G, Salvagno GL, Montagnana M, et al. Influence of the needle bore size used for collecting venous blood samples on routine clinical chemistry testing. Clin Chem Lab Med 2006; 44:1009–14.

73. Lippi G, Salvagno GL, Guidi GC. No influence of a butterfly device on routine coagulation assays and D-dimer measurement. J Thromb Haemost 2005; 3:389–91.

74. Kim HK, Song KS, Lee ES, et al. Optimized flow cytometric assay for the measurement of platelet microparticles in plasma: pre-analytic and analytic considerations. Blood Coagul Fibrinol 2002; 13:393–7.

75. Rand ML, Leung R, Packham MA. Platelet function assays. Transfus Apher Sci 2003; 28:307–17.

76. Wu YP, de Groot PG, Sixma JJ. Shear-stress-induced detachment of blood platelets from various surfaces. Arterioscler Thromb Vasc Biol 1997; 17:3202–7.

77. Cox D. Methods for monitoring platelet function. Am Heart J 1998; 135 (5 Pt 2 Su):S160–9.
78. Kurata M, Horii I. Blood coagulation tests in toxicological studies—review of methods and their significance for drug safety assessment. J Toxicol Sci 2004; 29:13–32.
79. Kurata M, Ishizuka N, Matsuzawa M, et al. A comparative study of whole-blood platelet aggregation in laboratory animals: its species differences and comparison with turbidimetric method. Comp Biochem Physiol C Pharmacol Toxicol Endocrinol 1995; 112:359–65.
80. Matzdorff A. Platelet function tests and flow cytometry to monitor antiplatelet therapy. Semin Thromb Hemost 2005; 31:393–9.
81. Kratzer MA, Born GV. Simulation of primary haemostasis in vitro. Haemostasis 1985; 15:357–62.
82. Hayward CP, Harrison P, Cattaneo M, et al. Platelet function analyzer (PFA)-100 closure time in the evaluation of platelet disorders and platelet function. J Thromb Haemost 2006; 4:312–9.
83. Nemmar A, Hoylaerts MF, Hoet PH, et al. Diesel exhaust particles enhance experimental peripheral thrombosis up to 24 h after their deposition in the lung. Am J Respir Crit Care Med 2003; 167:A107.
84. Heilmann EJ, Kundu SK, Sio R, et al. Comparison of four commercial citrate blood collection systems for platelet function analysis by the PFA-100 system. Thromb Res 1997; 87:159–64.
85. Baccarelli A, Zanobetti A, Martinelli I, et al. Effects of exposure to air pollution on blood coagulation. J Thromb Haemost 2007; 5:252–60.

17

Pulmonary and Cardiovascular Effects of Nanoparticles

Ken Donaldson

ELEGI Colt Laboratory, Medical Research Council/University of Edinburgh Centre for Inflammation Research, Queen's Medical Research Institute, Edinburgh, U.K.

David E. Newby

Cardiovascular Research, Division of Medical and Radiological Sciences, University of Edinburgh, Edinburgh, U.K.

William MacNee

ELEGI Colt Laboratory, Medical Research Council/University of Edinburgh Centre for Inflammation Research, Queen's Medical Research Institute, Edinburgh, U.K.

Rodger Duffin

ELEGI Colt Laboratory, Medical Research Council/University of Edinburgh Centre for Inflammation Research, Queen's Medical Research Institute, Edinburgh, U.K.

Andrew J. Lucking

Cardiovascular Research, Division of Medical and Radiological Sciences, University of Edinburgh, Edinburgh, U.K.

Nicholas L. Mills

Cardiovascular Research, Division of Medical and Radiological Sciences, University of Edinburgh, Edinburgh, U.K.

INTRODUCTION

The production of new forms of engineered nanoparticles (NP) is of increasing concern as nanotechnology continues to develop and manufacture them (1). These form a spectrum of particle types that includes nanotubes, fullerenes, quantum dots (QD), and compound particles of various types. While information on the toxicity of new types of NP is accumulating these are mostly in vitro studies, with few animal or human studies. The existing toxicology knowledge regarding NPs is almost entirely based on combustion-derived nanoparticles (CDNP) in environmental air. Evolving from the "ultrafine hypothesis" (2,3) this strand of research has focused on CDNP like diesel soot since this component of particulate matter (PM) is central in mediating the adverse health effects of environmental air pollution. The mechanism at the cellular level is understood in terms of the ability of particles to cause oxidative stress and inflammation and translocate from the site of deposition (4). This review builds on environmental NPs and their mechanisms, as a basic paradigm and then moves on to discuss toxicology of engineered NPs.

The portal of entry for NPs discussed here is the lungs and the toxic effects seen there are discussed. The lungs and cardiovascular system are intimately linked and the literature indicates that the majority of deaths occurring as a consequence of exposure to particulate air pollution are due to cardiovascular disease. For that reason the cardiovascular effects of NP are also discussed here.

COMBUSTION-DERIVED NANOPARTICLES IN THE ENVIRONMENTAL PARTICLE CLOUD

PM_{10} and Its Adverse Effects

The adverse health effects of air pollution have been recognized throughout much of recorded time and are now documented in large international epidemiological studies (Table 1). In the United Kingdom, fossil fuel combustion in towns and cities, during periods of cold weather, where there is little mixing of air have been associated with the generation of smog episodes. These smogs consisted largely of sulfur dioxide and particles and could very high concentrations in urban air. The particles component or PM represents a key part of the air pollution cocktail present in ambient air, which also comprises gases such as ozone, nitrogen dioxide, etc. Particulate material in ambient air (PM) is measured as the mass of particles collected

Table 1   Adverse Health Effects Due to PM

Mortality from cardiovascular and respiratory causes
Admission to hospital for cardiovascular causes
Exacerbations of asthma in preexisting asthmatics
Symptoms and use of asthma medication in asthmatics
Exacerbations of chronic obstructive pulmonary disease
Lung function decrease
Lung cancer

Abbreviation: PM, particulate matter.
Source: From Ref. .

using the PM_{10} or $PM_{2.5}$ sampling conventions (5). The adverse health effects of PM are seen at the levels that pertain in U.K. and other cities today and there is often no threshold. In other words there is a background of ill health being caused by PM that increases when the ambient particle cloud increases in concentration and goes down when the amount of particles in the air decreases (6).

These adverse health effects of air pollution have been measured in hundreds of studies and there is good coherence between the acute effects seen in time series and panel studies, and the chronic effects seen in environmental studies.

Within 1 or 2 days following an increase in PM concentrations there are increases in:

■ all-cause mortality;
■ asthma attacks and usage of asthma medication;
■ chronic obstructive pulmonary disease (COPD) deaths;
■ COPD exacerbations;
■ hospitalizations for cardiovascular disease and cardiac deaths (7).

The adverse cardiovascular effects associated with increases in PM are well-documented and in fact represent the greatest adverse health impact. Panel studies have documented associations between elevated levels of particles and:

■ onset of myocardial infarction (8);
■ increased heart rate (9);
■ altered heart rate variability (HRV) (10).

Studies exposing subjects to concentrated airborne particles (CAPs) are difficult to perform and the effects of weather and wind direction are likely to alter the composition of the particle component (11). These studies have shown modest increases in lung inflammation (12) and brachial artery vasoconstriction following exposure to CAPs (13). A recent epidemiological study in the United States measured carotid intima-media thickness (CIMT) in life (14), a measure of atherosclerosis, and demonstrated an association between atherosclerosis and ambient air pollution level. Living in an area with higher levels of $PM_{2.5}$ ($10\,\mu g/m^3$) was associated with a CIMT increase of 5.9% (95% confidence interval, 1–11%) with an even larger effect, 15.7%, seen in older women.

Nanoparticles as the Most Toxic Component of PM_{10}

PM is a complex mixture of particle types that vary widely depending on season, time of day, or the sampling site. CDNP are present in PM from conurbations and is a toxicologically important component (see below). CDNP originates principally from automobile tailpipes although there are other sources (4). The common components of PM are shown in Table 2

Table 2 Common Components of PM and Comments on their Origin, Nature, and Likely Toxic Potency

PM_{10} component	Comment	Toxic potency
Combustion-derived nanoparticles	Nanoparticles containing metals and organic volatiles; derived from combustion e.g. vehicle exhaust particles	High
Sodium/magnesium compounds	Derived from sea spray	Low
Sulfate	Predominantly ammonium sulfate	Low
Nitrate	Predominantly ammonium nitrate	Low
Calcium/potassium compounds and insoluble minerals	Derived from the earth's crust, e.g., clay	Low
Biologically derived materials	e.g., endotoxin	High

along with an indication of their toxic potency. Sulfates are very low in toxicity in experimental studies (15), but do show a relationship with adverse effects in some epidemiological studies (e.g., (16)); this apparent anomaly may be explained by a correlation between sulfates and a more potent component of the air pollution mix, such as fine particles, which may actually be responsible for the adverse effects associated with sulfate exposures.

NP numbers, likely to be principally CDNP numbers, ranged from 15,000 to 18,000 particles per cm^3 in three European cities (17) and 10,000 to 50,000 particles per cm^3 in a busy London street (18). In a study on U.S. highways exposure in a vehicle traveling in busy traffic was reported to be 200 to 560×10^3 particles per cm^3 (predominantly NPs) (19,20). Indoor air also contains NP and cooking, vacuuming and burning wax candles produce NPs of soot (21). NPs are also produced during combustion of domestic gas and in one study three gas rings produced around 50,000 particles per cm^3, which underwent rapid aggregation within a few minutes, as evidenced by increases in particle size and decrease in apparent number (22). Secondary NPs also arise from environmental chemistry (e.g., nitrates); but these are unlikely to be as toxicologically potent as CDNPs. The molecular mechanisms of the adverse effects of CDNPs has been extensively reviewed by the authors (4,23,24) and the proinflammatory mechanism is summarized in Figure 1.

CDNP AND THE LUNGS

The present understanding of CDNP activity in the lungs is that the surfaces, organics, and metals can all produce of free radicals with the

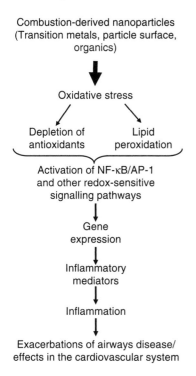

Combustion-derived nanoparticles
(Transition metals, particle surface,
organics)

Oxidative stress

Depletion of antioxidants / Lipid peroxidation

Activation of NF-κB/AP-1
and other redox-sensitive
signalling pathways

Gene expression

Inflammatory mediators

Inflammation

Exacerbations of airways disease/
effects in the cardiovascular system

Figure 1 Hypothetical series of events leading from combustion-derived nanoparticles such as diesel soot interacting with lung cells leading to inflammatory gene expression.

potential to produce oxidative stress and contribute to inflammation. Diesel exhaust particles (DEP) are one of the main CDNP to which individuals are exposed. DEP causes inflammation in rat (25,26) and human lungs (27) following short-term, high-level exposure. Oxidative stress is demonstrable as increased level of 8 OH-dG, the oxidative adduct of hydroxyl radical, in the lungs of rats following exposure to DEP and in cells in culture treated with DEP (28,29). The component of DEP responsible for the oxidative stress and subsequent proinflammatory signaling is principally the organic fraction (30–33), although transition metals may also be involved especially for welding fume (34). The oxidative stress then causes activation of signaling pathways for proinflammatory gene expression, including MAPK (30,35–37) and NF-κB activation (30,38) and histone acetylation that favors proinflammatory gene expression (39). Activation of these pathways culminates in transcription of a number of proinflammatory genes such as IL-8 in epithelial cells treated in vitro (40) and in human lungs exposed by inhalation (41). TNF-alpha concentrations increase in macrophages exposed to DEP in vitro (42) and IL-6 is released by primed human bronchial epithelial cells exposed to DEP (43).

CARDIOVASCULAR EFFECTS OF PM AND CDNP

The adverse cardiovascular effects associated with increases in PM concentration (44,45) could plausibly be mediated through the effects of CDNP. In a mixture of studies using PM, CAPs, and model NP, evidence is accumulating that NP causes inflammation that could adversely affect the cardiovascular system. Increases in ambient PM concentrations may result in systemic inflammation, as shown by elevated C-reactive protein, blood leukocytes, platelets, fibrinogen, and increased plasma viscosity (reviewed in Ref. 46). Atherothrombosis, the colocalization of atherosclerotic plaque with superimposed thrombus, is characteristic of the pathogenesis of vascular disease and is the main cause of cardiovascular morbidity and mortality (47). Atherosclerosis is initiated via vascular endothelial injury and is propagated by chronic intimal inflammation. Indeed, increased concentrations of systemic inflammatory markers predict risk for myocardial and cerebral infarction (47–49). Therefore repeated exposure to PM_{10} may, by increasing systemic inflammation, exacerbate the vascular inflammation of atherosclerosis and promote plaque development or rupture. Experimental studies with animal models susceptible to atherosclerosis provide some support for this contention (50,51).

Potential Effects of PM-Induced Lung Inflammation on the Endothelium and on Atherosclerotic Plaque Stability

Normally the endothelial monolayer delicately balances regulatory pathways controlling vasomotion, thrombosis, cellular proliferation, inflammation, and oxidative stress. Atherosclerosis is known to be an inflammatory process that is associated with a dysfunctional vascular endothelium (Ross, 1999). Loss of endothelial function results in expression of leukocyte adhesion proteins, reduced anticoagulant activity and the release of growth factors, inflammatory mediators, and cytokines. Chronic inflammation results in leukocyte and monocyte recruitment, induction of atheroma formation, and further arterial damage. Plaque expansion and disruption can lead to angina, crescendo angina and acute coronary syndromes, including myocardial infarction (Blum et al., 1996; Brand et al., 1996; Ross, 1999).

Biomarkers of systemic inflammation are elevated in patients with overt cardiovascular disease (Haverkate et al., 1997) and in those with established cardiovascular risk factors (Lee et al., 1997). In apparently healthy individuals, elevated plasma concentrations of the acute-phase reactant CRP, have been shown to predict the development of ischemic heart disease (Kuller et al., 1996; Ridker et al., 2000), and in particular the risk of a first myocardial or cerebral infarction, independent of other risk factors (Ridker et al., 2000). Increases in markers of systemic inflammation such as CRP, serum amyloid A, and IL-6, accompany acute coronary events, and correlate with short-term prognosis (Liuzzo et al., 1994). Elevation in inflammatory markers precedes myocardial necrosis, suggesting that inflammation may be the primary trigger of coronary plaque instability.

Short-term exposure to increased levels of PM_{10} induces changes that are indicative of systemic inflammation, such as increases in white blood cells and platelets (Schwartz, 2001b), rises in CRP (Seaton et al., 1999; Pope, 2001), fibrinogen (Pekkanen et al., 2000; Prescott et al., 2000), and plasma viscosity (Peters et al., 1997) as well as alterations in Factor VII (Seaton et al., 1999). Experimental exposures mirror these clinical findings (van Eeden et al., 2001) and demonstrate evidence of combined systemic inflammation and endothelial dysfunction (Vincent et al., 2001; Ross, 1993; Bonetti et al., 2003).

Repeated exposure to PM_{10} may, therefore, induce or exacerbate the vascular inflammation of atherosclerosis and promote plaque expansion or rupture. Indeed, using a Watanabe hereditary hyperlipidemic rabbit model, Suwa and coworkers (Suwa et al., 2002) described plaque progression and destabilization following instillation of high doses of PM_{10} (Suwa et al., 2002). In the same model, PM_{10} exposure accelerated monocyte release from the bone marrow (Goto et al., 2004). The amount of particulate phagocytosed by alveolar macrophage correlated with both the bone marrow response (Goto et al., 2004) and plaque volume (Suwa et al., 2002). The New York group of Lippmann has also demonstrated more severe lesions in the vessels of Apo-E mice exposed to New York CAPs compared to Apo-E mice exposed to filtered air (11,51,52). These data taken together suggest that particulate-induced pulmonary inflammation is capable of systemic effects, which can contribute to the progression of atherosclerosis. A recent panel study in Los Angeles provides the first evidence of a link between chronic PM exposure and atherosclerosis in human (Kunzli et al, 2004). A $10 \mu g/m^3$ increase in $PM_{2.5}$ was associated with an increase in CIMT, an ultrasonic measure of atheroma, suggesting that long-term ambient PM exposure may affect the development of atherosclerosis in human.

Inhaled PM may influence the vasculature through indirect effects mediated by pulmonary inflammation or through the direct action of particles that have become blood-borne. Whether inhaled nanoparticulate can access the circulation is currently the subject of intense research (Nemmar et al., 2001; Kreyling et al., 2002; Oberdorster et al., 2002) and there is conflicting reports on whether Technegas—radioactive carbon NPs—can reach the blood following inhalation in humans (53,54). Certainly, injured arteries can take up blood-borne NPs (Guzman et al., 2000), a fact exploited by the nanotechnology industry for both diagnostic and therapeutic purposes in cardiovascular medicine. The intra-arterial infusion of carbon black NPs has a detrimental effect on the mouse microcirculation with upregulation of von Willebrand factor expression and enhanced fibrin deposition on the endothelial surface (Khandoga et al., 2004). These pro-thrombotic effects are in keeping with toxicological evidence from inhalation studies, which suggest particle exposure may promote thrombogenesis (Nemmar et al., 2003a,b).

Small areas of denudation and thrombus deposition are a common finding on the surface of atheromatous plaques and are usually subclinical. Endogenous fibrinolysis and "passification" of the lesion may therefore be able to prevent thrombus propagation and vessel occlusion (55). However, in the presence of an adverse proinflammatory state or an imbalance in the fibrinolytic system, such microthrombi may propagate, ultimately leading to arterial occlusion and tissue infarction (56). Thus, the initiation, modification, and resolution of unstable and inflamed atheromatous plaques may be critically dependent on the cellular activation and function of the surrounding endothelium and vascular wall.

The endothelium plays a vital role in the control of blood flow, coagulation, fibrinolysis, and inflammation. Following the seminal work of Furchgott and Zawadski (57), it is widely recognized that an array of mediators including cigarette smoking can influence vascular tone through endothelium-dependent actions, and there is now extensive evidence of abnormal endothelium-dependent vasomotion in patients with atherosclerosis (58–60). Mild systemic inflammation also causes a profound, but temporary, suppression of endothelium-dependent vasodilatation (61). However, while endothelium-dependent vasomotion is important, it may not be representative of other aspects of endothelial function, such as the regulation of fibrinolysis.

The fibrinolytic factor tissue plasminogen activator (t-PA) regulates the degradation of intravascular fibrin and is released from the endothelium through the translocation of a dynamic intracellular storage pool (61,62). If endogenous fibrinolysis is to be effective, then the rapid mobilization of t-PA from the endothelium is essential because thrombus dissolution is much more effective if t-PA is incorporated during, rather than after, thrombus formation (63,64). The efficacy of plasminogen activation and fibrin degradation is further determined by the relative balance between the acute local release of t-PA and its subsequent inhibition through formation of complexes with plasminogen activator inhibitor type 1 (PAI-1). This dynamic aspect of endothelial function and fibrinolytic balance may be directly relevant to the pathogenesis of atherothrombosis.

CDNP and Endothelial Dysfunction

In order to investigate the potential role of the endothelial dysfunction in mediating the observed increase in acute myocardial infarctions following exposure to road traffic we investigated the effects of diesel exhaust inhalation on vascular and endothelial function in humans (65). In a double-blind, randomized, cross-over study, 30 healthy men were exposed to diluted diesel exhaust at 300 mg/m^3 particulate, or air, for 1 h with intermittent exercise. Six hours after exposure to diesel exposure or air, forearm blood flow was measured in response to infusions of intra-arterial agonists as an assessment of vascular vasomotor function. Inflammatory mediators in blood were measured concomitantly. There were no differences in resting forearm blood flow or inflammatory markers after exposure to diesel exhaust or air. There was a dose-dependent increase in blood flow with each vasodilator but this vasomotor response was significantly attenuated with bradykinin (BK), acetylcholine (Ach), and sodium nitroprusside (SNP) ($p < .001$) infusions 2 h after exposure to diesel exhaust, and this persisted at 6 h (Fig. 2).

In addition BK caused a dose-dependent increase in plasma t-PA that was suppressed 6 h after exposure to diesel ($p < .001$; area under the curve decreased by 34%). We concluded that, at levels encountered in an urban environment, inhalation of dilute diesel exhaust impairs two important and complementary aspects of vascular function in humans: the regulation of vascular tone and endogenous fibrinolysis. We propose a plausible explanation for the effects of CDNP on vascular function in Figure 3.

Vasodilator drugs Ach and BK act on membrane-bound G-protein coupled receptors on the vascular endothelium to stimulate calcium influx and nitric oxide synthase (eNOS) activation. This increases local nitric oxide (NO) levels in the adjacent smooth muscle cells resulting in relaxation, vasodilatation, and an increase in forearm blood flow. The NO-donor SNP increases local NO concentrations via endothelial-independent pathways, while verapamil causes smooth muscle relaxation via a NO-independent pathway. The observed blunting of the vasomotor response to all vasodilators except verapamil suggests that NO consumption is central to the mechanism of air pollution mediated vascular and endothelial dysfunction. Oxidative stress may result from pulmonary inflammation or directly from particles that gain access to the bloodstream. In this scenario excess superoxide produced as a result of enhanced oxidative stress rapidly combines with NO in the vessel wall to form peroxynitrite ($ONOO^-$), thus limiting NO availability and blunting smooth muscle relaxation. This explanation combines the well-known oxidative and proinflammatory effects of CDNP with key endothelial functions and so provides a potential mechanism that links air pollution to the pathogenesis of atherothrombosis and acute myocardial infarction (65).

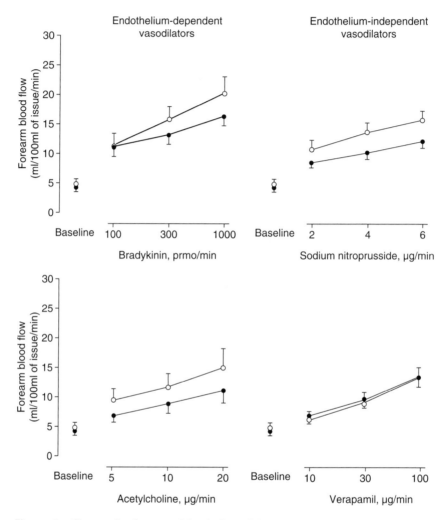

Figure 2 Change in forearm blood flow following infusion of endothelium-dependent (acetylcholine and bradykinin) and endothelium-independent (sodium nitroprusside and verapamil) vasodilators. Vasodilatation was significantly impaired following exposure to dilute diesel exhaust (closed circles) compared with filtered air (open circles). *Source*: From Ref. 66a.

CDNP and Effects on Thrombosis

In addition to investigating the effects of CDNP on endothelial function, we have conducted studies to assess their effect on thrombogenicity in human. While data from in vitro (66) and animal instillation studies (67) suggest that

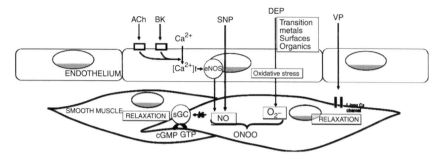

Figure 3 Hypothetical scheme to explain the observed effects of DEP exposure on vasomotor function. *Source*: Ref. 66.

exposure to CDNP is associated with increased thrombogenicity there are no data from inhalation studies in human.

We have used an established ex vivo model of thrombosis (68) to address the effects of CDNP following inhalation. The Badimon Chamber possesses a number of advantages over other techniques to assess thrombus formation in human. It allows the assessment of thrombus formation in unaltered whole blood. This is possible as the thrombus is generated just outside the body. It also allows the formation of thrombus under conditions of continual flow. Of particular relevance in this context, the morphology of the chamber is designed to produce flow conditions similar to those within patent or mild to moderately stenosed coronary arteries. The thrombogenic substrate is specially prepared strips of porcine aorta from which the intima has been removed, therefore exposing blood to the muscular layer of the vessel. Overall, the model is therefore one of deep coronary arterial injury.

In a small but robustly designed pilot study, inhalation of dilute diesel exhaust (1×10^6 particles/cm^3) for 2 h caused a modest increase in thrombus formation compared to filtered air (Lucking et al., abstract in press). While the underlying mechanism is at present unclear, thrombus formation was increased primarily following sheer stress in the chamber that reflects a moderately stenosed artery, suggesting the effect of diesel exhaust may be mediated by increased platelet activation. In vitro data suggest NPs associate preferentially with platelets and upregulate platelet p-selectin expression when added to human whole blood (McGuinnes et al., unpublished). Further human exposure studies in larger cohorts with assessments of thrombus formation and platelet activation in parallel are required to confirm these preliminary findings and elucidate the underlying mechanisms.

CDNP and the Heart

Epidemiologic and observational studies suggest that exposure to PM may worsen symptoms of angina (69), exacerbate exercise-induced myocardial ischemia (69,70), and trigger acute myocardial infarction (69,71). These observations are limited by imprecision in the measurement of pollution exposure, the effect of potential confounding environmental and social factors, and the lack of mechanistic data. Controlled exposures of air pollutants can help to address these shortcomings by providing a precisely defined exposure in a regulated environment that facilitates investigation with validated biomarkers and surrogate measures of cardiovascular health. We therefore assessed the effect of dilute diesel exhaust inhalation on myocardial function in an "at risk" population of patients with stable coronary heart disease.

Using a randomized double-blind cross-over study design, patients with previous myocardial infarction (>6 months previously) attended on two occasions at least 2 weeks apart for controlled exposure to dilute diesel exhaust ($300 \mu g/m^3$) or filtered air for 1 h (72). During each exposure, subjects performed two 15-min periods of exercise on a bicycle ergometer separated by two 15-min periods of rest. All subjects were fitted with 12-lead Holter electrocardiographic monitors and maximum ST-depression and ischemic burden were determined during each exercise period. Despite similar changes in heart rate, we documented painless myocardial ischemia that was increased up to threefold by diesel exhaust inhalation (Fig. 4). This reproducible effect was present despite a high use of maintenance β-blocker therapy in patients without limiting angina. It seems likely that the adverse effect of diesel exhaust inhalation will be even greater in other patient populations, such as those with limiting angina or those not receiving antianginal therapies. Thus we have established, for the first time, an immediate proischemic effect of diesel exhaust inhalation, and we believe this provides an important mechanism for the observed increase in myocardial infarction in the hour following exposure to traffic.

The precise mechanisms whereby diesel exhaust inhalation augments exercise-induced ischemic have yet to be established. There is an important relationship between autonomic regulation of the cardiac cycle and cardiovascular mortality (73). Variation in the interval between consecutive heart beats, or HRV, is controlled by the contrasting effects of the sympathetic and parasympathetic nervous systems. Reduction in HRV reflects either an increase in sym-pathetic drive or a decrease in vagal parasympathetic tone. Reduced HRV increases the risk of cardiovascular morbidity and mortality in both healthy individuals (74) and patients following myocardial infarction (75).

Although there is no data specifically on CDNP, a relatively large number of panel studies have reported a consistent association between

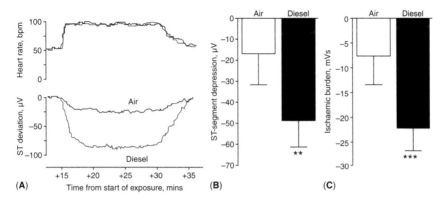

Figure 4 Myocardial ischemia during 15 min of exercise stress while exposed to diesel exhaust or filtered air. (**A**) Typical recording of change in heart rate and ST-segment. (**B**) Maximal ST-segment depression ($p = .003$, diesel exhaust versus filtered air), and (**C**) total ischemic burden ($p < .001$, diesel exhaust versus filtered air). *Abbreviation*: ST,

reduced HRV and high ambient PM (76–80). The finding of altered HRV in an elderly cohort exposed to concentrated ambient particles (CAPs) provides direct evidence of the effects of PM on autonomic activity (81). The importance of this effect in the presence of cardio-vascular pathology was demonstrated in a canine model of myocardial infarction, where exposure to residual oil fly ash (ROFA) reduced HRV and increased cardiac arrhythmia following infarction (82). Furthermore, in patients with implanted cardiac defibrillators there appears to be a relationship between ambient PM and the incidence of ventricular fibrillation (83). Experimental studies have also shown effects of PM and other pollution particles on heart rhythm (82, 84, 85). These effects could be caused by interstitialized particles directly irritating the nerve endings or by local inflammatory effects of cytokines released locally in response to the particles.

MANUFACTURED NANOPARTICLES

The Emerging Nanotechnologies project conducted by The Woodrow Wilson International Center for Scholars, along with the Pew Charitable Trusts, has identified over 200 consumer products into which newer nanotechnology, especially NPs are incorporated at April 2006 (http://www. nanotechproject.org/index.php?id = 44). The reasons for the rapid expansion in industrial use of this technology are its unique properties due to small size and large reactive surface area. NPs come in a wide variety of shapes, sizes, and chemical compositions. In addition to the spherical shapes observed for particles such as titanium dioxide (TiO_2), shape varieties also include carbon nanotubes (CNT), nanowhiskers, and nanofibers. Engineered NPs vary considerably in their size and composition and so would be anticipated to vary in toxicity. Nanotubes and nanowires can range from less than 100 nm diameter to tens of mm in length. The variety of chemical composition range from substances considered traditionally to be relatively inert (e.g., carbon and gold) to substances associated with significant toxicity (e.g., cadmium and other heavy metals). Since the NP size imparts heightened reactivity to the "inert" materials, it is interesting to consider the impact of small size on toxic materials, especially since reactivity might relate to toxicity.

Bulk-Manufactured Nanoparticles

Carbon black and TiO_2 along with alumina and silica have been studied for some time with regard to their proinflammatory effects but none of these has explicitly addressed effects on the cardiovascular system. Nanosize carbon black has been intensively studied with regard to the issue of low toxicity dust and the confounding effect of rat lung overload (extensively reviewed in Refs. 86–89). In view of the very high surface area per unit volume of NP and the identification of surface area as the driver for overload (90–92) attention focused on the nanopaticulate form of these nuisance dusts. These would be anticipated to produce lung overload at lower mass lung burdens than seen with the larger particles. This was indeed found to be the case (92,93). However even at low, nonoverload exposures to NPCB, there was a proinflammatory effect not seen with the larger CB particles (94).

Instillation studies have also shown that the nanoparticulate form of CB and TiO_2 produce more inflammation than an equal mass of larger, yet respirable, particles (95,96) of the same material and across a range of NPs of nuisance dust the surface are was found to be the driver of the inflam-mation (97). The molecular mechanism of the increased inflammatory effects of NP carbon black have demonstrated that they generate reactive oxygen species (ROS) in cell-free systems (98–100) and cause alterations in calcium signaling (101,102) in exposed cells. Oxidative stress from the CBNP can also activate the EGF receptor (103) and redox-responsive transcription factors such as NF-κB (102) and AP-1 (104) leading to the transcription of proinflammatory cytokines and lipid mediators (100,102).

Carbon Nanotubes

CNT are long sheets of graphite rolled in the form of a tube that can be a few nm thick (single-walled, SWCNT) or up to a few hundred nm thick (multiwalled, MWCNT). The needle-like structure implies that a paradigm relating to fibers such as asbestos might be appropriate in considering their toxicity. The potential pathogenicity of a conventional fiber is dictated by length greater than 20 mm, thinness and biopersistence (105). Biopersistence is an important determinant of mineral fiber and Synthetic Vitreous Fiber pathogenicity. Long biopersistent fibers are the biologically effective dose that drives pathogenic effects (105) while nonbiopersistent fibers undergo dissolution processes that can be enhanced at the acid pH of 5.0 existing inside macrophage phagolysosomes (106). Long biosoluble fibers undergo leaching of key structural molecules leading to breakage into short fibers that are readily phagocytosed by the macrophages (105,107).

One study (108) has addressed the important issue of biopersistence of CNT using both ungrounded and grounded nanotubes, 0.7 and 5.9 nm long, respectively. These were assessed for biopersistence and the longer, ungrounded nanotubes were more biopersistent than the short ones. This is consistent with the greater biopersistence of long fibers seen in studies with asbestos and other mineral fibers although these "long" nanotubes were much shorter than those mineral fibers defined as "long," which are in the region of 20 µm and greater (105). A 20 µm diameter rat macrophage is able to enclose and transport fibers less than its own diameter from the lungs (105), and the length-dependent inhibition of clearance seen with 5.9 µm long nanotubes is thus rather unexpected. It may be that the well-documented tendency for nanotubes to form bundles and wires (109) is important in impairment of clearance. Nanotubes have been used in a number of rat lung instillation studies (108,110–112). All of these used high dose and dose-rate and this raises questions about physiological relevance; no study has addressed the role of length by comparing long (>~20 µm) with short (<10 µm) nanotubes. However, all of the studies mentioned above showed an increased ability of CNT to cause granulomatous fibrosis in the absence of severe inflammation.

CNT have also been tested in a range of different cell types in vitro to assess their potential toxicity. Treatment of human keratinocytes have shown that both SWCNT and MWCNT are capable of being internalized and causing cellular toxicity (113,114). In a study with alveolar macrophages, SWCNT were more cytotoxic than MWCNT after exposure at equal mass dose (115). Human T cells exposed to oxidized MWCNT were killed in a time- and dose-dependent manner, with apoptosis being involved (116). As found also in kidney cells exposed to SWCNTs (117). Manna et al. demonstrated dose-dependent oxidative stress and NF-κB activation in human keratinocytes along with IκB depletion and MAPK phosphorylation (118). In vitro nanotubes can produce free radicals by the role of iron in causing Fenton-type reactions (119).

It is difficult to draw general conclusion on CNT toxicity because of the scarcity of data and CNT variability—they can very in length, and composition including metal contamination. CNT are often kinked and tangled into aggregates of varying size and shape. This kind of variability is found between and within samples. All of these factors could impact on toxicity. More rigid CNT are likely to disperse more efficiently than tangled CNT. However the tangles are more easily taken up by cells in culture and could thus be more readily cleared from the lungs by macrophages. A programme of research is warranted to define the factors that control CNT toxicity.

Fullerenes

Buckminster fullerene or C_{60} is a compact cage-like molecule comprising 60 carbon atoms. C_{60} can be viewed as a NP and has received some toxicological attention. The basic graphitic structure of fullerene can be functionalized in various ways to change the physical properties of the fullerene, for instance making it more dispersible/soluble (120). Carboxylated fullerenes are slightly less toxic than the native C_{60} and hydroxylated C_{60} are virtually nontoxic to human dermal fibroblasts (120). The toxicity of the native C_{60} appeared to be due to the ability to generate superoxide anion (120). Isakovic showed a similar effect with the native C_{60} being much more toxic on a mass basis than a soluble hydroxylated C_{60}. The authors concluded through the use of antioxidants and identifying different types of cell death with the two fullerenes, that unmodified C_{60} had strong pro-oxidant capacity responsible for the rapid necrotic cell death while polyhydroxylated C_{60} exerted mainly antioxidant/cytoprotective effects and produced modest apoptosis that was independent of oxidative stress (121). Unmodified C_{60} was not toxic to guinea pig alveolar macrophages in vitro in another study, while nanotubes were toxic at the same mass dose (115). Paradoxically, several studies have suggested that C_{60} is an antioxidant (122–125) and antinitrosating (122) agent. Clearly more research is warranted to resolve the issue as to the role of the C_{60} surface chemistry derivatization versus pristine C_{60} and the issue of antioxidant potential.

Quantum Dots

QD, also known as nanocrystals, are a unique class of semiconductor. At 2 to 10 nm, these are very small particle in which the electrons are strongly confined leading to emission of light. Emission wavelengths vary in response to size with smaller dots yielding "bluer" wavelengths an larger dots give "redder" wavelengths. To can achieve these properties because they are composed of an element each from different Periodic Table groups (126). Although there is little potential for inhalation exposure to QDs they have considerable potential for imaging and diagnosis in vivo and so there is potential for exposure of a number of target organs reached from the blood.

QDs can vary considerably in their elemental composition with cadmium, a toxic metal, commonly present. Cadmium QDs (127) have been found to kill cells in cultures and this effect was inhibited by the thiol *N*-acetyl cysteine, suggesting a role for oxidative stress. Other studies demonstrate low toxicity in some models of cellular toxicity (128,129). Animal studies have demonstrated similar lack of acute toxicity (128,130). Clearly more research is needed on QDs to fully understand their potential toxicity (see chap 19).

Other types of NP have been tested and have shown toxicity that might be reflected in lung effects or even cardiovascular effects. Striking differences were seen in the toxicity of a range of NPs with similar singlet particle size (average 20–50 nm) (131). This ranged from a virtually nontoxic rutile TiO_2 NP to highly toxic silver NPs; many NP however were intermediate in toxicity toward the RAW mouse macrophage cell line used in the study. When a panel of NP of similar size (30–45 nm) was tested in liver NP Cd were the most toxic followed by Ag while Mo, Al, Fe, and TiO_2 all had low toxicity cells (132). The mechanism of toxicity was assessed for Ag particles and suggested a role for oxidative stress. The toxicity of copper was tested in the form of copper ions, NP copper, and micron-sized copper. The greatest toxicity to the liver, kidney, and spleen was seen with the nano copper following oral dosing compared to the same mass dose of micron-sized copper (133). In a study by Dick et al a range of NP of different composition we compared for ability to induce ROS production in vitro versus ability to cause lung inflammation in rats (134). There was a good correlation between the two suggesting that the proinflammatory effects of these different NP were related to their ability to generate oxidative stress.

DO CDNP PROVIDE A MODEL FOR THE EFFECTS OF ENGINEERED NP ON THE LUNGS AND CARDIOVASCULAR SYSTEM?

Manufactured NP and the Lungs

If the environmental paradigm for CDNP was generalizable to new engineered NP we would anticipate that new NP would cause oxidative tress and inflammation in the lungs, affect the cardiovascular system to enhance atherothrombosis and also modulate HRV. To understand the impact that this might have it is necessary to hypothesize that the highest exposures to such NP would occur in the workplace and so the target population for acute effects of particles would not be affected. These are those with airways disease and those with severe cv disease; neither of these population is likely to be working in a dusty atmosphere. However the chronic exposure model of $PM_{10}/CDNP$ is that everyone is exposed and that chronic exposure renders them into the susceptible groups by causing COPD, cardiovascular disease and lung cancer. High workplace dust exposures are traditionally seen to cause lung fibrosis, COPD and lung cancer. Therefore we are most likely to see these kinds of endpoints in workplaces where there is high exposure to engineered NP (Fig. 5).

When materials undergo attrition in the environment and if NP are released then they might begin to cause acute effects. It should be noted, however, that there needs to he high enough exposure to produce these effects. So far studies with new NP have been almost completely confined to toxicity studies on cells and CNT have been used in animal studies. Little is known about their potential to affect the cardiovascular system. As described below, however, there are a wide range of composition and shape of NPs and these might be expected to impart considerable differences in toxicity.

Manufactured NP and the Cardiovascular System

Radomski et al. examined the role of new NP on the clotting system (66) studying the effects of MWCNT and SWCNT, C_{60} fullerenes, and mixed carbon black NPs on human platelet aggregation in vitro and rat vascular thrombosis in vivo. Standard urban PM was used as a control. Nanotubes and carbon black particles but not C_{60}, stimulated platelet aggregation and the same ranking was seen in ability to affect the rate of vascular thrombosis

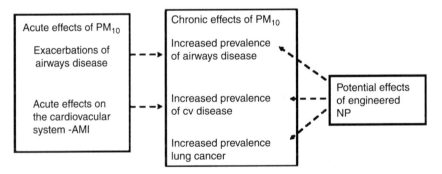

Figure 5 Possible relationships between acute and chronic effects of PM_{10} in relation to potential effects of manufactured nanoparticles. *Abbrebviation*: AMI, __; NP, nanoparticles; PM, particulate matter.

in rat carotid arteries; urban dust had low activity in these assays. Thus, there are differences between different carbon NPs to activate platelets and enhance vascular thrombosis. Yamawaki et al. have shown that carbon back of aggregate size 248 nm are cytostatic, cytotoxic, and proinflammatory in endothelial cells (135).

MANUFACTURED NP AND QUANTITATIVE STRUCTURE ACTIVITY RELATIONSHIPS

The numbers of new NP that are being produced pose a special problem in testing. NPs are relatively easy to alter in terms of physicochemistry—size, coating, composition, etc. and this makes for even more particles to be tested. Other factors are also important—the average small company that is developing a new NP type is unlikely to have the funds to carry out proper toxicology testing and the current climate against animal testing makes this type of testing not viable.

In the pharmacology and toxicology worlds the term quantitative structure activity relationship (QSAR) is used to describe the attempt to relate chemical structure to pharmacological or toxicological activity. This idea could be used to categorize NP on the basis of physicochemistry if physicochemical markers could be related to toxicity. The most obvious candidates for structural marker that could be related to toxicity markers at the moment are size/surface area and oxidative stress. For insoluble particles the surface area times the surface reactivity describes biologically effective dose (the dose that drives adverse effects) and so particle size is likely to be important. For NP the quantum effect changes in the physicochemical nature of the surface of a very small particle compared to a larger one could impact on toxicology. The dominant hypothesis for the action of harmful particles on cells is oxidative stress and the oxidative stressing activity of particles is a physicochemical parameter that may well be important in structure activity considerations. The QSAR idea is likely to be achievable for predicting lung inflammation and so could be predictive for cv effects if they are driven by pulmonary inflammation. For translocation from the lungs to the blood or for effects in the blood, a different QSAR may be important necessary.

POTENTIAL CARCINOGENIC EFFECTS OF MANUFACTURED NP

The ability of PM to cause cancer is well-documented and other types of particles, such as asbestos and silica, are also known to be carcinogenic. The mechanisms are, however, not completely well understood and may involve both direct genotoxic effects of the particles themselves and indirect

genotoxic effects mediated through the particles ability to cause inflammation. Direct genotoxic effects of particles involve the particles entering cells
and delivering damage to DNA. The chemical composition, as well as the
structural composition of the particles both play a role in this and so CDNP
certainly have the potential to mediate this type of effect (136). Transition
metals have been shown to redox cycle inside the cell and generate damaging
hydroxyl radicals that form mutagenic adducts with DNA (137). Organic
molecules adsorbed on to the surface of CDNP, such as polycyclic aromatic
hydrocarbons (PAHs), can also form adducts (138) while large surface areas
on NP are capable of generating oxidative stress (136). In addition, the
inflammatory effects of CDNP, as discussed above, can play an important
role in the genotoxic and carcinogenic processes and the products of the
leukocyte oxidative burst can form adducts within target cells (139). The
effects of oxidative stress inside the cell may cause lipid peroxide production
in the cell and the products of lipid peroxidation are longer-lived than the
ROS themselves and may therefore mediate adduct formation (Fig. 6) (140).

Certain types of NP appear to be able to enter the nucleus in cell
culture systems, to a much greater extent than larger particles of the same
material (141) and NPs in general seem to be cable of crossing biological
membranes (142). If NPs generally gain access to the nucleus rather than
being retained in the cytoplasm like larger particles, then by virtue of being
closer to the DNA, the oxidative products they produce may be more likely
to cause genotoxic effects; these potential effects are summarized in Figure 6.

CONCLUSION

A paradigm has evolved arising from experience with environmental,
CDNPs exemplified by diesel soot. In this paradigm oxidative stress and
inflammation are identified as key processes in the local effects in the lungs.
In addition inflammatory effects and blood translocation could explain
adverse cardiovascular effects seen in epidemiology studies with air
pollution particles. Support for this contention came from a number of
studies using model NP and CDNP, where adverse cardiovascular effects
such as clotting plaque development and endothelial dysfunction were
enhanced after NP exposures in a number of different models. In parallel
with these studies, an increasing number of toxicology studies used bulk
NP such as TiO_2 and carbon black and these identified a key role for the
large surface area and its ability to produce oxidative stress (100,134,143).
It is not known whether the same paradigm can be used for new engineered
NPs and nanotubes. In the limited studies so far published engineered NPs
such as the CNT are also reported to induce oxidative stress, cell death and
inflammation. However there are variations in the degree of the adverse
effects shown by NP in various models and so not all are likely to show the

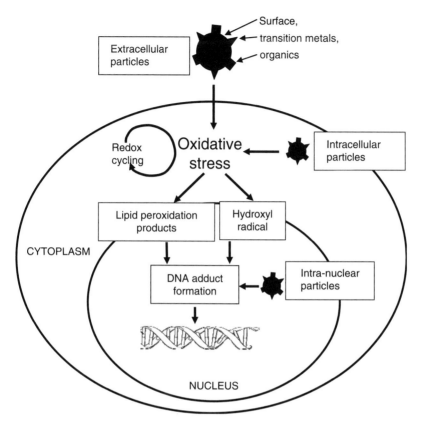

Figure 6 Diagram of likely interactions between nanoparticles and genotoxic effects.

same toxic potency. This is to be anticipated since the total toxicity of any particle sample is the complex sum of the surface reactivity times the surface area plus releasable toxic moieties, plus shape, all modified by biopersistence. There is a strong likelihood that all of these can vary considerably and so the total toxicity is very likely to vary between particle types.

The other variable is exposure. Even hazardous particles require some exposure and very little is known about exposure to the newer engineered NP—this data is urgently needed. Taken together the data suggest that, for some of the new engineered NP, sufficient exposure could lead to oxidative stress and a stimulation of the inflammatory response, and that this would be linked to adverse health effects similar to those seen with CDNP (Fig. 7).

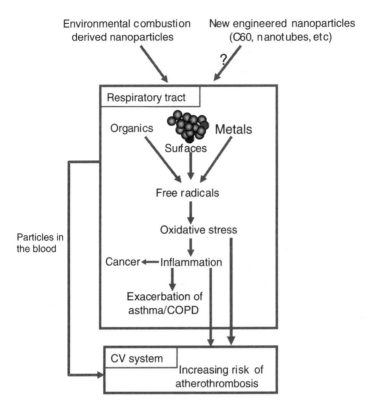

Figure 7 Figure summarizing the paradigm for the harmful effects of combustion-derived NP raising the question of whether new engineered nanoparticles—a very diverse group of materials—could conform to the same paradigm. *Abbreviations*: COPD, chronic obstructive pulmonary disease; CV, cardiovascular.

REFERENCES

1. Royal Society and Royal Academy of Engineering. Nanoscience and Nanotechnologies: Opportunities and Uncertainties. London: The Royal Society 2004.
2. Seaton A, MacNee W, Donaldson K, Godden D. Particulate air-pollution and acute health-effects. Lancet 1995; 345:176–8.
3. Utell MJ, Frampton MW. Acute health effects of ambient air pollution: the ultrafine particle hypothesis. J Aerosol Med 2000; 13:355–9.
4. Donaldson K, Tran L, Jimenez L, Duffin R, Newby DE, Mills N, et al. Combustion-derived nanoparticles: a review of their toxicology following inhalation exposure 1. Part Fibre Toxicol 2005; 2:10.
5. Quality of Urban Air Review Group. Airborne Particulate Matter in the United Kingdom. Third Report of the Quality of Urban Air Review Group. Quality of Urban Air Review Group, 1996.

6. Brunekreef B, Holgate ST. Air pollution and health. Lancet 2002; 360: 1233–42.
7. Pope CA, Dockery DW. Epidemiology of particle effects. In: Holgate ST, Samet JM, Koren HS, Maynard RL, eds. Air Pollution and Health. San Diego: Academic Press, 1999:673–705.
8. Peters A, Dockery DW, Muller JE, Mittleman MA. Increased particulate air pollution and the triggering of myocardial infarction. Circulation 2001; 103: 2810–5.
9. Gong HJr, Linn WS, Terrell SL, Clark KW, Geller MD, Anderson KR, et al. Altered heart-rate variability in asthmatic and healthy volunteers exposed to concentrated ambient coarse particles. Inhal Toxicol 2004; 16:335–43.
10. Devlin RB, Ghio AJ, Kehrl H, Sanders G, Cascio W. Elderly humans exposed to concentrated air pollution particles have decreased heart rate variability. Eur Respir J Suppl 2003; 40:76s–80.
11. Lippmann M, Ito K, Hwang JS, Maciejczyk P, Chen LC. Cardiovascular effects of nickel in ambient air. Environ Health Perspect 2006; 114:1662–9.
12. Ghio AJ, Kim C, Devlin RB. Concentrated ambient air particles induce mild pulmonary inflammation in healthy human volunteers. Am J Respir Crit Care Med 2000; 162:981–8.
13. Brook RD, Brook JR, Urch B, Vincent R, Rajagopalan S, Silverman F. Inhalation of fine particulate air pollution and ozone causes acute arterial vasoconstriction in healthy adults. Circulation 2002; 105:1534–6.
14. Kunzli N, Jerrett M, Mack WJ, Beckerman B, LaBree L, Gilliland F, et al. Ambient air pollution and atherosclerosis in Los Angeles. Environ Health Perspect 2005; 113:201–6.
15. Schlesinger RB, Cassee F. Atmospheric secondary inorganic particulate matter: the toxicological perspective as a basis for health effects risk assessment. Inhal Toxicol 2003; 15:197–235.
16. Pope CA, Thun MJ, Namboodiri MM, Dockery DW, Evans JS, Speizer FE, et al. Particulate air pollution as a predictor of mortality in a prospective study of U.S. adults. Am J Respir Crit Care Med 1995; 151:669–74.
17. de Hartog JJ, Hoek G, Mirme A, Tuch T, Kos GP, ten BrinkHM, et al. Relationship between different size classes of particulate matter and meteorology in three European cities. J Environ Monit 2005; 7:302–10.
18. Air Quality Expert Group. Particulate Matter in the United Kingdom. London: The Department of Environment, Food and Rural Affairs, 2005.
19. Elder A, Gelein R, Finkelstein J, Phipps R, Frampton M, Utell M, et al. On-road exposure to highway aerosols. 2. Exposures of aged, compromised rats. Inhal Toxicol 2004; 16(Suppl 1):41–53.
20. Kittelson DB, Watts WF, Johnson JP, Remerowki ML, Ische EE, Oberdorster G, et al. On-road exposure to highway aerosols. 1. Aerosol and gas measurements. Inhal Toxicol 2004; 16(Suppl 1):31–9.
21. Afshari A, Matson U, Ekberg LE. Characterization of indoor sources of fine and ultrafine particles: a study conducted in a full-scale chamber. Indoor Air 2005; 15:141–50.
22. Dennekamp M, Howarth S, Dick CA, Cherrie JW, Donaldson K, Seaton A. Ultrafine particles and nitrogen oxides generated by gas and electric cooking. Occup Environ Med 2001; 58:511–6.

23. Donaldson K, Jimenez LA, Rahman I, Faux SP, MacNee W, Gilmour PS, et al. Respiratory health effects of ambient air pollution particles: role of reactive species. In: Vallyathan V, Shi X, Castranova V, eds. Oxygen/Nitrogen Radicals: Lung Injury and Disease in Lung Biology in Health and Disease. New York: Marcel Dekker, 2004.

24. Donaldson K, Stone V, Borm PJ, Jimenez LA, Gilmour PS, Schins RP, et al. Oxidative stress and calcium signaling in the adverse effects of environmental particles (PM10). Free Radic Biol Med 2003; 34:1369–82.

25. Miyabara Y, Yanagisawa R, Shimojo N, Takano H, Lim HB, Ichinose T, et al. Murine strain differences in airway inflammation caused by diesel exhaust particles. Eur Respir J 1998; 11:291–8.

26. Tsurudome Y, Hirano T, Yamato H, Tanaka I, Sagai M, Hirano H, et al. Changes in levels of 8-hydroxyguanine in DNA, its repair and OGG1 mRNA in rat lungs after intratracheal administration of diesel exhaust particles. Carcinogenesis 1999; 20:1573–6.

27. Nordenhall C, Pourazar J, Blomberg A, Levin JO, Sandstrom T, Adelroth E. Airway inflammation following exposure to diesel exhaust: a study of time kinetics using induced sputum. Eur Respir J 2000; 15:1046–51.

28. Ichinose T, Yajima Y, Nagashima M, Takenoshita S, Nagamachi Y, Sagai M. Lung carcinogenesis and formation of 8-hydroxy-deoxyguanosine in mice by diesel exhaust particles. Carcinogenesis 1997; 18:185–92.

29. Arimoto T, Yoshikawa T, Takano H, Kohno M. Generation of reactive oxygen species and 8-hydroxy-2′-deoxyguanosine formation from diesel exhaust particle components in L1210 cells. Jpn J Pharmacol 1999; 80:49–54.

30. Bonvallot V, Baeza-Squiban A, Baulig A, Brulant S, Boland S, Muzeau F, et al. Organic compounds from diesel exhaust particles elicit a proinflammatory response in human airway epithelial cells and induce cytochrome p450 1A1 expression. Am J Respir Cell Mol Biol 2001; 25:515–21.

31. Hirano S, Furuyama A, Koike E, Kobayashi T. Oxidative-stress potency of organic extracts of diesel exhaust and urban fine particles in rat heart microvessel endothelial cells. Toxicology 2003; 187:161–70.

32. Li N, Venkatesan MI, Miguel A, Kaplan R, Gujuluva C, Alam J, et al. Induction of heme oxygenase-1 expression in macrophages by diesel exhaust particle chemicals and quinones via the antioxidant-responsive element. J Immunol 2000; 165:3393–401.

33. Nel AE, az-Sanchez D, Li N. The role of particulate pollutants in pulmonary inflammation and asthma: evidence for the involvement of organic chemicals and oxidative stress. Curr Opin Pulm Med 2001; 7:20–6.

34. McNeilly JD, Jimenez LA, Clay MF, MacNee W, Howe A, Heal MR, et al. Soluble transition metals in welding fumes cause inflammation via activation of NF-kappaB and AP-1. Toxicol Lett 2005; 158:152–7.

35. Marano F, Boland S, Bonvallot V, Baulig A, Baeza-Squiban A. Human airway epithelial cells in culture for studying the molecular mechanisms of the inflammatory response triggered by diesel exhaust particles. Cell Biol Toxicol 2002; 18:315–20.

36. Hiura TS, Kaszubowski MP, Li N, Nel AE. Chemicals in diesel exhaust particles generate reactive oxygen radicals and induce apoptosis in macrophages. J Immunol 1999; 163:5582–91.

37. Hashimoto S, Gon Y, Takeshita I, Matsumoto K, Jibiki I, Takizawa H, et al. Diesel exhaust particles activate p38 MAP kinase to produce interleukin 8 and RANTES by human bronchial epithelial cells and N-acetylcysteine attenuates p38 MAP kinase activation. Am J Respir Crit Care Med 2000; 161: 280–5.

38. Takizawa H, Ohtoshi T, Kawasaki S, Kohyama T, Desaki M, Kasama T, et al. Diesel exhaust particles induce NF-kappa B activation in human bronchial epithelial cells in vitro: importance in cytokine transcription. J Immunol 1999; 162:4705–11.

39. Gilmour PS, Rahman I, Donaldson K, MacNee W. Histone acetylation regulates epithelial IL-8 release mediated by oxidative stress from environmental particles. Am J Physiol Lung Cell Mol Physiol 2003; 284:L533–40.

40. Terada N, Hamano N, Maesako KI, Hiruma K, Hohki G, Suzuki K, et al. Diesel exhaust particulates upregulate histamine receptor mRNA and increase histamine-induced IL-8 and GM-CSF production in nasal epithelial cells and endothelial cells. Clin Exp Allergy1999; 29:52–9 [see comments].

41. Salvi SS, Nordenhall C, Blomberg A, Rudell B, Pourazar J, Kelly FJ, et al. Acute exposure to diesel exhaust increases IL-8 and GRO-alpha production in healthy human airways. Am J Respir Crit Care Med 2000; 161:550–7.

42. Yang HM, Ma JC, Castranova V, Ma JH. Effects of diesel exhaust particles on the release of interleukin-1 and tumor necrosis factor-alpha from rat alveolar macrophages. Exp Lung Res 1997; 23:269–84.

43. Steerenberg PA, Zonnenberg JJ, Dormans JA, Joon PT, Wouters IM, vanBree L, et al. Diesel exhaust particles induced release of interleukin 6 and 8 by (primed) human bronchial epithelial cells (BEAS 2B) in vitro. Exp Lung Res 1998; 24:85–100.

44. Brook RD, Franklin B, Cascio W, Hong Y, Howard G, Lipsett M, et al. Air pollution and cardiovascular disease: a statement for healthcare professionals from the Expert Panel on Population and Prevention Science of the American Heart Association. Circulation 2004; 109:2655–71.

45. Brook RD, Brook JR, Rajagopalan S. Air pollution: the "Heart" of the problem. Curr Hypertens Rep 2003; 5:32–9.

46. Donaldson K, Mills N, MacNee W, Robinson S, Newby D. Role of inflammation in cardiopulmonary health effects of PM. Toxicol Appl Pharmacol 2005; 207:483–8.

47. Viles-Gonzalez JF, Anand SX, Valdiviezo C, Zafar MU, Hutter R, Sanz J, et al. Update in atherothrombotic disease. Mt Sinai J Med 2004; 71:197–208.

48. Libby P, Ridker PM, Maseri A. Inflammation and atherosclerosis. Circulation 2002; 105:1135–43.

49. Van Lente F. Markers of inflammation as predictors in cardiovascular disease. Clin Chim Acta 2000; 293:31–52.

50. Suwa T, Hogg JC, Quinlan KB, Ohgami A, Vincent R, van Eeden SF. Particulate air pollution induces progression of atherosclerosis. J Am Coll Cardiol 2002; 39:935–42.

51. Sun Q, Wang A, Jin X, Natanzon A, Duquaine D, Brook RD, et al. Long-term air pollution exposure and acceleration of atherosclerosis and vascular inflammation in an animal model. JAMA 2005; 294:3003–10.

52. Lippmann M, Gordon T, Chen LC. Effects of subchronic exposures to concentrated ambient particles in mice. IX. Integral assessment and human

health implications of subchronic exposures of mice to CAPs. Inhal Toxicol 2005; 17:255–61.

53. Nemmar A, Hoet PH, Vanquickenborne B, Dinsdale D, Thomeer M, Hoylaerts MF, et al. Passage of inhaled particles into the blood circulation in humans. Circulation 2002; 105:411–4.

54. Mills N, Amin N, Robinson S, Davies J, de la Fuent JM, Boon NA, et al.: Inhaled ^{99m}Technetium-labeled carbon nanoparticles do not translocate into the circulation in man. Am J Resp Crit Care Med 2005, submitted.

55. Davies MJ. Coronary disease: the pathophysiology of acute coronary syndromes. Heart 2000; 83:361–6.

56. Rosenberg RD, Aird WC. Vascular-bed-specific hemostasis and hyper-coagulable states. N Engl J Med 1999; 340:1555–64.

57. Furchgott RF, Zawadzki JV. The obligatory role of endothelial cells in the relaxation of arterial smooth muscle by acetylcholine. Nature 1980; 288:373–6.

58. Ludmer PL, Selwyn AP, Shook TL, Wayne RR, Mudge GH, Alexander RW, et al. Paradoxical vasoconstriction induced by acetylcholine in atherosclerotic coronary arteries. N Engl J Med 1986; 315:1046–51.

59. Celermajer DS, Adams MR, Clarkson P, Robinson J, McCredie R, Donald A, et al. Passive smoking and impaired endothelium-dependent arterial dilatation in healthy young adults. N Engl J Med 1996; 334:150–4.

60. Newby DE, Wright RA, Labinjoh C, Ludlam CA, Fox KA, Boon NA, et al. Endothelial dysfunction, impaired endogenous fibrinolysis, and cigarette smoking: a mechanism for arterial thrombosis and myocardial infarction. Circulation 1999; 99:1411–5.

61. Hingorani AD, Cross J, Kharbanda RK, Mullen MJ, Bhagat K, Taylor M, et al. Acute systemic inflammation impairs endothelium-dependent dilatation in humans. Circulation 2000; 102:994–9.

62. Eijnden-Schrauwen Y, Kooistra T, de Vries RE, Emeis JJ. Studies on the acute release of tissue-type plasminogen activator from human endothelial cells in vitro and in rats in vivo: evidence for a dynamic storage pool. Blood 1995; 85: 3510–7.

63. Brommer EJ. The level of extrinsic plasminogen activator (t-PA) during clotting as a determinant of the rate of fibrinolysis; inefficiency of activators added afterwards. Thromb Res 1984; 34:109–15.

64. Fox KA, Robison AK, Knabb RM, Rosamond TL, Sobel BE, Bergmann SR. Prevention of coronary thrombosis with subthrombolytic doses of tissue-type plasminogen activator. Circulation 1985; 72:1346–54.

65. Mills NL, Tornqvist H, Robinson SD, Gonzalez M, Darnley K, MacNee W, et al. Diesel exhaust inhalation causes vascular dysfunction and impaired endogenous fibrinolysis. Circulation 2005; 112:3930–6.

66. Radomski A, Jurasz P, onso-Escolano D, Drews M, Morandi M, Malinski T, et al. Nanoparticle-induced platelet aggregation and vascular thrombosis. Br J Pharmacol 2005.

66a. Circulation article (details TK).

67. Nemmar A, Nemery B, Hoet PH, Vermylen J, Hoylaerts MF. Pulmonary inflammation and thrombogenicity caused by diesel particles in hamsters: role of histamine. Am J Respir Crit Care Med 2003; 168:1366–72.

68. Badimon JJ, Lettino M, Toschi V, Fuster V, Berrozpe M, Chesebro JH, et al. Local inhibition of tissue factor reduces the thrombogenicity of disrupted human atherosclerotic plaques: effects of tissue factor pathway inhibitor on plaque thrombogenicity under flow conditions. Circulation 1999; 99:1780–87.
69. Pope CA, III, Muhlestein JB, May HT, Renlund DG, Anderson JL, Horne BD. Ischemic heart disease events triggered by short-term exposure to fine particulate air pollution 1. Circulation 2006: 114:2443–8.
70. Lanki T, de Hartog. JJ, Heinrich J, Hoek G, Janssen NA, Peters A, et al. Can we identify sources of fine particles responsible for exercise-induced ischemia on days with elevated air pollution? The ULTRA study. Environ Health Perspect 2006; 114:655–60.
71. Miller KA, Siscovick DS, Sheppard L, Shepherd K, Sullivan JH, Anderson GL, et al. Long-term exposure to air pollution and incidence of cardiovascular events in women 1. N Engl J Med 2007; 356:447–58.
72. Mills NL, Tornqvist H, Gonzalez M, Robinson SD, MacNee W, Blomberg A, et al. Adverse cardiovascular effects of air pollution in patients with coronary heart disease. J Am Coll Cardiol, abstract (in press).
73. Task Force of the European Society of Cardiology and the North American Society of Pacing and Electrophysiology. Heart rate variability. Standards of measurement, physiological interpretation, and clinical use. Eur Heart J 1996; 17:354–81.
74. Tsuji H, Venditti FJ, Jr., Manders ES, Evans JC, Larson MG, Feldman CL, et al. Reduced heart rate variability and mortality risk in an elderly cohort. The Framingham Heart Study. Circulation 1994; 90:878–83.
75. Kleiger RE. Heart rate variability and mortality and sudden death post infarction. J Cardiovasc Electrophysiol 1995; 6:365–7.
76. Pope CA, III, Verrier RL, Lovett EG, Larson AC, Raizenne ME, Kanner RE, et al. Heart rate variability associated with particulate air pollution [see comments]. Am Heart J 1999; 138:890–9.
77. Liao D, Creason J, Shy C, Williams R, Watts R, Zweidinger R. Daily variation of particulate air pollution and poor cardiac autonomic control in the elderly. Environ Health Perspect 1999; 107:521–5.
78. Magari SR, Hauser R, Schwartz J, Williams PL, Smith TJ, Christiani DC. Association of heart rate variability with occupational and environmental exposure to particulate air pollution. Circulation 2001; 104:986–91.
79. Creason J, Neas L, Walsh D, Williams R, Sheldon L, Liao D, et al. Particulate matter and heart rate variability among elderly retirees: the Baltimore 1998 PM study. J Expo Anal Environ Epidemiol 2001; 11:116–22.
80. Gold DR, Litonjua A, Schwartz J, Lovett E, Larson A, Nearing B, et al. Ambient Pollution and Heart Rate Variability. Circulation 2000; 101:1267–73.
81. Devlin RB, Ghio AJ, Kehrl H, Sanders G, Cascio W. Elderly humans exposed to concentrated air pollution particles have decreased heart rate variability 14. Eur Respir J Suppl 2003; 40:76s–80s.
82. Wellenius GA, Saldiva PH, Batalha JR, Krishna Murthy GG, Coull BA, Verrier RL, et al. Electrocardiographic changes during exposure to residual oil fly ash (ROFA) particles in a rat model of myocardial infarction. Toxicol Sci 2002; 66:327–35.

83. Peters A, Liu E, Verrier RL, Schwartz J, Gold DR, Mittleman M, et al. Air pollution and incidence of cardiac arrhythmia [see comments]. Epidemiology 2000; 11:11–7.

84. Campen MJ, Nolan JP, Schladweiler MC, Kodavanti UP, Costa DL, Watkinson WP. Cardiac and thermoregulatory effects of instilled particulate matter-associated transition metals in healthy and cardiopulmonary-compromised rats. J Toxicol Environ Health A 2002; 65:1615–31.

85. Godleski JJ, Verrier RL, Koutrakis P, Catalano P, Coull B, Reinisch U, et al. Mechanisms of morbidity and mortality from exposure to ambient air particles. Res Rep Health Eff Inst 2000; 5–88.

86. Bellmann B, Muhle H, Creutzenberg O, Mermelstein R. Irreversible pulmonary changes induced in rat lung by dust overload. Environ Health Perspect 1992; 97:189–91.

87. Morrow PE. Dust overloading of the lungs: update and appraisal. Toxicol Appl Pharmacol 1992; 113:1–12.

88. Mauderly JL, Cheng YS, Snipes MB. Particle overload in toxicological studies: friend or foe. J Aerosol Med 1990; 3(Suppl 1):S169–87.

89. Morrow PE. Possible mechanisms to explain dust overloading of the lungs. Fundam Appl Toxicol 1988; 10:369–84.

90. Tran CL, Buchanan D, Cullen RT, Searl A, Jones AD, Donaldson K. Inhalation of poorly soluble particles. II. Influence of particle surface area on inflammation and clearance. Inhal Toxicol 2000; 12:1113–26.

91. Cullen RT, Tran CL, Buchanan D, Davis JM, Searl A, Jones AD, et al. Inhalation of poorly soluble particles. I. Differences in inflammatory response and clearance during exposure. Inhal Toxicol 2000; 12:1089–11.

92. Driscoll KE. Role of inflammation in the development of rat lung tumors in response to chronic particle exposure. Inhal Toxicol 1996; 8(Suppl): 139–53.

93. Oberdorster G, Ferin J, Soderholm S, Gelein R, Baggs R, Morrow PE. Increased pulmonary toxicity of inhaled ultrafine particles: due to overload alone? Inhal Toxicol 1999; 38:295–302.

94. Gilmour PS, Ziesenis A, Morrison ER, Vickers MA, Drost EM, Ford I, et al. Pulmonary and systemic effects of short-term inhalation exposure to ultrafine carbon black particles. Toxicol Appl Pharmacol 2004; 195:35–44.

95. Renwick LC, Brown D, Clouter A, Donaldson K. Increased inflammation and altered macrophage chemotactic responses caused by two ultrafine particle types. Occup Environ Med 2004; 61:442–7.

96. Hohr D, Steinfartz Y, Schins RP, Knaapen AM, Martra G, Fubini B, et al. The surface area rather than the surface coating determines the acute inflammatory response after instillation of fine and ultrafine TiO_2 in the rat. Int J Hyg Environ Health 2002; 205:239–44.

97. Duffin R, Clouter A, Brown D, Tran CL, MacNee W, Stone V, et al. The importance of surface area and specific reactivity in the acute pulmonary inflammatory response to particles. Ann Occup Hyg 2002; 46(Suppl 1):242–5.

98. Wilson MR, Lightbody JH, Donaldson K, Sales J, Stone V. Interactions between ultrafine particles and transition metals in vivo and in vitro. Toxicol Appl Pharmacol 2002; 184:172–9.

99. Stone V, Shaw J, Brown DM, MacNee W, Faux SP, Donaldson K. The role of oxidative stress in the prolonged inhibitory effect of ultrafine carbon black on epithelial cell function. Toxicol In Vitro 1998; 12:649–59. 1998.
100. Beck-Speier I, Dayal N, Karg E, Maier KL, Schumann G, Schulz H, et al. Oxidative stress and lipid mediators induced in alveolar macrophages by ultrafine particles. Free Radic Biol Med 2005; 38:1080–92.
101. Stone V, Tuinman M, Vamvakopoulos JE, Shaw J, Brown D, Petterson S, et al. Increased calcium influx in a monocytic cell line on exposure to ultrafine carbon black. Eur Respir J 2000; 15:297–303.
102. Brown DM, Donaldson K, Borm PJ, Schins RP, Dehnhardt M, Gilmour P, et al. Calcium and ROS-mediated activation of transcription factors and TNF-alpha cytokine gene expression in macrophages exposed to ultrafine particles. Am J Physiol Lung Cell Mol Physiol 2004; 286:L344–53.
103. Tamaoki J, Isono K, Takeyama K, Tagaya E, Nakata J, Nagai A. Ultrafine carbon black particles stimulate proliferation of human airway epithelium via EGF receptor-mediated signaling pathway. Am J Physiol Lung Cell Mol Physiol 2004; 287:L1127–33.
104. Timblin CR, Shukla A, Berlanger I, Berube KA, Churg A, Mossman BT. Ultrafine airborne particles cause increases in protooncogene expression and proliferation in alveolar epithelial cells. Toxicol Appl Pharmacol 2002; 179: 98–104.
105. Donaldson K, Tran CL. An introduction to the short-term toxicology of respirable industrial fibers. Mutat Res 2004; 553:5–9.
106. Nyberg K, Johansson U, Rundquist I, Camner P. Estimation of pH in individual alveolar macrophage phagolysosomes. Exp Lung Res 1989; 15: 499–510.
107. Hesterberg TW, Miiller WC, Musselman RP, Kamstrup O, Hamilton RD, Thevenaz P. Biopersistence of man-made vitreous fibers and crocidolite asbestos in the rat lung following inhalation. Fundam Appl Toxicol 1996; 29: 267–79.
108. Muller J, Huaux F, Moreau N, Misson P, Heilier JF, Delos M, et al. Respiratory toxicity of multi-wall carbon nanotubes. Toxicol Appl Pharmacol 2005; 207:221–31.
109. Maynard AD, Baron PA, Foley M, Shvedova AA, Kisin ER, Castranova V. Exposure to carbon nanotube material: aerosol release during the handling of unrefined single-walled carbon nanotube material. J Toxicol Environ Health A 2004; 67:87–107.
110. Lam CW, James JT, McCluskey R, Hunter RL. Pulmonary toxicity of single-wall carbon nanotubes in mice 7 and 90 days after intratracheal instillation. Toxicol Sci 2004; 77:126–34.
111. Warheit DB, Laurence BR, Reed KL, Roach DH, Reynolds GA, Webb TR. Comparative pulmonary toxicity assessment of single-wall carbon nanotubes in rats. Toxicol Sci 2004; 77:117–25.
112. Shvedova AA, Kisin ER, Mercer R, Murray AR, Johnson VJ, Potapovich AI, et al. Unusual inflammatory and fibrogenic pulmonary responses to single-walled carbon nanotubes in mice. Am J Physiol Lung Cell Mol Physiol 2005; 289:L698–708.

113. Monteiro-Riviere NA, Nemanich RJ, Inman AO, Wang YY, Riviere JE. Multi-walled carbon nanotube interactions with human epidermal keratinocytes. Toxicol Lett 2005; 155:377–84.
114. Shvedova AA, Castranova V, Kisin ER, Schwegler-Berry D, Murray AR, Gandelsman VZ, et al. Exposure to carbon nanotube material: assessment of nanotube cytotoxicity using human keratinocyte cells. J Toxicol Environ Health A 2003; 66:1909–26.
115. Jia G, Wang H, Yan L, Wang X, Pei R, Yan T, et al. Cytotoxicity of carbon nanomaterials: single-wall nanotube, multi-wall nanotube, and fullerene. Environ Sci Technol 2005; 39:1378–83.
116. Bottini M, Bruckner S, Nika K, Bottini N, Bellucci S, Magrini A, et al. Multi-walled carbon nanotubes induce T lymphocyte apoptosis. Toxicol Lett 2006; 160:121–6.
117. Cui D, Tian F, Ozkan CS, Wang M, Gao H. Effect of single wall carbon nanotubes on human HEK293 cells. Toxicol Lett 2005; 155:73–85.
118. Manna SK, Sarkar S, Barr J, Wise K, Barrera EV, Jejelowo O, et al. Single-walled carbon nanotube induces oxidative stress and activates nuclear transcription factor-kappaB in human keratinocytes. Nano Lett 2005; 5: 1676–84.
119. Kagan VE, Tyurina YY, Tyurin VA, Konduru NV, Potapovich AI, Osipov AN, et al. Direct and indirect effects of single walled carbon nanotubes on RAW 264.7 macrophages: role of iron. Toxicol Lett 2006; 165:88–100.
120. Sayes CM, Fortner JD, Guo W, Lyon D, Colvin VL, et al. The differential cytotoxicity of water-soluble fullerenes. Nano Lett 2004; 4:1881–7.
121. Isakovic A, Markovic Z, Todorovic-Markovic B, Nikolic N, Vranjes-Djuric S, Mirkovic M, et al. Distinct cytotoxic mechanisms of pristine versus hydroxylated fullerene. Toxicol Sci 2006.
122. Mirkov SM, Djordjevic AN, Andric NL, Andric SA, Kostic TS, Bogdanovic GM, et al. Nitric oxide-scavenging activity of polyhydroxylated fullerenol, $C_{60}(OH)_{24}$. Nitric Oxide 2004; 11:201–7.
123. Corona-Morales AA, Castell A, Escobar A, Drucker-Colin R, Zhang L. Fullerene C60 and ascorbic acid protect cultured chromaffin cells against levodopa toxicity. J Neurosci Res 2003; 71:121–6.
124. Gharbi N, Pressac M, Hadchouel M, Szwarc H, Wilson SR, Moussa F. [60]fullerene is a powerful antioxidant in vivo with no acute or subacute toxicity. Nano Lett 2005; 5:2578–85.
125. Lee YT, Chiang LY, Chen WJ, Hsu HC. Water-soluble hexasulfobutyl[60]-fullerene inhibit low-density lipoprotein oxidation in aqueous and lipophilic phases. Proc Soc Exp Biol Med 2000; 224:69–75.
126. Hardman R. A toxicologic review of quantum dots: toxicity depends on physicochemical and environmental factors. Environ Health Perspect 2006; 114:165–72.
127. Lovric J, Bazzi HS, Cuie Y, Fortin GR, Winnik FM, Maysinger D. Differences in subcellular distribution and toxicity of green and red emitting CdTe quantum dots. J Mol Med 2005; 83:377–85.
128. Ballou B, Lagerholm BC, Ernst LA, Bruchez MP, Waggoner AS. Noninvasive imaging of quantum dots in mice. Bioconjug Chem 2004; 15:79–86.

129. Dubertret B, Skourides P, Norris DJ, Noireaux V, Brivanlou AH, Libchaber A. In vivo imaging of quantum dots encapsulated in phospholipid micelles. Science 2002; 298:1759–62.
130. Larson DR, Zipfel WR, Williams RM, Clark SW, Bruchez MP, Wise FW, et al. Water-soluble quantum dots for multiphoton fluorescence imaging in vivo. Science 2003; 300:1434–6.
131. Soto KJ, Carrasco A, Powell TG, Garza KM, Murr LE. Comparative in vitro cytotoxicity assessment of some manufactured nanoparticulate materials characterised by transmission electron microscopy. J Nanoparticle Res 2005; 7:145–69.
132. Hussain SM, Hess KL, Gearhart JM, Geiss KT, Schlager JJ. In vitro toxicity of nanoparticles in BRL 3A rat liver cells. Toxicol In Vitro 2005; 19:975–83.
133. Chen Z, Meng H, Xing G, Chen C, Zhao Y, Jia G, et al. Acute toxicological effects of copper nanoparticles in vivo. Toxicol Lett 2005.
134. Dick CA, Brown DM, Donaldson K, Stone V. The role of free radicals in the toxic and inflammatory effects of four different ultrafine particle types. Inhal Toxicol 2003; 15:39–52.
135. Yamawaki H, Iwai N. Mechanisms underlying nano-sized air-pollution-mediated progression of atherosclerosis: carbon black causes cytotoxic injury/inflammation and inhibits cell growth in vascular endothelial cells. Circ J 2006; 70:129–40.
136. Don Porto CA, Hoet PH, Verschaeve L, Schoeters G, Nemery B. Genotoxic effects of carbon black particles, diesel exhaust particles, and urban air particulates and their extracts on a human alveolar epithelial cell line (A549) and a human monocytic cell line (THP-1). Environ Mol Mutagen 2001; 37:155–63.
137. Schins RP. Mechanisms of genotoxicity of particles and fibers. Inhal Toxicol 2002; 14:57–78.
138. de Kok TM, Hogervorst JG, Briede JJ, van Herwijnen MH, Maas LM, Moonen EJ, et al. Genotoxicity and physicochemical characteristics of traffic-related ambient particulate matter. Environ Mol Mutagen 2005; 46:71–80.
139. Knaapen AM, Borm PJ, Albrecht C, Schins RP. Inhaled particles and lung cancer. Part A: Mechanisms. Int J Cancer 2004; 109:799–809.
140. Esterbauer H, Schaur RJ, Zollner H. Chemistry and biochemistry of 4-hydroxynonenal, malonaldehyde and related aldehydes. Free Radic Biol Med 1991; 11:81–128.
141. Chen M, von Mikecz A. Formation of nucleoplasmic protein aggregates impairs nuclear function in response to SiO_2 nanoparticles. Exp Cell Res 2005; 305:51–62.
142. Geiser M, Rothen-Rutlshauser B, Kapp N, Schurch S, Kreyling W, Schulz H, et al. Ultrafine particles cross cellular membranes by non-phagocytic mechanisms in lungs and in cultured cells. Environ Health Perspect 2005, in press.
143. Donaldson K, Beswick PH, Gilmour PS. Free radical activity associated with the surface of particles: a unifying factor in determining biological activity? Toxicol Lett 1996; 88:293–8.
144. Pope CA, III, Dockery DW. Epidemiology of particle effects. In: Holgate ST, Samet JM, Koren HS, Maynard RL. eds. Air Pollution and Health. San Diego: Academic Press, 1999:673–705.

18

Understanding the Potential Neurotoxicology of Nanoparticles

Rosemary M. Gibson

Health Effects Division, Health and Safety Laboratory, Derbyshire, U.K.

INTRODUCTION

Humans have been exposed to ultrafine particles in the atmosphere for centuries, from combustion as well as natural sources such as sea spray. Since the industrial revolution, the levels of ambient particles have increased significantly, and with the recent expansion of nanotechnology, we are likely to be exposed to manufactured as well as ambient nanoparticles. Organs such as the lungs are obvious targets for exposure to airborne agents via inhalation. The potential for nanoparticles to reach the brain and nervous systems seems, at first glance, to be unlikely, since they have well-developed barriers that are effective against many xenobiotics. However, very small agents and hydrophobic molecules can penetrate these barriers, to gain access to the elaborate networks of functional cells, the neurons and glia, within the nervous systems. Some agents can also take a direct route into the brain, from the olfactory epithelium in the nasal cavity, along the olfactory neurons and into the olfactory bulb. If they can cross synapses, access to distant structures within the brain is then plausible. There is the potential therefore for nanoparticles to access and affect the functions of the neurons within the central nervous system (CNS). Acute toxicity may be unlikely, except in extreme circumstances, but chronic toxicity might occur, and indeed, the etiology of many neurodegenerative diseases is considered to involve interaction between environmental agents, genetic factors, and aging (1). Furthermore, symptoms frequently only manifest themselves when a large proportion of a particular population of neurons has been lost or is no longer functional; for example, the symptoms of Parkinson's disease only become apparent when 60 to 80% of dopaminergic neurons in the motor coordination centers of the brain have died. Therefore, chronic exposure to even very low levels of nanoparticles might modulate neuronal function or induce cell death, and lead eventually to neurological problems.

Studying these phenomena is very difficult, since the systems are complex and mimicking the multifactorial elements of neurodegenerative disease in the laboratory, even in vivo, is extraordinarily challenging. However it is not impossible, although it is critical that the limitations of the model systems are borne in mind. In this chapter, after considering the routes by which nanoparticles may access the CNS, the evidence that so far implicates nanosized particles in potentially neuropathological changes will be summarized, and then methods for analyzing the effects of nanoparticles in nervous tissue will be reviewed.

PENETRATION OF NANOPARTICLES INTO THE CENTRAL NERVOUS SYSTEM

In contrast to large (fine- or micron-sized) particles, which are taken up into cells by phagocytosis, a process that depends on the actin-myosin network within cells, smaller particles of less than 100 nm may enter cells passively. Therefore, when inhaled into the respiratory tract, it is feasible that they penetrate into cells and surrounding tissues, including the blood circulation. They can then be transported around the body, and gain access to extrapulmonary organs. This route of entry into the brain requires transfer across the blood–brain barrier (BBB), but other routes exist. Nanoparticles may enter the CNS where the BBB is absent or limited, such as the circumventricular organs, or after pathophysiological changes to the BBB, induced by injury, disease, or aging. Alternatively, following inhalation, nanoparticles may gain access to the brain via an olfactory nerve pathway.

The olfactory system represents a unique interface between the nervous system and the external environment, since there is an intimate association between the nasal epithelium and olfactory neurons. Thus it is possible for inhaled agents to be taken up directly by olfactory neurons, a route that was originally recognized for 30 nm poliovirus particles (e.g., Ref. 2) and has been investigated considerably for solvents and metals such as manganese (3). Studies have shown that manganese is taken up into olfactory neurons following inhalation or instillation in a number of species (e.g., rat, mouse, freshwater pike), and can accumulate in the olfactory bulb. Furthermore, although the highest levels are observed in the olfactory bulb, manganese is also found in distal structures such as the striatum, suggesting that the metal successfully traverses synapses, albeit slowly (4). More soluble forms of manganese result in higher concentrations in the olfactory bulb than insoluble forms such as manganese phosphate (5). Recent studies in monkeys using magnetic resonance imaging (MRI) have also shown that following inhalation of manganese, the metal can be detected in the olfactory epithelium, olfactory bulb, and distant brain regions including the globus pallidus (6).

Inhalation of manganese in humans, via occupational exposure to welding fumes for example, can lead to respiratory symptoms and with chronic occupational exposure, to neurotoxicity (3). The symptoms of manganese-induced neurotoxicity or manganism, progress from initial psychiatric problems to Parkinson's-like disease, characterized by muscular contractions and rigidity, reduced muscle movement, and muscular tremors. The disease is marked by elevated concentrations of manganese in midbrain regions such as the globus pallidus and substantia nigra, and it has been proposed that the output pathways of the nigrostriatal pathway are damaged, distinguishing the disease clinically from Parkinson's disease, in which the nigrostriatal pathway itself degenerates. The neurological symptoms associated with chronic inhalation of high levels of manganese suggests that transport of this metal into the brain is significantly neurotoxic, and potentially points to the involvement of olfactory transport in the development of neurological diseases. However, the mechanisms of manganese-induced neurotoxicity are unknown. Oxidative stress in the brain has been proposed as a potential mechanism, but reports that both support and reject this hypothesis can be found in the literature (7).

The potential role of olfactory transport of inhaled nanosized particles was demonstrated as early as 1970 by De Lorenzo (8). Translocation of gold nanoparticles (50 nm diameter) was followed along olfactory neurons to the olfactory bulb following intranasal instillation in the monkey. The particles were visualized by electron microscopy and it was noted that they crossed synapses in the olfactory glomerulus and had reached the mitral cell dendrites as soon as 1 h after administration, suggesting movement at 2.5 mm/h. More recently, Oberdorster's group has demonstrated uptake and movement of nanoparticles of carbon and manganese oxide along this olfactory route. Following inhalation of ^{13}C nanoparticles (36 nm diameter) for 6 h in the rat, the distribution of the particles was analyzed for up to 7 days later (9). The levels of ^{13}C in the olfactory bulb increased on the first day and remained elevated for the duration of the experiment. Further studies from this group have shown that while manganese oxide nano-particles (31 nm diameter) accumulate in the lung, striatum, and cortex of the rat following inhalation or intranasal instillation, the largest increases are seen in the olfactory bulb (10). If one nostril is occluded, the accumulation of manganese oxide is restricted to one side of the olfactory bulb; transport via the lung and systemic circulation continues, demonstrating that the olfactory pathway is the source of the accumulation in the olfactory bulb. The authors suggest that about 11.5% of manganese deposited on the nasal epithelium translocates to the olfactory bulb.

Overall therefore, the olfactory pathway represents an alternative route to systemic circulation and crossing the BBB for penetration of agents into the brain, and one which should not be overlooked for nanoparticles, particularly since nasal deposition increases with decreasing size. The extent of deposition and importance of the different routes into the brain will also depend on characteristics of the nanoparticles in addition to size. The importance of the olfactory route for humans is debated and has yet to be conclusively demonstrated, their nasal anatomy being considerably different to rodents, but the demonstration of olfactory transport in nonhuman primates argues that it may play an important role.

EFFECTS OF NANOPARTICLES WITHIN THE CNS

Little is known to date of the downstream consequences of manufactured nanoparticles reaching the CNS. In the periphery, exposure to nanoparticles can lead to elevation of inflammatory markers. The CNS was viewed for many years as a site of immune privilege, which neither contributes to nor is affected by peripheral inflammatory events; it is now realized however that inflammatory responses both affect and occur within the CNS (11). The responses of the CNS to inflammation are nevertheless different to the periphery; e.g., leukocyte recruitment is delayed, although activation of resident brain inflammatory cells (microglia) is very rapid. Increases in inflammatory parameters may accompany aging and may be further elevated in both acute and chronic neurodegenerative disorders. Therefore if exposure to ambient pollution and nanomaterials leads to both peripheral and/or CNS inflammation, it can be hypothesized that they might contribute to CNS disease.

One seminal and frequently cited study suggests that ambient pollution can induce neuropathological changes in the brain. Calderon-Garciduenas and coworkers compared the nasal mucosae and brains of dogs from two Mexican cities (12): Southwest Metropolitan Mexico City (SWMMC), an urban area with high levels of pollutants including particulate matter and ozone, both of which exceed the U.S. National Ambient Air Quality Standards (USNAAQS), and Tlaxcala, a city at a similar altitude, but with pollution levels below USNAAQS. Significant changes were observed in the older dogs from SWMMC, including pathological changes in the nasal and olfactory mucosae, reactive astrocytosis, apoptosis of glia in white matter, and early activation in neurons and glia of the transcription factor NF-κB, which is involved in the expression of a number of proinflammatory genes such as inducible nitric oxide synthase (iNOS). Neuropathological changes included neuronal degeneration, and formation of neurofibrillary tangles and plaques. These changes suggest that the dogs living in the more polluted city have signs of inflammation and neurodegenerative disease, although there are no data on the contributions of individual agents or ultrafine particles.

Evidence of brain inflammation in response to ambient fine and ultrafine particles has been obtained with a more homogeneous population of animals. Increases in the transcription factor NF-κB and the proinflammatory cytokines interleukin-1 (IL-1) β and tumor necrosis factor (TNF) α have been observed in mice exposed to concentrated ultrafine airborne particles (13).

Exposure to ultrafine particulate matter in pollution may also induce inflammation and neurological effects in humans. Further work from the group of Calderon-Garciduenas suggests that children living in the heavily polluted SWMMC show signs of chronic inflammation of the respiratory tract, and damage to the nasal epithelium, which may exacerbate effects of pollutants by increasing access to the systemic circulation and the brain (14,15). Further studies in human subjects living in Mexico City or Monterrey, both heavily polluted cities, showed elevations of messenger RNA for the enzyme cyclooxygenase (Cox) 2, which is involved in the generation of proinflammatory prostaglandins, in the cortex of brains taken at autopsy, and specifically in blood vessel endothelia (16). There was also significant accumulation of the amyloid β peptide (A-β42), associated with Alzheimer's disease, in the cortex and hippocampus of individuals in the high exposure group. Cox-2 and A-β42 were also significantly increased in the olfactory bulbs of some subjects.

Further evidence comes from studies of mice with a deletion of the gene for apolipoprotein (Apo) E; this gene is often mutated in Alzheimer's disease, and these mice have been shown to manifest increased levels of oxidative stress. The animals were exposed to either air or concentrated ambient particles, and their brains were analyzed for markers of dopaminergic neurons and activated glia in areas that control motor function and are significantly affected in diseases such as Parkinson's disease (PD). There was a significant reduction in the numbers of dopaminergic neurons in the ApoE deleted mice after exposure to ambient particles, and an increase in glial activation (16). The precise mechanism underlying the selective nature of the neurotoxicity is unclear, but one hypothesis arises from the observation that when exposed to concentrated ambient particles in vitro, microglial cells release proinflammatory cytokines and generate an oxidative burst (17). Furthermore, it has been shown that the dopaminergic neurotoxicity of diesel exhaust particles requires microglia and is prevented in cocultures of cells from mice that lack a catalytic subunit of NADH oxidase and hence lack a respiratory burst (18). The brain is very sensitive to oxidative stress, at least partly because of its high energy requirements and low levels of endogenous free radical scavengers. It can be hypothesized therefore that in response to ambient particles, microglia become activated and generate a respiratory burst, which leads to secondary neuronal loss in areas with a sufficiently high density of microglia and neurons, and that are particularly sensitive to oxidative stress, such as the mesencephalon, involved in motor control and targeted in Parkinson's disease (PD).

Despite the evidence that links ambient ultrafine particles, brain inflammation and neurological effects, a direct contribution from individual components of ambient pollution is difficult to prove. Recent studies suggest, however, that pure nanoparticles can induce inflammation in the brain. Intranasal instillation of carbon black (CB) nanoparticles into mice leads to increases in the messenger RNA for specific cytokines and chemokines (IL-1β, TNFα, macrophage inflammatory protein [MIP]-1 α and monocyte chemoattractant protein [MCP]-1), as well as the chemokine ligand CXCL9; these changes are only seen in response to 14 nm and not 95 nm particles, and they are only observed in the olfactory bulb, not the hippocampus (19). Inflammatory changes have also been observed in the olfactory bulb, cortex, midbrain, and striatum of the rat following inhalation or intranasal instillation of manganese oxide nanoparticles (31 nm diameter): increases in messenger RNA for TNFα and MIP-2 were noted, as well as increases in glial fibrillary acidic protein (GFAP), a marker for astrocyte activation (10).

APPROACHES FOR STUDYING THE EFFECTS OF NANOPARTICLES IN THE CNS

The regulatory guidelines (approved by the U.S. Environmental Protection Agency and Organization for Economic Cooperation and Development) for evaluating the neurotoxicity of a chemical recommend extensive testing in animals (20,21). The aim is to provide a thorough analysis of any nervous system effects to inform risk assessment. The first stage usually involves identifying whether a particular chemical displays neurotoxicity. Acute and subchronic exposures are administered, usually at three different doses, and a wide range of observations are made, including changes in behavior, signs of convulsions, measurement of body weight, and a range of histological stains are applied to tissue sections. If the chemical displays signs of neurotoxicity in these studies, a second stage will involve more extensive characterization of the effect(s).

Since the number of new nanoparticles emerging is increasing exponentially, this strategy for evaluating neurotoxicity may not be feasible except for representative particles. Oberdorster et al. (22) have proposed a tiered testing strategy for nanoparticles consisting of in vitro investigations followed by two tiers of animal tests; in the first tier, rats or mice would be exposed by an inhalation route (inhalation, intratracheal instillation, or pharyngeal or laryngeal aspiration), to an aerosol of three different doses of the nanoparticle. Endpoints would focus on pulmonary inflammation and cytotoxicity, but effects in secondary organs such as the brain would be examined. As well as histological staining of secondary organs, tissue-specific endpoints are also proposed, e.g., immunohistochemical staining for the viability of specific subsets of neurons or for GFAP, an indicator of astrocyte activation and potential CNS injury. The second tier of studies would then evaluate in greater detail any effects observed in tier 1, and if necessary, analyze the effects of the nanoparticles in animal models of susceptible subpopulations, such as the elderly or those predisposed to cardiovascular disease.

Broadly therefore, Oberdorster and comembers of the International Life Sciences Institute (ILSI) working group recommend a somewhat simplified version of the current regulatory testing strategy (22). Animal models have been used effectively for exploring the potential toxicity of nanoparticles; a recent review of the literature suggests that about 60 studies have been published in the last 6 years, looking at the effects of engineered and pure nanoparticles in animal models of human exposure. Only a few of these studies, however, have examined neurotoxicity; some of those, as highlighted above, have concentrated on investigating the olfactory route of uptake into the CNS. Little is therefore known about the neurological effects of engineered nanoparticles.

Specific questions about the neurotoxicity of nanoparticles can be at least partially addressed using in vitro methods, proposed by Oberdorster and coworkers as one tier of their testing strategy (22). Neurotoxicity risk assessment guidelines propose that analyzes using in vitro systems can highlight a potential effect, but provide inadequate evidence of neurotoxicity, although they can enhance the reliability of in vivo data (20). Thus they could provide a useful first-stage screening tool for new manufactured nano-particles, and could reduce the numbers of animals needed for full-scale testing by pointing to particles that have potential neurotoxic effects. However, prevalidation and validation exercises will be required to demonstrate whether these in vitro tests have acceptable sensitivity and specificity.

IN VITRO MODEL SYSTEMS FOR STUDYING NEUROTOXICITY

There are four basic types of nervous system models that can be employed for analyzing nanoparticle neurotoxicity: organotypic cultures, reaggregated cell cultures, primary cells isolated from animals or humans, and cell lines (23).

Organotypic Cultures

Organotypic cultures are typically slices of embryonic brain, but whole organs can be used, and they preserve, at least initially, the three-dimensional organization of the tissue and hence the cellular interactions and microenvironment. Depending on culture conditions, the slices can survive for weeks or even months, and they have been used extensively for electrophysiological recordings of receptor and channel activity, and hence investigating excitotoxic and convulsive activities of chemicals. Typically, slices are taken from the hippocampus, but they can successfully be cultured from other brain regions such as the cerebellum or cortex. Slices would be well suited for investigation of the persistence of nanoparticles within neural tissue, and their effects on specific aspects of neuronal function, such as electrical activity and neurotransmission, particularly during chronic or repeated exposures. These cultures do suffer from several disadvantages however, and cannot be regarded as retaining perfectly and indefinitely the in vivo organization of the brain. Firstly, cutting slices damages the tissue, and hypoxia and necrosis may occur during prolonged culture. Secondly, synaptic rearrangement results from the loss of afferent and efferent innervations and the flattening of the slice that occurs during culture (23).

Reaggregated Cultures

Reaggregated cultures generally consist of primary brain tissue that has been dissociated and the cells then allowed to reaggregate in suspension culture, usually under gently rotating conditions to prevent adhesion. The cultures can be maintained for quite long periods (up to months). The cells differentiate in the spheres, re-forming cellular interactions and synapses, replicating the structural organization of the intact tissue. These cultures have, for example, been used for generating retina-like tissue from neonatal animals for a range of purposes including toxicological analysis (24,25). Reaggregating cultures can suffer from some of the same problems as organotypic cultures, such as hypoxia, but they are promising for neuro-toxicological testing since they are quite robust, and can be used for acute and chronic testing.

Aggregates of neural stem cells can also be grown in suspension as "neurospheres." These dynamic structures are generated from dissociated embryonic CNS tissue, and they are being explored for many purposes including implantation in animal models of neurodegenerative disease (26). They can be propagated in vitro for several months, and then upon plating out on suitable substrates, the cells differentiate into neurons and glia. These cultures offer several advantages for testing the toxicity of nanoparticles, not least the possibility to culture large numbers of CNS cells.

Dissociated Primary CNS Cells

Dissociated primary CNS cells are widely used for a variety of experimental purposes. The cells are derived from dissected embryonic or early postnatal tissue, which is dissociated either mechanically or enzymatically. Cultures of different types of CNS cells can be obtained from an initial mixture of dissociated cells. Primary neurons are prepared by plating the cells on to an appropriate adhesive substrate (frequently poly-lysine) in the presence of mitotic inhibitors to eliminate the dividing glial cells. Neurons of more than 95% purity can be isolated in this way from a variety of brain regions, including the cortex, cerebellum, and hippocampus (e.g., Ref. 27). Alternatively mixed glia (astrocytes, microglia, and oligodendrocytes) can be cultured from dissociated brain tissue in the absence of the mitotic inhibitors; separate cultures of individual glial types can be subsequently obtained, taking advantage of their differential adhesion properties. For example, after 2 weeks in culture, flasks of mixed glia can be shaken to dislodge the microglia (within a few hours) and oligodendrocytes (after more than 12 h) from the underlying astrocytes. Successful culture of the different cell types depends heavily on optimization of the culture conditions (serum concentration, seeding density, media) as well on the age of the donor tissue. These types of culture are well suited for analysis of the toxicity of nanoparticles since the effects of particles on defined populations of cells can be compared with those on cocultures prepared from mixing different populations. This approach allows dissection of the contribution of individual cells to a neurotoxic effect; for example, neurotoxicity may require the presence of particular glia as demonstrated by Block et al. (18), who have shown that the microglial respiratory burst induced by inhaled ambient particles is neurotoxic to neighboring dopaminergic neurons.

Cell Lines

Cell lines represent the most amenable source of human cells for analysis of the potential neurotoxicity of nanoparticles. A range of types is available from the European and American stock centers (Table 1), and they are largely but not exclusively tumor-derived. Large numbers of the cells can be obtained for toxicity analysis, and many lines express selected neuronal and glial markers and display appropriate morphologies following differ-entiation. The stem cell-like lines offer particular promise for developmental and adult toxicity studies since they can be induced to differentiate irreversibly into neural and other CNS cell types; they have been implanted into injured rodent and even human brain, where they can integrate into the existing circuitry and survive for more than a year (e.g., Refs. 28,29). These results highlight their similarities to cells in vivo. However, irreversible differentiation of Ntera2 cells into neurons can take up to a month, even by a suspension aggregation method, while differentiation of some of the other neural lines is faster, and therefore may be more amenable for "high-throughput" nanoparticle toxicity testing. There has been considerable effort put into investigating how representative neural cell lines are of animal dose-responses to chemicals, with the general conclusion that more work is needed. The most promising routes are to investigate combinations

Table 1 Examples of Commonly Used Cell Lines Available for Neurotoxicity Analysis

Name	Major cell type	Source
Ntera2	Neural and glial "stem-like"	Human embryonal carcinoma (derived from lung metastasis of testicular tumor)
C17.2	Neural and glial "stem-like"	Mouse neonatal cerebellar precursor cells
HCN-1A	Neural	Human cortical tissue, removed during surgery
IMR-32	Neural	Human abdominal neuroblastoma
SH-SY5Y	Neural	Derived from SK-N-SH, from bone metastasis of human neuroblastoma
Neuro2A	Neural	Spontaneous mouse tumor
N1E-115	Neural	Mouse neuroblastoma
MN9D	Neural	Mouse rostral mesencephalic tegmentum
PC12	Neural	Rat adrenal phaeochromocytoma
NG108-15	Neural	Fusion of mouse neuroblastoma and rat glioma cells
U-373 MG	Glial	Human astrocytoma
C6	Glial	Rat glioma induced by N-nitrosomethylurea
N9	Microglial	Mouse embryonic brain
SCL 4.1/F7	Schwann	Rat neonatal Schwann cells

of cell types to mimic more closely the in vivo situation (e.g., using neural and liver cells; (30)), and to explore differentiated stem-like cell lines.

In vitro systems have both advantages and disadvantages. One advantage of dissociated cultures (primary or cell lines) is the ability to add a nanoparticle to a specific cell type and observe its *direct* effects on a wide variety of endpoints (discussed below) including viability or neuronal function. However this also highlights one of the major disadvantages from the point of view of the nervous system, where neurons exist in complex relationships with glia that may significantly alter or even induce a neurotoxic response. Modeling chronic or repeated exposures is also particularly difficult in vitro, and neurotoxicity of nanoparticles may require their accumulation and persistence in the tissue. These issues can be at least partially avoided in explant or slice cultures where the complex cellular environment of most of the cells is maintained. Most in vitro culture systems preclude study of the effects of metabolism on the form of the agent, and although this may be less relevant for nanoparticles, particularly ones taken up into olfactory neurons, contact with physiological fluids e.g., blood, may result in significant adsorption to proteins and changes in nanoparticle behavior. Similarly, contact between nanoparticles and cell culture medium may lead to adsorption to proteins (if present), or other changes, which may not be representative of what would occur in vivo and means that it is challenging to determine toxicologically relevant doses. Characterization of the nanoparticles as delivered to the cells will be critical.

ENDPOINTS FOR TESTING THE NEUROTOXICITY OF NANOPARTICLES

Endpoints for neurotoxicity testing of nanoparticles can be divided into two types: generic ones, which are applicable to any cell type, such as cell death and oxidative stress, and those specific to cells of the nervous system, such as effects on neurotransmission.

It has been proposed that the large surface area and high surface reactivity of nanoparticles is likely to induce oxidative stress, reactive oxygen species (ROS) and inflammation (31). The nervous system is very sensitive to oxidative stress, and Nel and coauthors (31) have proposed a hierarchical stress model that provides a useful paradigm for investigating neurotoxicity either in vivo or in vitro. Oxidative stress can be monitored in a number of ways (32). Reduced glutathione (GSH) is one of the most important oxidant defenses in the body, and the balance of GSH and its oxidized form (GSSG) provides a good indication of the level of oxidative stress. Fluorescent approaches are becoming increasingly popular for measuring ROS. For example, when the nonfluorescent diacetate form of 2'-7'-dichlorofluorescein (DCF-DA) is taken up by cells, it is esterified and then in the presence of ROS, it is oxidized to fluorescent DCF. Another fluorescent assay for ROS is based on dihydrorhodamine 123 (DHR), which penetrates cells, and acts as a sensitive indicator of mitochondrial membrane potential, and can be oxidized by ROS to the fluorophore rhodamine 123. Assays based on these reagents could provide semiquantitative indications of the ability of nanoparticles to induce oxidative stress and ROS in cultured CNS cells or tissue slices.

Oxidative stress can lead to inflammation through activation of signaling cascades involving enzymes such as mitogen-activated protein kinases and the transcription factors nuclear factor kappa B (NF-κB) and activator protein 1 (AP-1), and their downstream target genes (e.g., iNOS). As previously discussed, the nervous system is not immune-privileged as once thought, and although inflammation in the brain differs from that in the periphery, certain features can be assessed either in vivo or in vitro. Microglia are the brain's resident immune cells, and upon activation, they convert from their resting ramified form into round, migratory macrophages, and generate cytokines and other inflammatory mediators. Most inflammatory mediators such as cytokines and chemokines are virtually undetectable in healthy CNS tissue, but their levels increase in response to a variety of peripheral or CNS scenarios, including injury and infection (11), and most recently, it has been shown that messenger RNA for several proinflammatory mediators including TNFα and IL-1β increase in the brain in response to exposure of animals by inhalation to nanosized manganese oxide or CB (10,19). Activation of signaling cascades and generation of inflammatory mediators can be followed in several ways; they can be detected in situ using immunological methods on tissue sections, a time-consuming approach, frequently used for detecting c-*fos* transcription, considered to be a marker of neuronal activation (33), but this method can give useful information about the cells expressing the mediators. Other more quantitative immunological methods include analysis of individual mediators by enzyme-linked immunosorbent assays (ELISA), bead-based multiplex immunoassay systems or slide antibody arrays, the latter two approaches offering the advantage of efficiently screening for many different mediators in one sample. Tin Tin Win et al. (19) used an RNA-based quantitative approach, in which reverse transcribed RNA, extracted from dissected brain samples, was analyzed by quantitative real-time polymerase chain reaction (PCR). All these approaches can be applied to either brain tissue following in vivo or slice experiments, or isolated cells after in vitro exposure to nanoparticles, although when applied to homogenized tissues, there will be no information about which cells expressed these mediators. The problem of potential interference with the assays by the nanoparticles needs to be checked using carefully chosen controls.

In response to high levels of oxidative stress or cellular damage, apoptosis or necrosis may result. Cell death can be identified in brain sections (either following an in vivo experiment or in a tissue slice) by histological staining methods, as used for many years to analyze, for example, areas of infarcted tissue following experimental stroke in animals (34). A wide variety of cell death endpoints can be used on isolated cells. These include the classic membrane permeability assays that make use of the fact that dead and dying cells take up dyes such as trypan blue or propidium iodide, or release enzymes such as lactate dehydrogenase (LDH). LDH assays can be done quantitatively and semiautomatically.

Energy balance is critical in nervous tissue, and furthermore, some of the first studies on olfactory uptake of gold nanoparticles found them specifically in mitochondria (8). Enzyme-based ATP assays can be used to analyze energy production in cells, and the MTT (3-(4,5-dimethylthiazoyl-2)-2,5-diphenyltetrazolium bromide) assay, in which mitochondrial dehydrogenases reduce tetrazolium substrates to colored formazan products, is commonly used to monitor mitochondrial activity and cellular viability. Other mitochondrial changes that accompany apoptotic cell death can be followed in vitro: some fluorophores such as dihydrorhodamine accumulate in these organelles in proportion to the mitochondrial membrane potential, and their fluorescence decreases early in apoptosis (35). Many of these assays can be effectively carried out in high-throughput format on cells grown in vitro and will yield valuable information about the ability of nanoparticles to target mitochondria and compromise the energy production of brain tissue and cells.

Two specific functions of the nervous system could potentially be targeted by nanoparticles: axonal transport and synaptic transmission. Neuronal viability and function requires transport of cellular components and organelles along the cytoskeleton of axons, often for very long distances, a process that is energy-dependent. Nanoparticles might interfere with generation of the energy required for this, as noted above, or with the molecular motors participating in transport itself. A wide range of tracers has been employed for following transport and mapping neuronal pathways in vivo (36). In vitro, organelle transport can be followed using the powerful technique of video-enhanced differential interference contrast microscopy, in which the number of organelles crossing a transverse line is scored. The cytoskeleton regulates the architecture and stability of axons and dendrites, and is critical for transport. Aberrations of cytoskeletal components and axonal degeneration have been linked with a number of neurological diseases (37), and might be induced by nanoparticles, since free radical generation can disrupt the cytoskeleton (38). Cytoskeletal as well as overall neuronal integrity and process formation can be followed using immunological methods such as immunostaining or Western blotting analysis of neurofilaments and other proteins in neuronal or tissue extracts.

Communication between neurons is complex and depends on the integrity of many processes both inside and outside of cells, including cell surface receptor and channel activity, signal transduction, neurotransmitter synthesis, and vesicle dynamics. There are a concomitantly large number of endpoints that can be used to analyze neurotransmission experimentally (Table 2). These methods are most easily used on dissociated cells in culture (either primary cells or cell lines) or cells within tissue slices. Recently, the effects of manganese nanoparticles on dopaminergic transmission were studied in the PC12 cell line (39). Both the 40 nm manganese nanoparticles and larger agglomerates adhered to and were taken up by the cells, and this led to a decrease in the levels of dopamine and its metabolites, measured by high-performance liquid chromatography (HPLC), which equalled (on a mass basis) that seen with soluble Mn^{2+}, and was greater than that seen with silver nanoparticles (15 nm).

CONCLUSIONS

Nanotechnology has the potential to bring a wealth of benefits for society and many of these are already being realized, examples being stain-resistant clothing, sunscreens, and cosmetics. Nanomaterials are also being developed for a range of medicinal purposes, including grafting materials and drug delivery. From a neurological viewpoint, nanomaterials may be able to

Table 2 Summary of Potential Endpoints for Analyzing Effects of Nanoparticles on Neurotransmission

Endpoint	Methods for analysis
Calcium signaling	Fluorescent imaging with probes such as Fura-2
Membrane channel activity	Electrophysiological recordings on cells/tissue slices in vitro
	Measurements of calcium levels using Fura-2
Neurotransmitter synthesis	Levels of synthetic enzymes such as tyrosine hydroxylase (e.g., by immunological methods)
	Levels or release of neurotransmitters (e.g., by HPLC)
Vesicle dynamics	Fluorescent dyes (e.g., FM1-43) that facilitate monitoring of vesicle release, reuptake and trafficking

Abbreviation: HPLC, high-performance liquid chromatography.

promote neuronal regeneration following injury, since a self-assembling peptide nanofiber scaffold has been shown to create a permissive environment for axonal regeneration, and restore some function after severing of the optic nerve in the hamster (40). Nanomaterials also have the potential to revolutionize many aspects of biological imaging; dextran-coated iron oxide has been used to image axonal transport and visualize functional nerves in vivo by MRI (41), and nanocrystals of fluorophores have been used to label radial glia in the olfactory bulb (42). MRI also has potential for monitoring occupational exposure to some nanoparticles; it has been used to detect manganese, which is paramagnetic, in the CNS of monkeys following subchronic inhalation (43).

Although this chapter has focused on the potential neurotoxicity of nanoparticles, many nanomaterials may not have detrimental effects, and it will be as important for researchers to report experiments that demonstrate a *lack* of effect of nanoparticles as those that demonstrate toxicity. Indeed, two recent studies highlight protective effects of nanoparticles: cerium and yttrium oxide nanoparticles are not toxic to the neuronal cell line HT22, and in fact, they act as antioxidants and can protect cells from oxidative stress induced by glutamate (44). The fullerene DF-1 also has antioxidant properties and has now been shown to reduce radiation-induced toxicity (including neurotoxicity) in zebra fish embryos (45).

Reports of the health effects (or lack of effects) of manufactured nanoparticles directly in humans are scarce. Evidence however from ambient ultrafine particles suggests that there may be neurological consequences of their inhalation, giving some credence to the hypothesis that environmental factors can contribute to neurodegenerative disease. Although still very limited, data on the neurotoxic effects of manufactured nanoparticles are now starting to be generated, using a range of in vivo and in vitro systems. Studying the toxicity of nanoparticles presents unique challenges, in terms of effective delivery of the particles to the animals or cells, and problems of interactions between nanoparticles and cell culture reagents, assay substrates, or endpoints. Carefully selected controls are therefore critical. Agglomeration is often perceived as a problem in toxicological analysis of nanoparticles. However, humans may be exposed to an aggregated form of nanoparticles rather than a single particle dust or aerosol; indeed Maynard et al. (46) have shown that generation of dust of single carbon nanotubes is difficult.

In summary therefore, manufactured nanoparticles present both unique possibilities but also potentially unique human health concerns. These concerns are not restricted to effects in the lungs, where they will lodge initially upon inhalation, but may also apply to the CNS, which they may reach either via the systemic circulation or the olfactory nerves. However, a variety of simple and complex in vitro models can provide useful information of the potential neurotoxicity of nanoparticles, and their likely mechanism of action. They can inform and hence reduce the extent of the animal studies that will be required to ensure safe handling and use of these exciting new chemicals.

REFERENCES

1. Campbell A. Inflammation, neurodegenerative diseases, and environmental exposures. Ann N Y Acad Sci 2004; 1035:117–32.
2. Bodian D, Howe HA. The rate of progression of poliomyelitis virus in nerves. Bull Johns Hopkins Hosp1941; LXIX:79–85.
3. Aschner M, Erikson KM, Dorman DC. Manganese dosimetry: species differences and implications for neurotoxicity. Crit Rev Toxicol 2005; 35:1–32.
4. Tjalve H, Henriksson J, Talkvist J, Larsson BS, Lindquist NG. Uptake of manganese and cadmium from the nasal mucosa into the central nervous system via olfactory pathways in rats. Pharmacol Toxicol 1996; 79:347–56.
5. Dorman DC, Brenneman KA, McElveen AM, Lynch SE, Roberts KC, Wong BA. Olfactory transport: a direct route of delivery of inhaled manganese phosphate to the rat brain. J Toxicol Environ Health A 2002; 65:1493–511.
6. Dorman DC, Struve MF, Marshall MW, Parkinson CU, James RA, Wong BA. Tissue manganese concentrations in young male rhesus monkeys following subchronic manganese sulfate inhalation. Toxicol Sci 2006; 92:201–10.
7. Taylor MD, Erikson KM, Dobson AW, Fitsanakis VA, Dorman DC, Aschner M. Effects of inhaled manganese on biomarkers of oxidative stress in the rat brain. Neurotoxicology 2006; 27:788–97.
8. De Lorenzo AJD. The olfactory neuron and the blood–brain barrier. In: Wolstenholme GEW, Knight J, eds. Taste and Smell in Vertebrates. London: J & A. Churchill, 1970:151–76.
9. Oberdorster G, Sharp Z, Atudorei V, et al. Translocation of inhaled ultrafine particles to the brain. Inhal Toxicol 2004; 16:437–45.

10. Elder A, Gelein R, Silva V, et al. Translocation of inhaled ultrafine manganese oxide particles to the central nervous system. Environ Health Perspect 2006; 114:1172–8.
11. Lucas SM, Rothwell NJ, Gibson RM. The role of inflammation in CNS injury and disease. Br J Pharmacol 2006; 147(Suppl 1):S232–40.
12. Calderon-Garciduenas L, Azzarelli B, Acuna H, et al. Air pollution and brain damage. Toxicol Pathol 2002; 30:373–89.
13. Campbell A, Oldham M, Becaria A, et al. Particulate matter in polluted air may increase biomarkers of inflammation in mouse brain. Neurotoxicology 2005; 26:133–40.
14. Calderon-Garciduenas L, Mora-Tiscareno A, Fordham LA, et al. Respiratory damage in children exposed to urban pollution. Pediatr Pulmonol 2003; 36:148–61.
15. Calderon-Garciduenas L, Valencia-Salazar G, Rodriguez-Alcaraz A, et al. Ultrastructural nasal pathology in children chronically and sequentially exposed to air pollutants. Am J Respir Cell Mol Biol 2001; 24:132–8.
16. Peters A, Veronesi B, Calderon-Garciduenas L, et al. Translocation and potential neurological effects of fine and ultrafine particles a critical update. Part Fibre Toxicol 2006; 3:13.
17. Veronesi B, Makwana O, Pooler M, Chen LC. Effects of subchronic exposures to concentrated ambient particles. VII. Degeneration of dopaminergic neurons in Apo E–/– mice. Inhal Toxicol 2005; 17:235–41.
18. Block ML, Wu X, Pei Z, et al. Nanometer size diesel exhaust particles are selectively toxic to dopaminergic neurons: the role of microglia, phagocytosis, and NADPH oxidase. FASEB J 2004; 18:1618–20.
19. Tin Tin Win S, Yamamoto S, Ahmed S, Kakeyama M, Kobayashi T, Fujimaki H. Brain cytokine and chemokine mRNA expression in mice induced by intranasal instillation with ultrafine carbon black. Toxicol Lett 2006; 163:153–60.
20. US EPA. Guidelines for neurotoxicity risk assessment. Fed Regis 1998; 63:26926–54.
21. OECD. Guidance Document for Neurotoxicity Testing. OECD Series on Testing and Assessment 2004; 20.
22. Oberdorster G, Maynard A, Donaldson K, et al. Principles for characterizing the potential human health effects from exposure to nanomaterials: elements of a screening strategy. Part Fibre Toxicol 2005; 2:8.
23. Harry GJ, Billingsley M, Bruinink A, et al. In vitro techniques for the assessment of neurotoxicity. Environ Health Perspect 1998; 106(Suppl 1):131–58.
24. Paraoanu LE, Mocko JB, Becker-Roeck M, Smidek-Huhn J, Layer PG. Exposure to diazinon alters in vitro retinogenesis: retinospheroid morphology, development of chicken retinal cell types, and gene expression. Toxicol Sci 2006; 89:314–24.
25. Rothermel A, Biedermann T, Weigel W, et al. Artificial design of three-dimensional retina-like tissue from dissociated cells of the mammalian retina by rotation-mediated cell aggregation. Tissue Eng 2005; 11:1749–56.
26. Meissner KK, Kirkham DL, Doering LC. Transplants of neurosphere cell suspensions from aged mice are functional in the mouse model of Parkinson's. Brain Res 2005; 1057:105–12.

27. Moore JD, Rothwell NJ, Gibson RM. Involvement of caspases and calpains in cerebrocortical neuronal cell death is stimulus-dependent. Br J Pharmacol 2002; 135:1069–77.
28. Miyazono M, Nowell PC, Finan JL, Lee VM, Trojanowski JQ. Long-term integration and neuronal differentiation of human embryonal carcinoma cells (NTera-2) transplanted into the caudoputamen of nude mice. J Comp Neurol 1996; 376:603–13.
29. Nelson PT, Kondziolka D, Wechsler L, et al. Clonal human (hNT) neuron grafts for stroke therapy: neuropathology in a patient 27 months after implantation. Am J Pathol 2002; 160:1201–6.
30. Mannerstrom M, Toimela T, Ylikomi T, Tahti H. The combined use of human neural and liver cell lines and mouse hepatocytes improves the predictability of the neurotoxicity of selected drugs. Toxicol Lett 2006; 165:195–202.
31. Nel A, Xia T, Madler L, Li N. Toxic potential of materials at the nanolevel. Science 2006; 311:622–7.
32. Tarpey MM, Wink DA, Grisham MB. Methods for detection of reactive metabolites of oxygen and nitrogen: in vitro and in vivo considerations. Am J Physiol Regul Integr Comp Physiol 2004; 286:R431–44.
33. Lawrence CB, Williams T, Luckman SM. Intracerebroventricular galanin-like peptide induces different brain activation compared with galanin. Endocrinology 2003; 144:3977–84.
34. Loddick SA, Wong ML, Bongiorno PB, Gold PW, Licinio J, Rothwell NJ. Endogenous interleukin-1 receptor antagonist is neuroprotective. Biochem Biophys Res Commun 1997; 234:211–5.
35. Degli Esposti M. Measuring mitochondrial reactive oxygen species. Methods 2002; 26:335–40.
36. Vercelli A, Repici M, Garbossa D, Grimaldi A. Recent techniques for tracing pathways in the central nervous system of developing and adult mammals. Brain Res Bull 2000; 51:11–28.
37. Bauer P, Schols L, Riess O. Spectrin mutations in spinocerebellar ataxia (SCA). Bioessays 2006; 28:785–7.
38. Allani PK, Sum T, Bhansali SG, Mukherjee SK, Sonee M. A comparative study of the effect of oxidative stress on the cytoskeleton in human cortical neurons. Toxicol Appl Pharmacol 2004; 196:29–36.
39. Hussain SM, Javorina AK, Schrand AM, Duhart HM, Ali SF, Schlager JJ. The interaction of manganese nanoparticles with PC-12 cells induces dopamine depletion. Toxicol Sci 2006; 92:456–63.
40. Enochs WS, Schaffer B, Bhide PG, et al. MR imaging of slow axonal transport in vivo. Exp Neurol 1993; 123:235–42.
41. Petropoulos AE, Schaffer BK, Cheney ML, Enochs S, Zimmer C, Weissleder R. MR imaging of neuronal transport in the guinea pig facial nerve: initial findings. Acta Otolaryngol 1995; 115:512–6.
42. Puche AC, Shipley MT. Radial glia development in the mouse olfactory bulb. J Comp Neurol 2001; 434:1–12.
43. Dorman DC, Struve MF, Wong BA, Dye JA, Robertson ID. Correlation of brain magnetic resonance imaging changes with pallidal manganese concentrations in rhesus monkeys following subchronic manganese inhalation. Toxicol Sci 2006; 92:219–27.

44. Schubert D, Dargusch R, Raitano J, Chan SW. Cerium and yttrium oxide nanoparticles are neuroprotective. Biochem Biophys Res Commun 2006; 342: 86–91.
45. Daroczi B, Kari G, McAleer MF, Wolf JC, Rodeck U, Dicker AP. In vivo radioprotection by the fullerene nanoparticle DF-1 as assessed in a zebrafish model. Clin Cancer Res 2006; 12:7086–91.
46. Maynard A D, Baron P A, Foley M, Shvedova A A, Kisin E R, Castranova V. Exposure to carbon nanotube material: aerosol release during the handling of unrefined single-walled carbon nanotube material. J Toxicol Environ Health. Part A 2004; 67:87–107.

19

Dermal Effects of Nanomaterials

Nancy A. Monteiro-Riviere, Alfred O. Inman, and
Jessica P. Ryman-Rasmussen
*Center for Chemical Toxicology Research and Pharmacokinetics,
North Carolina State University, Raleigh, North Carolina, U.S.A.*

INTRODUCTION

Nanomaterials have been proposed for use in many biological applications, although little is known of their toxicity, potential mutagenic, carcinogenic or teratogenic effects, or overall risk to human health. To avoid past-mistakes made with new technological innovations when chemicals or drugs were released prior to a broad-based risk assessment, information is needed regarding the potential toxicological impact and biological effects of exposure for their medical, occupational health and environmental effects (1).

Nanomaterials have structural features between 1 and 100 nm. By definition, nanoparticles must have at least one dimension smaller than 100 nm. Engineered and manufactured nanoparticles have been engineered to exploit properties and functions associated with size. Nanostructured particles have a substructure greater than atomic/molecular dimensions but less than 100 nm and exhibit physical, chemical and biological characteristics associated with nanostructures. This chapter will focus on the nature of interactions between manufactured nanoparticles and the skin. Skin is unique because it is a potential route for exposure to nanoparticles during their manufacture and also provides an environment within the avascular epidermis where particles could potentially lodge and not be susceptible to removal by phagocytosis. What are the toxicological consequences of nanoparticles (catalyst residue) becoming lodged in the epidermal layers of skin? In fact, it is this relative biological isolation in the lipid domains of the epidermis that has allowed the delivery of drugs to the skin using lipid nanoparticles and liposomes. Larger particles of zinc and titanium oxide used in topical skin-care products have been shown to be able to penetrate the stratum corneum barrier of rabbit skin (2), with the highest absorption occurring from water and oily vehicles. The skin is a primary route of potential exposure to toxicants, including novel nanoparticles. However, there is no information on whether carbon-based nanoparticles are absorbed across the stratum corneum barrier or whether systemically administered particles can accumulate in dermal tissue. Studies are on going to investigate this in our lab. This chapter will review all the current literature regarding the toxicity and nanomaterial interactions with the skin cells (keratinocytes) or with intact skin.

Carbon-Based Nanomaterials

Carbon nanotubes (CNT), commonly known as buckytubes, are made up of seamless, cylindrical shells of graphitic carbon in the range of one to tens of nanometers in diameter and up to several micrometers in length. CNT can be either single-walled nanotubes (SWNT) or multi-walled nanotubes (MWNT). They have been utilized for their extraordinary electrical and mechanical properties, and are 100 times stronger than steel. They can be flexible, yet their hardness provides wear resistance (3,4). One of the principal attributes of SWNTs that makes their development such a breakthrough is their unique catalytic properties. For example, pure SWNT are capable of reacting with many organic compounds due to their carbon chemistry base. Modifications including end-of-tube (e.g., via reaction with carboxyl groups at the SWNT open tip ends) or sidewall derivatization would modify their physical properties and alter solubility or dispersion. The physicochemical and toxicological implications of these properties have not been studied.

Data is limited on the toxicology and the biological effects of manufactured carbon nanotubes (1), especially for dermal effects. Lung toxicity with multifocal granulomas was present after intratracheal instillation of SWNT at high doses of 5 mg/kg in rats for 24 hours. However, the 15% mortality rate resulted from mechanical blockage of the upper airways by the instillate and not the SWNT particulate (5). Mice exposed intratracheally to SWNT that were synthesized with three different methods and catalysts showed dose-dependent epithelioid granuloma formation (6). It must be stressed that inhalational exposure of particulate matter such as SWNT is fundamentally different than dermal or oral exposure, as the lung is designed to trap particulate matter.

SWNT in Skin Cells

Functionalized carbon nanotubes have the potential for therapeutic drug delivery. Derivatized single-walled carbon nanotubes such as

6-aminohexanoic acid (AHA-SWCNT) (7) are soluble in aqueous solutions but their interactions with skin cells (keratinocytes) and their biological compatibility has recently been studied (8). Human epidermal keratinocytes (HEK) dosed with AHA-SWNT at a range of concentrations (0.00000005–0.05 mg/ml) showed a significant decrease in viability ($p <$ 0.05) from 0.00005 to 0.05 mg/ml after 24 hours. Cytokines, an early marker of inflammation were also evaluated. Interleukin-6 (IL-6) increased in cells treated with 0.05 mg/ml from 1 to 48 hours, while interleukin-8 (IL-8) showed a significant increase at 24 and 48 hours. Expression of other cytokines such as TNF-α, IL-10 and IL-1β was not significant. Ultrastructural evaluation showed that the AHA-SWNT were localized within intracytoplasmic vacuoles in HEK. Studies with the surfactant 1% Pluronic® F127 helped to disperse the AHA-SWNT aggregates in the culture medium and caused less toxicity (8).

There are a few reports of dermal irritation in humans such as carbon fiber dermatitis and hyperkeratosis that suggest nanoparticles may gain entry into the viable epidermis after topical exposure. Immortalized HaCaT cells, which are non-tumorigenic human epidermal cells, exposed to nonfunctionalized SWNT showed oxidative stress, a decrease in glutathione levels, and a depletion of vitamin E. Higher concentrations of the SWNT altered the morphology of cytoplasmic organelles (9). However, this study was conducted in immortalized cells and did not evaluate for inflammation. Previously, our laboratory found significant differences in the toxicological response to jet fuels between immortalized versus primary keratinocytes (10). Recently, it has been shown that SWNT can activate NF-κB in a dose-dependent manner in HEK (11). Gene expression profiling conducted in HEK exposed to 1.0 mg/ ml of SWNT showed a similar profile to alpha-quartz or silica, considered to be the main cause of silicosis in humans. Also, genes not previously associated with these particulates from the structural protein and cytokine families were significantly expressed (12; see Cunningham Chapter 12).

MWNT in Skin Cells

The dermal toxicity of MWNT has been studied in HEK. Cells exposed to 0.1, 0.2 and 0.4 mg/ml of MWNT for 1, 2, 4, 8, 12, 24 and 48 hours depicted MWNT within the cytoplasmic vacuoles of HEK (Fig. 1). These are classified as MWNT because they exhibit a base mode growth; very little disordered carbon, and are well ordered and aligned. Transmission electron microscopy found numerous vacuoles within the cytoplasm containing MWNT of various sizes, up to 3.6 µm in length (Figs. 1 and 2). At 24 hours, 59% of the HEK contained MWNT, compared to 84% by 48 hours at the 0.4 mg/ml dose. Viability decreased with an increase in MWNT concentration, and IL-8, an early biomarker for irritation, increased with time and concentration (13). This data showed that MWNT, neither derivatized nor

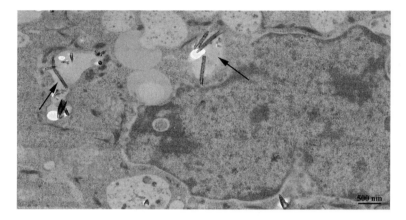

Figure 1 Transmission electron micrograph of an HEK depicting numerous intracytoplasmic vacuoles containing MWNT. Arrows indicate individual MWNT. *Abbreviations*: HEK, human epidermal keratinocytes; MWNT, multi-walled nanotubes.

optimized for biological applications, were capable of both localizing and initiating an irritation response in skin cells. These initial data are suggestive of a significant dermal hazard after topical exposure to select nanoparticles should they be capable of penetrating the stratum corneum barrier.

Cell culture techniques remain a powerful tool to study chemical or nanoparticle interaction with most cell types. Localization of nanotubes in the cell, such as HEK discussed above, may be limited by the substantial van der Waals attractions that cause them to readily agglomerate in aqueous culture medium. To obtain the optimum effect as in drug delivery studies, a permeation enhancer such as a surfactant could be used to disperse the MWNT and to alter the membrane permeability, thus increasing the effective concentration of the MWNT. There are several classes of surfactants (anionic, cationic, amphoteric, and nonionic) that are categorized by their polar functional groups. The nonionic surfactants are known to be less irritating and can affect the permeability of biological membranes by solubilizing the lipid membrane. Also, some have been shown to function as penetration enhancers in transdermal delivery systems because they are considered nonirritating and have low toxicity. Occupational exposure can occur during the manufacturing process to both manufactured nano-materials as well as surfactants. In contrast, the surfactants used to prevent aggregation in cell culture safety protocols cannot be toxic or irritating to the HEK, otherwise false indicators of toxicity may occur. Suspension of individual nanoparticles in aqueous solution is needed to understand the potential biomedical applications and to understand the mechanisms of toxicity.

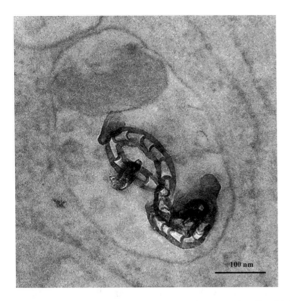

Figure 2 Transmission electron micrograph of a high magnification of MWNTs within an intracytoplasmic vacuole of a keratinocyte. *Abbreviation*: MWNT, multi-walled nanotube.

MWNT and surfactant effects: We studied the effects of five commonly used nonionic surfactants: Pluronic® L61, Pluronic® L92, Pluronic® F127, Tween® 20, and Tween® 60 on the toxicity of HEK. Only Pluronic® F127, a bifunctional block copolymer surfactant, caused minimal toxicity and therefore was assessed to determine the dispersal effects of MWNT and toxicity to HEK. HEK viability, proportional to surfactant concentration, ranged from 27.1% to 98.5% with Pluronic® F127; viability with other surfactants was less than 10%. Surfactants dispersed MWNT and reduced aggregation in media. MWNT at 0.4 mg/ml in 5% or 1% F127 were incubated with HEK and assayed for IL-8. MWNT were cytotoxic to HEK independent of surfactant exposure. In contrast, MWNT-induced IL-8 release was reduced when exposed to 1% or 5% F127 ($p < 0.05$). However, both MWNT and surfactant, alone or in combination, increased IL-8 release compared to control exposures at 12 and 24 hours. Our results suggest that the surfactant-MWNT interaction is more complex than simple dispersion alone and should be investigated to determine the mode of interaction (14).

Proteomic analysis was also conducted in HEK exposed to MWNT to determine the effect on the HEK proteome. This study showed an increase and decrease in expression of many proteins relative to controls. HEK dosed with 0.4 mg/ml of MWNT altered the expression of 36 proteins after 24 hours and 106 proteins by 48 hours, compared to controls. Various protein identities reflected complex cellular responses that suggested dysregulation of intermediate filament expression, cell cycle inhibition, altered vesicular trafficking/exocytosis and membrane scaffold protein down-regulation (15, see Witzmann and Monteiro-Riviere Chapter 13).

Studies with hat-stacked carbon nanofibers that resembled MWNT implanted in rat subcutaneous tissue depicted granulation and an inflammatory response that was similar to foreign body granulomas. These carbon nanofibers were found within the macrophages without severe inflammation, necrosis or degeneration of tissue (16).

These data suggest a significant dermal hazard after topical exposure to MWNT or SWNT nanotubes should they penetrate the stratum corneum barrier. One may question that the exposure level ranging from 0.1 to 0.4 mg/ml is quite high. However, studies involving the handling of SWNT in four different field sites showed that estimated exposure to SWNT on left- and right-hand glove samples ranged from 0.2 to 6.0 mg of CNT per glove (17). Also, the amount of CNT deposited on the glove was so vast that they remained visible on the glove at the end of the sampling period. Therefore, the exposure levels studied above are realistic and within the range noted after occupational exposure.

Fullerenes or buckyball effects in skin cells: Fullerenes or buckyballs (C_{60}) are molecular structures made up of 60 or more carbon atoms. The fullerenes are used in materials science, superconductivity applications, electronic circuits, nonlinear optics, pharmaceuticals, and in everyday items such as clothing, tennis rackets, bowling balls and numerous other applications. They have been added to the resin coatings of bowling balls to improve controllability. The cost to produce fullerenes and to purchase them is quite expensive. They have been considered to be a commercial success for some companies and thus are being made in multi-ton quantities (18). Fullerenes have been used in many biological applications, although little is known of their toxicity, potential carcinogenic effects or overall health risk, especially the dermal effects of these nanomaterials.

Information regarding the biodistribution and metabolism of C_{60} in skin is limited, probably due to the fact that C_{60} is insoluble in aqueous solutions coupled with a paucity of sensitive analytical techniques. Since skin is the largest organ of the body, it will probably come into contact with fullerenes, especially during the manufacturing process. The dermal toxicity of fullerenes has also been the focus of some studies. Topical administration of 200 µg of fullerenes to mouse skin over 72 hours found no effect on either DNA synthesis or ornithine decarboxylase activity. The ability of fullerenes to act as a tumor promoter was also investigated. Studies have shown repeated application to mouse skin after initiation with dimethlybenzan-thracene for 24 weeks did not result in benign or malignant skin tumor formation, but promotion was observed with 12-0-tetradecanoylphorbol-13-acetate resulting in benign skin tumors (19).

In vitro studies using ^{14}C-labelled underivatized C_{60} exposed to immortalized HEK showed cellular incorporation of the label at various times. By 6 hours, approximately 50% of the radiolabeled was taken up, but it was unclear whether particles actually entered the cell or were associated with the cell surface. These investigators also found no effect of C_{60} on the proliferation of immortalized HEK and fibroblasts (20).

Four types of water-soluble fullerenes were assessed in human liver carcinoma cells and dermal fibroblasts for their toxicity in biomedical technologies. Water-soluble functional groups on the surface of fullerenes can dramatically decrease the toxicity of pristine C_{60}. The least derivatized and most aggregated form of C_{60} was more toxic than the highly soluble derivatives such as C_3, Na^+_{2-3} $[C_{60}O_{7-9}$ $(OH)_{12-15}]$, and C_{60} $(OH)_{24}$ (21,22). There are conflicting reports as to the potential toxicity of C_{60}. While C_{60} itself has essentially no solubility in water, it has been shown to aggregate with either organic solvent inclusion or partial hydrolysis to create water-soluble species n-C_{60}. These aggregates have exceptionally low mobility in aqueous solutions but have been proposed to have high cellular toxicity.

A series of fullerene substituted phenylalanine derivatives were prepared to compare to related functionalized fullerenes. The presence of the C_{60} substituent has been shown to alter the conformation of the native peptide (e.g., from a random coil to a β-sheet), making the conditions under which conversion to an alpha helix occurs important. Studies have shown there is no apparent toxicity to the cells; however, early studies did not confirm that the peptide was incorporated into the cells (23). We have shown that agglomerates of derivatized C_{60} (Baa) at 0.4 mg/ml exposed to HEK can become localized within large cytoplasmic vacuoles similar to the MWNT. Also, agglomerates of nonderivatized C_{60} at 0.4 mg/ml has also been shown to be located along the periphery of the nucleus in large vacuoles. HEK exposed to the phenylalanine-based fullerene amino acid solutions ranging from 0.04 to 0.004 mg/ml depicted a significant decrease in viability and a statistically significant increase in IL-8 for the 0.04 mg/ml dose by 8, 12, and 24 hours. IL-6 and IL-1β were greater at 24 and 48 hours but there was no significant TNF-α or IL-10 expression (24). In addition, TEM showed this Bucky amino acid fullerene (Baa) was taken up into the HEK and at times appears to be phagocytized by the HEK (Fig. 3).

When HEK were exposed to nano-C_{60} ranging from 0.0000025 to 0.0005 mg/ml and $C_{60}(OH)_{24}$ ranging from 0.000005 to 0.001 mg/ml for 24 and 48 hours, MTT viability showed nano-C_{60} ranging from 0.00025 to 0.0005 mg/ml decreased HEK viability significantly ($p < 0.05$) by 24 hours. IL-8 and IL-6 were significantly ($p < 0.05$) greater than controls, while IL-10, IL-1β, and TNF-α were below detectable limits. However, $C_{60}(OH)_{24}$ showed no toxicity to HEK at all concentrations. These results show that

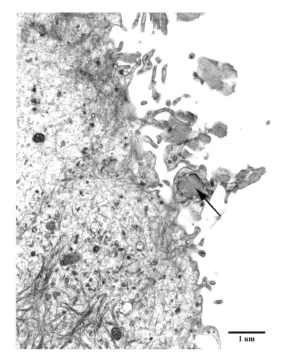

1 um

Figure 3 Transmission electron micrograph of an HEK depicting a fullerene-based amino acid (Baa) nanoparticle. Arrow indicates the Baa fullerene surrounded by the cell's plasma membrane. *Abbreviation*: HEK, human epidermal keratinocytes.

derivatized C_{60} $(OH)_{24}$ is nontoxic in the tested range, and nano-C_{60} is toxic at concentrations as low as 0.00025 mg/ml in HEK (25).

The incorporation of a fullerene with an amino acid analog has been used in drug delivery studies. When HEK were exposed to concentrations ranging from 0.4 to 0.001 mg/ml of a fullerene C_{60} peptide with a fluorescently tagged nuclear localization signal (NLS-FITC) for 24 and 48 hours, MTT viability decreased and was statistically significant ($p < 0.05$) at 0.4 mg/ml at both 24 and 48 hours. IL-8 and IL-6 statistically increased at 0.2 and 0.4 mg/ml. IL-1β (0.4mg/ml) was low but was significantly different from controls, while IL-10 and TNF-α were below detectable limits. TEM showed the C_{60} -NLS-FITC to be located within large cytoplasmic vacuoles in close proximity to the nucleus (Fig. 4). In addition, 4.4 μg and 1.1 μg/cm^2 of C_{60} -NLS-FITC was topically applied to porcine skin in flow-through diffusion cells for 24 hours with and without 1% Pluronic® F127 surfactant or NLS-FITC alone, confocal microscopy for C_{60}-NLS-FITC and NLS-FITC depicted penetration of the label through all epidermal layers. TEM showed that the C_{60}-NLS-FITC localized within the intercellular bi-lipid

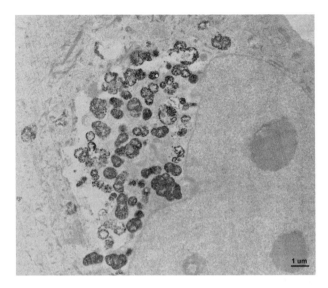

Figure 4 Transmission electron micrograph of an HEK showing numerous electron-dense C_{60}-NLS-FITC nanoparticles in close proximity to the nuclear membrane. *Abbreviation*: HEK, human epidermal keratinocytes.

layers of the stratum corneum cell layers (Fig. 5). Surfactant greatly enhanced the permeability for all treatments. These results show that substituted fullerenes can penetrate through intact skin and can elicit an inflammatory response (26).

Previously, it has been shown that carbon nanotubes still remain visible on the gloves of workers and in some cases workers may not wear the proper personal protection equipment when handling nanomaterials. Therefore, dermal handling could increase under different conditions. In an occupational environment, repetitive motion that accentuates naturally occurring biomechanical forces may alter the body's ability to perform certain physiological functions. Therefore, the effects of mechanical flexion on the penetration of fullerene amino acid-derivatized peptide was studied in porcine skin in our laboratory. The thought was that mechanical stimulation caused by repetitive motions could alter the skin's morphology that would lead to a defect in the permeability barrier of the stratum corneum, thereby increasing the penetration of particles through the lipid bilayers. Studies in our lab have shown a direct correlation between particle penetration and flexion. A fullerene-substituted peptide, Baa-Lys (FITC)-NLS was synthesized (22,27), and its penetration determined through flexed and unflexed skin. Dermatomed porcine skin of 400 μm was dosed with 20 μL of Baa-Lys (FITC)-NLS (3.5 nm) in 1% PBS (33.5 mg/ml), and the dosed areas were

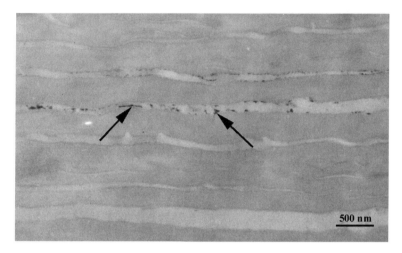

500 nm

Figure 5 Transmission electron micrograph showing the intercellular localization of C_{60} -NLS-FITC (arrows) nanoparticles within the bi-lipid layers of the stratum corneum cells.

subsequently flexed for 60 min or 90 min or left unflexed (control). The skin was then fixed to a flexing apparatus designed to flex skin at ±45° at a frequency of 20 flexes/min prior to placing on the flow-through diffusion cells (28,29) for 8 and 24 hours. This showed an increase in penetration and TEM depicted the Baa-Lys (FITC)-NLS present within the intercellular space of the stratum corneum layers and after 90 min in the stratum granulosum layers. Initial studies in our lab using flexed skin for 60 and 90 min, placed on diffusion cells and then topical application of Baa-Lys (FITC)-NLS did not show an increase in penetration. In addition, when skin was flexed for only 15 min or 30 min and then dosed with radiolabeled methyl parathion, there was no evidence of increased penetration compared to unflexed skin. These results suggest the action of a flexing procedure and length of time can increase the rate by which fullerenes can penetrate through the skin. Furthermore, as the flexing time increased, the amount of fullerenes that penetrated into the dermal layers of skin also increased, indicated by the higher fluorescence intensity of fullerenes for both 60 and 90 min flexed skin (30).

The toxicology of fullerenes and its derivatives have been presented to overview what little is known of their potential to cause adverse effects in skin or skin cells. However, fullerenes also have beneficial effects. Numerous studies have also been published that show functionalized fullerenes may be therapeutically useful in the treatment of a number of diseases. A balanced benefit-risk assessment must be made before these substances are released for human use.

POTENTIAL PITFALLS IN ASSESSING THE TOXICITY OF CARBON-BASED NANOMATERIALS IN CULTURES

Ultrafine carbon black (CB) commonly used for in vivo inhalation studies with gross and microscopic endpoints may not be suitable for use in cell culture due to their interference with viability and cytokine assays (31). Nanosize CB has been recommended to serve as a negative control when conducting viability assays in cell culture. However, caution must be exercised when utilizing CB since we have observed carbon can adsorb the viability marker dyes such as neutral red (NR) to interfere with the quantitative absorption spectra to cause false positive and negative results. Our laboratory was the first to report that dye-based assays provided false viability and cytokine data in a series of experiments that studied the effects of CB on HEK (31).

As discussed previously, CNT have been studied to determine their in vitro effects on a number of different cell types. Our laboratory has shown that chemically unmodified MWNT within the cytoplasmic vacuoles of HEK can cause mortality and the release of the proinflammatory cytokine IL-8 in a dose-dependent manner (13). These results may even be greater than what we reported due to the possible adsorbance of the dye to carbon nanomaterials. Studies have recently shown that CNT causes cytotoxicity in other cell types such as the guinea pig alveolar macrophages (32), human fibroblasts (33), human lung tumor cells (34), cells derived from human cervical cancer and lung carcinoma (11), and HEK (11). However, other investigators have found no cytotoxic effects from CNT in rat alveolar macrophages (35), human umbilical vein endothelial cells (36), human osteoblasts and fibroblasts (37), and human colon and lung cells (38). These differences in cell viability may be explained by the adsorption capabilities of carbon based nanomaterials that could interfere with in vitro cytotoxicity assays. CB are non porous materials engineered to be sorbents, but by virtue of their very small primary particle sizes can possess significant surface areas for adsorption.

The NR assay is a widely utilized viability test in cell culture experiments (39,40). We have observed that CB can adsorb the viability marker dyes such as NR (3-amino-7-dimethylamino-2-methylphenazine hydrochloride) from cell culture media, and interfere with the quantitative absorption assay to cause false readings. The presence of NR indicates active lysosomes, with the uptake of NR into cells being proportional to the number of viable cells. Our laboratory found that when NR assay protocol was used with 75 nm (Cabot), 68 nm (Fisher), and 14 to −16 nm (Degussa) CB varieties and of different sizes in the absence of HEK, a false positive signal was generated inaccurately indicating the presence of viable cells. The CB was found to adsorb NR dye and generate a signal in the assay suggesting high cell viability when in fact cells were not even present (31).

Our studies have found that other classical dye-based assays used to determine cell viability may also produce incorrect results due to interactions between the CNT and MTT (3-[4,5-dimethyl-2-thiazol]-2,5-diphenyl-2H-tetrazolium bromide). This colorimetric metabolic assay is based on the mitochondrial dye conversion to assess viability. The tetrazolium salt is used to assess the activity of various dehydrogenase enzymes where the tetrazolium ring is cleaved in active mitochondria, demonstrating the presence of living cells. We found that in the presence of CB, the tetrazolium dye desorbed from the cells was adsorbed by the CB, thereby reducing the absorbance reading and giving a false positive signal for reduced viability and thus cytotoxicity (31). Similar observations were also noted that nanotubes reduce the color of aromatic dyes, causing assays using MTT, alamar blue, and propidium iodide to provide incorrect results (41). Other investigators using the MTT viability studies with MWNT, carbon nanofibers, and CB, found that CB exhibited the highest cytotoxicity at all concentrations and time points (34). Studies with human fibroblasts in culture showed a direct relationship exists between the surface area of carbon materials and their effect on cell survival (33).

All of these studies have shown that carbon adsorbents may also interfere with in vitro cytokine assays (e.g. ELISA). CB attached to the plasma membrane may adsorb the chromagen or even the IL-8 protein as it is released from the cells in to the culture medium. CB may also adsorb the constituents of the growth media as well as other proteins, thereby preventing the cells from receiving proper nutrients and growth factors. CB may adsorb other soluble components that could alter pH and cell viability. Ultrafine CB may act as an adsorbent that could potentially bind compounds during the manufacturing process (31). The type of CB used in a study and its characterization and composition is extremely important. For instance, ultrafine CB commonly used for in vivo inhalation studies with gross and microscopic endpoints may not be suitable for use in cell culture studies because it interferes with viability and cytokine assays. Because of the possible limitations in assessing cell viability with quantitative assays, the viability or toxicity must also be confirmed with TEM analysis of the cells (8,31).

Titanium Dioxide and Skin

Titanium dioxide (TiO_2) is a naturally occurring mineral that is widely used in sunscreens and cosmetics due to its ability to filter ultraviolet radiation. Nanoscale TiO_2 is proposed for use in sunscreens due to greater UV filtering ability and greater transparency, the latter of which is important aesthetically. These potential benefits are countered with concerns of increased depth of skin penetration, increased reactivity, and increased toxicity.

The ability of TiO_2 in sunscreen preparations to penetrate the protective stratum corneum barrier is controversial. Plastic surgery candidates applied sunscreen with 8% microfine TiO_2 to skin surrounding a lesion scheduled for surgical excision twice daily for 2 to -6 weeks. After biopsy, the stratum corneum was stripped with two applications of cyanoacrylate ester, the skin digested, and titanium levels measured by mass spectrometry. Higher titanium levels were observed in the patients than in sunscreen-free skin from cadaver controls (42). However, a significant difference between these two groups was obtainable only after exclusion of a control sample with unexplainably high titanium levels. In a more rigorously controlled study, healthy volunteers had a sunscreen emulsion with UV-Titan M 160 TiO_2 microparticles ca. 17 nm in size (www. kemra.com) applied to the left forearm and an emulsion-only control applied to the right forearm for several days prior to tape stripping 15 times to remove individual skin layers. Titanium in each strip was measured by X-ray fluorescence and each strip correlated to horny layer depth. TiO_2 microparticles were detected only in the upper horny layers, with fewer microparticles observable in hair follicles and none present in the viable skin layers (43). This result is supported by a more recent study in which TiO_2 was observable by light microscopy and TEM only on the outer stratum corneum of healthy volunteers that had been treated with TiO_2 having different surface coatings, sizes, and shapes: T805 (20 nm, cubic), Eusolex T-2000 (10–15 nm, 100 nm aggregate needles), and Tioveil AQ-10P (100 nm needles) (44). Other studies have shown that larger particles of zinc and titanium oxide used in topical skin-care products are able to penetrate the stratum corneum barrier of rabbit skin (2), with the highest absorption occurring from water and oily vehicles.

Exposure to the viable layers of skin resulting from topically applied TiO_2 may result in cytotoxicity and immunotoxicity. Nano-sized particles are expected to have greater inflammatory potential than larger particles due to a large surface area to volume ratio (45). However, a recent study indicates surface area may be a less important factor than phase composition in the cytotoxicity and immunotoxicity of TiO_2 (46). Phase composition influences the surface catalytic properties of TiO_2. Anatase-phase TiO_2 catalytically dissociates water to form hydroxyl radicals under illumination, whereas rutile-phase TiO_2 has comparatively little catalytic activity. Anatase-phase TiO_2 exhibits significantly greater cytotoxicity and release of the inflammatory cytokine, IL-8, than rutile-phase TiO_2 in primary human dermal fibroblasts and lung A549 cells, and cytotoxicity is potentiated in the presence of UV light (46).

In summary, preliminary studies thus far indicate that nano-sized TiO_2 does not penetrate the viable layers of skin in healthy adults. However, more study on exposure to TiO_2 via the dermal route is needed, with careful attention paid to the effects of size, shape, surface properties, emulsion composition, and skin disposition on the depth of penetration. The role of TiO_2 phase composition should also be investigated for any cytotoxicity and immunotoxicity resulting from dermal exposures.

Quantum Dots and Skin

Semiconductor nanocrystals, or quantum dots (QD), are a diverse class of engineered nanostructures that are highly variable in chemical composition, size, and shape. Unlike most nanomaterials, QD are easily detected due to intense and photostable fluorescence. QD have been proposed for use in the biomedicine, electronics, and security industries. Biomedical applications include targeted drug delivery, diagnostics, and imaging. The chemical composition of QD is highly variable and tuned to the intended application. QD are comprised of a heterogeneous, colloidal core of inorganic atoms (e.g. CdSe, CdTe, InAs, GaN,) in which the core is surrounded by a shell or "cap", such as ZnS (47) or tri-*n*-octylphosphine oxide or TOPO (48). Surface coatings in one or more layers are often applied to the core or core/shell complex. These coatings increase solubility in biological media and/or contain reactive groups that allow quantum dots to be bioconjugated to antibodies or receptor ligands for "targeted" drug delivery and diagnostics (49).

QD can be obtained commercially in liquid and powder form, to which both producers and consumers may be exposed and therefore the skin or skin cells could be directly evaluated. If utilized in nanomedicine as image contrast or drug delivery agents, QD may be administered by injection. Therefore, toxicity resulting from all potential routes of exposure (injection, inhalation, dermal, and ingestion) should be evaluated. There are no published reports to date of *in vivo* studies specifically designed to assess QD toxicity. Rather, the interaction of QD with biological systems has been most described in the context of pre-clinical studies using QD for diagnostic imaging. Ballou et al. (50) intravenously injected Balb/C and athymic nude mice with CdSe core/ZnS shell QD coated with methoxy-capped polyethylene glycol (mPEG-750). Fluorescence imaging of intact and dissected animals showed accumulation in the liver, lymph nodes, and bone marrow within 24 hours that remained 132 days, with no obvious signs of adverse health effects. Others have used athymic nude mice with prostate-specific membrane antigen (PMSA)-positive tumor xenografts to investigate the diagnostic utility of CdSe core/TOPO-capped QD coated with PMSA. Six hours after intravenous injection, these QD localized to the liver and spleen, as well as the tumor. Experiments with similar QD of carboxylic acid or polyethylene glycol (PEG) coatings showed similar results (48). Ackerman et al. (51) also reported nonselective accumulation of CdSe core/ZnS shell QD coated with targeting peptides in the liver and spleen of nude mice with tumor xenografts within 20 min of intravenous injection. This nonselective accumulation could be reduced (although not eliminated) by co-adsorbing PEG onto the QD surface. Together, these data indicate that intravenously administered QD with diverse coatings can accumulate in unintended organs, where they may remain for months.

We have evaluated skin as a route of unintended exposure to QD with different core sizes and surface coatings. We topically applied commercially available QD 565 and 655 with three different surface coatings (PEG, PEG-amines, or carboxylic acids) to porcine skin in flow-through diffusion cells and found penetration of the intact stratum corneum to the viable layers of the epidermis (and, in some cases, the dermis) within 8 to 24 hours (52) (Fig. 6). Further evaluation of the potential hazard of QD skin exposure in HEK showed that QD of both sizes and all surface coatings are efficiently taken up by the cells within 24 hours at a low 2 nM concentration, with cytoplasmic localization and in the nucleus. Cell viability assays and evaluation of cytokine release revealed coating-dependent effects, with cytotoxicity and irritancy being greatest for carboxylic acid-coated QD. These coating-dependent effects were consistent across size (53).

Routes of exposure to QD other than intravenous injection and topical application have not been described. The hazards of QD are largely unknown, but there are increasing reports of QD cytotoxicity in cultured cells. Comparison of studies is frustrated by the diversity of QD, the use of different cell lines, and a variety of endpoints of cytotoxicity (see (54) for review). We observed that surface coating was a more important determinant than size for cytotoxicity and immunotoxicity of CdSe core/ZnS shell QD in HEK. However, all QD tested localized to the

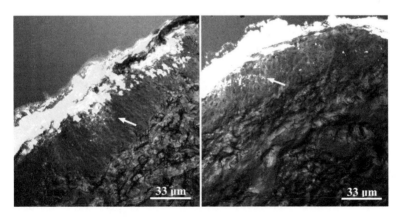

Figure 6 Laser confocal microscopy showing skin penetration of carboxylic acid-coated QD 565 (*left*) at 8 hours and carboxylic acid-coated QD 655 (*right*) at 24 hours. Arrows show penetration of QD through the epidermal layers of intact skin. *Abbreviation*: QD, quantum dots.

cellular interior by 24 hours, regardless of surface coating (53). This finding differs from another study in N9 neuroblastoma and PC12 pheochromo-cytoma cells which showed that green, cationic cysteineamine CdTe QD of 2.3 nm core size were more cytotoxic than similarly coated red CdTe QD of 5.2 nm core size, indicating a role for QD size in cytotoxicity (55). This study also reported that these QD localize to the interior of PC12 and N9 cells, with an effect of size on the cellular localization of these QD in the N9 cell line. A different study reported that the cytotoxic effects of CdSe core QD in primary human hepatocytes was related to both QD composition and environmental conditions. Cytotoxicity of QD that had been oxidized by air or UV light was correlated with release of Cd^{+2} into the culture medium. Cytotoxicity and Cd^{+2} release were attenuated when the CdSe core was synthetically capped with a ZnS shell to prevent leaching of core metals under oxidizing conditions (47). Together, these three studies illustrate that the physical properties of QD (e.g., size, surface coatings, and chemical composition), the cell type of interest, and environmental factors (pH, light, etc.) may work alone, or in combination, to influence cytotoxicity. These factors will influence the mechanisms of QD toxicity, which are not well understood. Hypothesized mechanisms of toxicity include leaching of core metals into the culture medium (47), oxidative stress as a result of QD-mediated ROS production (56), and coating-related mechanisms (53). The pathways of QD uptake and endocytic trafficking in cells may also be an important mechanistic component (53,56).

QD have a great potential for use in medicine and industry and has been shown to interact with cells. There is experimental evidence that intravenously administered QD can accumulate in unintended tissues and that exposure to QD may occur through intact skin. Accumulating *in vitro* evidence indicates that exposure to QD such as in the manufacturing and handling may be hazardous, depending upon the physicochemical compo-sition of the QD, the cell types involved, and environmental factors.

EXPOSURE AND RISK ASSESSMENT

This chapter has reviewed the literature relating to the dermal effects of different types of nanomaterials with skin. General principles governing the safety of all nanomaterials needs to be evaluated to establish specific nanotoxicology safety and testing guidelines after occupational exposure during manufacture, exposure in academic research laboratories, or environmental exposure from manufacturing waste or post-consumer use (57). Risk is defined as "exposure" times "hazard." The studies reviewed that many types of nanomaterials such as fullerenes, derivatized fullerenes, single-walled and multi-walled carbon nanotubes, or derivatized nanotubes produce biological effects; hence hazard exists. Exposure is a function of both source and portal of entry into the body. Other chapters in this book show that injection, dermal, inhalation, and oral absorption occurs, hence exposure occurs. What is our risk of toxicity to nanomaterials?

There is a great deal of attention directed to the inhalational toxicology of carbon nanomaterials due to their particulate nature and their anthropogenic occurrence in diesel exhaust. However, it is obvious that many of these nanomaterials mentioned in the book are produced for biomedical or cosmetic applications and do not result in inhalational exposure. Since many engineered nanomaterials are prepared and processed in liquids, there is a high probability that dermal absorption and oral ingestion may be the more relevant exposure route during the manufacturing process or during accidental spills, shipping and handling (58). Prevention of dermal exposure by the use of gloves is underscored by a study indicating that some workers had as much as 7 mg of nanotube material deposited on gloves in areas directly contacting nanotubes (59). This study had shown that gloves could offer dermal protection from nanotube material, with the caveat that the permeability of different types of gloves to specific nanomaterials is unknown.

CONCLUSION

Many of the dermal toxicology studies presented in this chapter indicate that nanomaterials can interact with biological systems such as HEK. The composition, size and surface properties are important attributes that are needed to predict biological effects. It is intriguing that materials of vastly different chemical compositions have similar interactions with biological systems; the clearest example being preferential cellular uptake of QD. Size also seems to be an important factor. The precise nature of toxicity seen is a function of the chemistry of the nanoparticle. The physical and chemical properties of many nanoparticle surface modifications may be the factor that determines their ultimate safety. Comparisons of particles across different compositions, size and densities in cell culture is inherently different since without particle characterization, dose is difficult to define due to differences in particle settling, binding and diffusion (60). There is a dearth of literature that exists with nanomaterials having commercial applications, including TiO_2 particles for sunscreens and iron oxide particles or QD for imaging. Similarly, pivotal disposition and cell targeting data is often available for those nanomaterials intended for use in drug delivery, such as seen with QD, fullerenes and carbon nanotubes. There is a serious lack of information about human health and environmental implications of manufactured nanomaterials. This emerging field of nanotoxicology will continue to grow as new products are continuously produced. Then there will be even a greater need for toxicological studies to be conducted with well-characterized nanoparticles that can be used in risk assessment. Knowledge of exposure and hazard are needed for understanding risks associated with nano-materials. This chapter has explored the beginning threads of nanomaterial toxicology on skin cells and in skin for several types of nanomaterials.

REFERENCES

1. Dagani R. Nanomaterials: safe or unsafe? Chem Eng News 2003; 81:30–3.
2. Lansdown ABG, Taylor A. Zinc and titanium oxides: promising UV-absorbers but what influence do they have on intact skin. Int J Cosmetic Sci 1997; 19: 167–72.
3. Dai H, Hafner JH, Rinzler AG, Colbert DT, Smalley RE. Nanotubes as nanoprobes in scanning probe microscopy. Nature 1996; 384:147–50.
4. Moloni K, Lal A, Lagally MG. Sharpened carbon nanotube probes. Proc. SPIE 2000; 4098:76–83.
5. Warheit DB, Laurence BR, Reed KL, Roach DH, Reynolds GAM, Webb TR. Comparative pulmonary toxicity assessment of single wall carbon nanotubes in rats. Tox Sci 2004; 77:117–25.
6. Lam CW, James JT, McCluskey R, Hunter RL. Pulmonary toxicity of single wall carbon nanotubes in mice 7 and 90 days after intratracheal instillation. Tox Sci 2004; 77:126–34.
7. Zeng L, Zhang L, Barron AR. Tailoring aqueous solubility of functionalized single-wall carbon nanotubes over a wide pH range through substituent chain length. Nano Lett 2005; 5(10):2001–4.
8. Zhang L, Zeng L, Barron AR, Monteiro-Riviere NA. Biological interaction of functionalized single-walled carbon nanotubes in human keratinocytes. Int J Toxicol 2007; 26:103–113.
9. Shvedova AA, Kisin ER, Murray AR, Gandelsman VZ, Maynard A, Baron P. Exposure to carbon nanotube material: Assessment of nanotube cytotoxicity using human keratinocyte cells. J Toxicol Environ Health A 2003; 66:1909–26.
10. Allen DG, Riviere JE, Monteiro-Riviere NA. Cytokine induction as a measure of cutaneous toxicity in primary and immortalized porcine keratinocytes exposed to jet fuels, and their relationship to normal human epidermal keratinocytes. Tox Lett 2001; 119:209–17.
11. Manna SK, Sarkar S, Barr J, Wise K, Barrera EV, Jejelowo O, Rice-Ficht AC, Ramesh GT. Single-walled carbon nanotube induces oxicative stress and activates nuclear transcription factor-kB in human keratinocytes. Nano Lett 2005; 5:1676–84.
12. Cunningham MJ, Magnuson SR, Falduto MT. Gene expression profiling of nanoscale materials using a systems biology approach. The Toxicologist 2005; 84(S-1):9.
13. Monteiro-Riviere NA, Nemanich RA, Inman AO, Wang YY, Riviere JE. Multi-walled carbon nanotube interactions with human epidermal keratinocytes. Tox Lett 2005; 155:377–84.
14. Monteiro-Riviere NA, Inman AO, Wang YY, Nemanich RJ. Surfactant effects on carbon nanotube interactions with human epidermal keratinocytes. Nanomed: Nanotechnol Biol Med 2005; 1:293–9.

15. Witzmann FA, Monteiro-Riviere NA. Multi-walled carbon nanotube exposure alters protein expression in human keratinocytes. Nanomed: Nanotechnol Biol Med 2006; 2:158–68.
16. Yokoyama A, Sato Y, Nodasaka Y, Yamamoto S, Kawasaki T, Shindoh M, Kohgo T, Akasaka T, Uo M, Watari F, Kazuyuki T. Biological behavior of hat-stacked carbon nanofibers in the subcutaneous tissue in rats. Nano Lett 2005; 5:157–61.
17. Maynard AD, Baron PA, Foley M, Shvedova AA, Kisin ER, Castranova V. Exposure to carbon nanotube material: aerosol release during the handling of unrefined single-walled carbon nanotube material. J Toxicol Environ Health Part A 2004; 67:87–107.
18. Tremblay JF. Fullerenes by the ton. Chem Eng News 2003; 81:13–14.
19. Nelson MA, Frederick ED, Bowden GT, Hooser SB, Fernando Q, Carter DE. Effects of acute and subchronic exposure of topically applied fullerene extracts on the mouse skin. Tox Industr Health 1993; 9:623–30.
20. Scrivens WA, Tour JM, Creek KE, Pirisi L. Synthesis of 14C-labeled C_{60}, its suspension in water, and its uptake by human keratinocytes. J Am Chem Soc 1994; 116:4517–18.
21. Sayes CM, Fortner JD, Guo W, Lyon D, Boyd AM, Ausman KD, Tao YJ, Sitharaman B, Wilson LJ, Hughes JB, West JL, Colvin VL. The differential cytotoxicity of water-soluble fullerenes. Nano Lett 2004; 4:1881–7.
22. Sayes CM, Liang F, Hudson JL, Mendez J, Guo W, Beach JM, Moore VC, Doyle CD, West JL, Billups WE, Ausman KD, Colvin VL. Functionalization density dependence of single-walled carbon nanotubes cytotoxicity in vitro. Tox Lett 2006; 161:135–42.
23. Yang J, Barron AR. A new route to fullerene substituted phenylalanine derivatives. Chem Commun 2004; 24:2884–5.
24. Rouse JG, Yang J, Barron AR, Monteiro-Riviere NA. Fullerene based amino acid nanoparticle interactions with human epidermal keratinocytes. Tox In Vitro 2006; 20:1313–20.
25. Inman AO, Sayes CM, Colvin VL, Monteiro-Riviere NA. Nano-C_{60} and derivatized C_{60} toxicity in human epidermal keratinocytes. Tox Sci 2006; 90 (S-1):167.
26. Monteiro-Riviere NA, Yang J, Inman AO, Ryman-Rasmussen J, Barron AR, Riviere JE. Skin penetration of fullerene substituted amino acids and their interactions with human epidermal keratinocytes. Tox Sci 2006; 90(S-1):168.
27. Yang J, Alemany LB, Driver J, Hartgerink JD, Barron AR. Fullerene-derivatized amino acids: synthesis, characterization, antioxidant properties, and solid phase peptide synthesis. Chem Eur J 2007, in press.
28. Chang SK, Riviere JE. Percutaneous absorption of parathion *in vitro* in porcine skin. Effects of dose, temperature, humidity and perfusate composition on absorptive flux. Fundam Appl Toxicol 1991; 17:494–504.
29. Bronaugh RL, Stewart RF. Methods for in vitro percutaneous absorption studies IV: The flow-through diffusion cell. J Pharm Sci 1985; 74:64–7.
30. Rouse JG, Yang J, Ryman-Rasmussen JP, Barron AR, Monteiro-Riviere NA. Effects of mechanical flexion on the penetration of fullerene amino acid-derivatized peptide nanoparticles through skin. Nano Lett 2007; 7:155–60.

31. Monteiro-Riviere NA, Inman AO. Challenges for assessing carbon nano-material toxicity to the skin. Carbon 2006; 44:1070–8.
32. Jia G, Wang H, Yan L, Wang X, Pei R, Yan T, Zhoa Y, Guo X. Cytotoxicity of carbon nanomaterials: single-wall nanotube, multi-wall nanotube, and fullerene. Environ Sci Technol 2005; 39:1378–83.
33. Tian F, Cui D, Schwartz H, Estrada GG, Kobayashi H. Cytotoxicity of single-wall carbon nanotubes on human fibroblasts. Tox in Vitro 2006; 20:1202–12.
34. Magrez A, Kasas S, Salicio V, Pasquier N, Seo JW, Celio M, Catsicas S, Schwaller B, Forró L. Cellular toxicity of carbon-based nanomaterials. Nano Lett 2006; 6(6):1121–5.
35. Pulskamp K, Diabaté S, Krug HF. Carbon nanotubes show no sign of acute toxicity but induce intracellular reactive oxygen species in dependence on contaminants. Tox Lett 2007; 168:58–74.
36. Flahaut E, Durrieu MC, Remy-Zolghadri M, Bareille R, Baquey CH. Investigation of the cytotoxicity of CCVD carbon nanotubes towards human umbilical vein endothelial cells. Carbon 2006; 44:1093–9.
37. Chlopek J, Czajkowska B, Szaraniec B, Frackowiak E, Szostak K., Béguin F. In vitro studies of carbon nanotubes biocompatibility. Carbon 2006; 44: 1106–11.
38. Panessa-Warren BJ, Warren JB, Wong SS, Misewich JA. Biological cellular response to carbon nanoparticle toxicity. J Phys Condens Matter 2006; 18: S2185–201.
39. Borenfreund E, Puerner J. A simple quantitative procedure using monolayer cultures for cytotoxicity assays (HTD/NR-90). J Tissue Culture Method 1984; 9:7–9.
40. Borenfreund E, Puerner J. Toxicity determined in vitro by morphological alterations and neutral red absorption. Tox Lett 1985; 24:119–24.
41. Isobe H, Tanaka T, Maeda R, Noiri E, Solin N, Yudasaka M, Iijima S, Nakamura E. Preparation, purification, characterization, and cytotoxicity assessment of water-soluble, transition-metal-free carbon nanotube aggre-gates. Angew Chem Int Ed 2006; 45:6676–80.
42. Tan M-H, Commens CA, Burnett L, Snitch PJ. A pilot study on the percutaneous absorption of microfine titanium dioxide from sunscreens. Aust J Dermatol 1996; 37:185–7.
43. Lademann J, Weigmann H-J, Rickmeyer C, Barthelmes H, Schaefer H, Mueller G, Sterry W. Penetration of titanium dioxide microparticles in a sunscreen formulation in to the horny layer and the follicular orifice. Skin Pharmacol Appl Skin Physiol 1999; 12:247–56.
44. Schulz J, Hohenberg H, Pflucker F, Gartner E, Will T, Feiffer S, Wepf R, Wendel V, Gers-Barlag H, Wittern K-P. Distribution of sunscreens on skin. Adv Drug Deliv Rev 2002; 54(S1):S157–63.
45. Oberdörster G, Oberdörster E, Oberdörster J. Nanotoxicology: an emerging discipline evolving from studies of ultrafine particles. Environ Health Perspect 2005; 113:823–39.
46. Sayes CM, Wahi R, Kurian PA, Liu Y, West JL, Ausman KD, Warheit DB, Colvin VL. Correlating nanoscale titania structure with toxicity: a cytotoxic and inflammatory response study with human dermal fibroblasts and human lung epithelial cells. Tox Sci 2007; 92(1): 174–85.

47. Derfus AM, Chan WCW, Bhatia S. Probing the cytotoxicity of semiconductor nanocrystals. Nano Lett 2004; 4:11–18.
48. Gao X, Levenson RM, Chung LWK, Nie S. In vivo cancer targeting and imaging with semiconductor quantum dots. Nature Biotech 2004; 22(8): 969–76.
49. Michalet X, Pinaud FF, Bentolila LA, Tsay JM, Doose S, Li JJ, Sundaresan G, Wu AM, Gambhir SS, Weiss S. Quantum dots for live cells, in vivo imaging, and diagnostics. Science 2005; 307(5709):538–44.
50. Ballou B, Lagerholm C, Ernst LA, Bruchez MP, Waggoner AS. Noninvasive imaging of quantum dot in mice. Bioconjugate Chem 2004; 15:79–86.
51. Ackerman ME, Chan WCW, Laakkonen P, Bhatia SN, Ruoslahti E. Nanocrystal targeting in vivo. Proc Natl Acad Sci 2002; 99(20):12617–21.
52. Ryman-Rasmussen JP, Riviere JE, Monteiro-Riviere NA. Penetration of intact skin by quantum dots with diverse physicochemical properties. Tox Sci 2006; 91:159–65.
53. Ryman-Rasmussen JP, Riviere JE, Monterio-Riviere NA. Surface coatings determine cytotoxicity and irritation potential of quantum dot nanoparticles in epidermal keratinocytes. J Invest Dermatol 2007; 127:143–53.
54. Hardman R. A toxicologic review of quantum dots: toxicity depends on physicochemical and environmental factors. Environ Health Perspect 2006; 114:165–72.
55. Lovric J, Bazzi HS, Cuie Y, Fortin GR, Winnik FM, Maysinger D. Differences in subcellular distribution and toxicity of green and red emitting CdTe quantum dots. J Mol Med 2005; 83(5): 377–85.
56. Lovric J, Cho SJ, Winnik FM, Maysinger D. Unmodified cadmium telluride quantum dots induce reactive oxygen species formation leading to multiple organelle damage and cell death. Chem Biol 2005; 12:1227–34.
57. Monteiro-Riviere NA, Ryman-Rasmussen JP. Toxicology of nanomaterials. In: Riviere JE, ed. Biological Concepts and Techniques in Toxicology: An Integrated Approach, Chapter 12 New York: Taylor and Francis Publishers, 2006.
58. Colvin VL. The potential environmental impact of engineered nanomaterials. Nature Biotech 2003; 21:1166–70.
59. Baron PA, Maynard A, Foley M. Evaluation of aerosol release during the handling of unrefined single walled carbon nanotube material. NIOSH 2002, Dart-02-191.
60. Teeguarden JG, Hinderliter PM, Orr G, Thrall BD, Pounds JG. Particokinetics in vitro nanoparticle toxicity assessments. Tox Sci 2007; 95: 300–12.

20

Toxicity of Nanoparticles in the Eye

Tarl Prow and Gerard A. Lutty

Wilmer Ophthalmological Institute, Johns Hopkins Hospital, Baltimore, Maryland, U.S.A.

INTRODUCTION

The eye is a superb organ in which to utilize therapeutic nanomaterials. Some of the disease processes that occur in the eye are defects in basement membrane, ischemic events, neovascularization, inflammatory events, and neuronal degenerations. Ocular diseases affect a myriad of cell types including cells of fibroblast origin, endothelial cells, glia, monocyte origin dendritic cells, and neurons. The eye also has a clear medium allowing light to enter the eye and stimulate sensory retinal neurons, photoreceptors, and finally the brain (Fig. 1). In being a clear medium, the investigator can assess the effects of therapeutic nanomaterials in vivo in real time. The most common diseases of the eye are conjunctivitis, cataracts, glaucoma, ischemic retinopathies (ex. diabetic and sickle cell retinopathies) and age-related macular degeneration (AMD).

Common Eye Diseases

The conjunctiva is the mucous membrane between the eyelid and the anterior sclera, or the white collagenous outer surface of the eye. By virtue of its location, this tissue is exposed to many potential pathogens. Both bacteria and viruses can cause infection of the conjunctiva. Most cases are not serious, but some severe cases can cause blindness. The most common treatment for bacterial conjunctivitis is topical antibiotics. Viral conjunctivitis can be treated if it is caused by the Herpes virus, but is untreatable when caused by the more common Adenovirus. The major application of

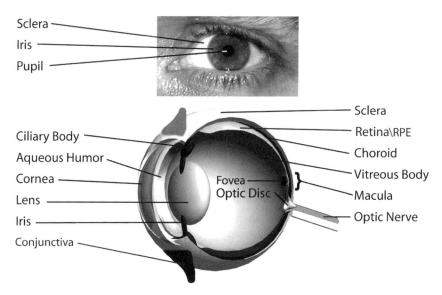

Figure 1 Anatomy of the eye. The upper panel shows the exposed surfaces of the eye. The lower panel identifies some of the major structures of the eye. The two fluid-filled chambers of the eye are filled with aqueous humor (anterior to the lens) and vitreous (posterior to the lens). The center of the macula region of retina is the fovea.

nanotechnology for conjunctivitis may be through controlled, continuous antibiotic/antiviral delivery.

There are two optically clear lenses in the eye, the cornea and the lens. The lens is a colorless, crystalline structure that focuses light on the sensory retina. The clarity of the lens is crucial for light to be focused on the retina. A cataract is a condition where the lens becomes colored, opaque, or cloudy. Cataracts decrease the passage of light through the lens and increase light scattering that result in poor visual acuity and low light vision. The current therapy for cataracts is extraction of the crystalline lens and replacement with an artificial lens. Without surgery, the patient can become blind. Nanomaterials may provide better lens prostheses in the future.

One of the leading causes of blindness is glaucoma. This disease is caused by a buildup of excess aqueous humor in the anterior chamber of the eye. The fluid buildup causes a dangerous increase of intraocular pressure that can cut off the delivery of nutrients and removal of waste from the anterior chamber. Chronic glaucoma can lead to the death of retinal neurons and the optic nerve, resulting in total blindness.

The leading cause of vision loss in senior citizens is AMD. The lens focuses light on the macula, the center of vision, which possesses more cones (photoreceptor cells that see colors) than any area of retina. The fovea is the small pit in the center of macula, which is the center of the visual axis.

The macula photoreceptors then send visual signals to the brain. Macular degeneration can be caused by neural atrophy (dry AMD) or through severe hemorrhagic or serous exudation after growth of neovascularization (wet AMD). Macular degeneration can cause visual acuity to decrease to 20/400, while leaving the rest of the retina unaffected and peripheral vision intact.

Routes of Delivery

Ocular diseases affect all tissues of the eyes. Delivery route for nanoparticles (NP) will vary by tissue affected and diffusability of the drug or gene to the affected tissue. For corneal diseases, which include corneal neovascularization, ulceration, inflammation, and loss of corneal endothelial cells, the NP suspension can simply be delivered topically by eye drops. If the drug is small enough and/or hydrophobic, a topical route may be sufficient for delivery to any part of the eye if the drug can diffuse through the cornea. The evaluation of toxic effects from NP delivered by this route would follow the criterion of the Draize test: usually 4 hours exposure and then evaluate changes in cornea for up to 14 days. The other extra-ocular route is injection into the space between the conjunctiva and the globe, i.e., sub-conjunctival injection. As in topical delivery to cornea, this route is acceptable for delivery to the surface of the eye but only some drugs can diffuse across eye wall to penetrate intraocular tissues. However, Ambati and associates found that some IgG could traverse the eye wall when delivered sub-conjunctivally (1,2).

For diseases affecting retina, the most common route is injection into the vitreous, the gel that fills the large chamber of the eye behind the lens (Fig. 2, Left panel). The needle is inserted just posterior to the iris and anterior to peripheral limit of the retina (ora serrata) in the area called the pars plana. For diseases of the choroid or retina, a sub-retinal injection may be used. A small hole or retinotomy is made in sensory retina, and 50 µl or less of fluid can be injected behind the retina, between the retinal photoreceptors and the retinal pigment epithelium (RPE) in the sub-retinal space (Fig. 2, Right panel, and Fig. 3A). The fluid causes the retina to bleb out into the vitreous but with resorption of the NP solution, the retina will reattach. This is known as a sub-retinal injection.

In Vivo Versus in Vitro

Most of the cells in the eye can be maintained in culture, so the first line of evaluation of the nanoparticle can be done in vitro in cell culture systems. The in vitro systems simplify the experiments so that only one cell type is evaluated for effect of the therapy and toxicity of the NP. However, the in vitro analysis excludes the complexity of the tissue and the interactions of

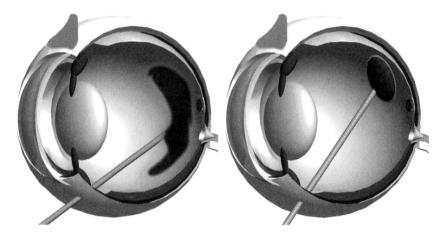

Figure 2 Intravitreal and sub-retinal injection routes. The left panel is a schematic of an intravitreal injection. The right panel shows a sub-retinal injection resulting in a bleb. In both panels the needle punctures the eye just posterior to the ciliary body, an area called the pars plana. The sub-retinal injection causes the retina to bleb out.

neighboring cells. In vitro analysis also excludes the reaction of the immune system to NP. In vivo and in vitro toxicity analysis will be included in this chapter, when available, and the pros and cons of such approaches will also be highlighted. We have not included ex vivo tissue experiments in the following discussion because they are usually short term and, therefore, may not be of sufficient duration to judge toxicity.

Payloads

The number of materials made into nanoparticles has increased greatly in recent years. The diversity of the NP materials permit systemic and targeted delivery of both drugs and genes. This chapter attempts to include all therapeutic uses of NP in the eye including drugs and genes. The payload will be determined by the capabilities of the NP material as well as the target tissue and disease. In some examples, only the NP itself was delivered without payload as a preliminary feasibility study.

Although the above are common diseases of the eye, there are many more ocular diseases. Nanotechnology has the potential to prevent or treat most ocular diseases, but this can only be accomplished if the nanomaterials used are nontoxic. Unfortunately, very few toxicity studies have been done on nanomaterials in the eye or ocular cells. One reason for the lack of data on the toxicity of nanomaterials in the eye is the potential for negative toxicity results to not be published. Most studies are focused on showing positive effects of a nanomaterial on a disease state. The following sections

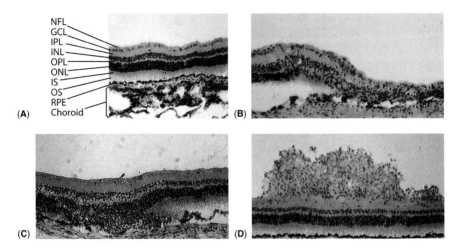

Figure 3 Anatomy of the retina, RPE, and choroid and appearance of toxicity from nanoparticles. (**A**) The retina is divided into eight distinct layers: nerve fiber layer (NFL), ganglion cell layer (GCL), inner plexiform layer (IPL), inner nuclear layer (INL), outer plexiform layer (OPL), inner segments (IS), and outer segments (OS). Beneath the retina lay the RPE and the choroid. Panels b, c, and d are photos of retinas exposed to toxic nanomaterials and constituents. Panel (**B**) illustrates retinal degeneration and abnormal RPE as a result of a sub-retinal injection of PCEP. Panel (**C**) shows a disorganized ONL and abnormal RPE caused by an intravitreal injection of chitosan. Finally, panel (**D**) is an example of inflammation generated from an intravitreal injection of impure plasmid DNA. *Abbreviations*: PCEP, poly [[(cholesteryl oxocarbonylamido ethyl); RPE, retinal pigment epithelium.

summarize the available data on both in vitro and in vivo ocular studies of nanomaterials and their toxicity.

TOXICITY OF NANOMATERIALS IN THE EYE

Metallic Nanoparticles

Magnetic nanoparticles have been used as contrast agents for MRI and are FDA approved for such use systemically (3). Krause and associates used them to perform blood volume measurements of choroidal melanoma, an important measurement for tracking growth of such tumors lying in a highly pigmented tissue like choroid and evaluating effectiveness of therapies for the tumors (4,5).

We have evaluated the feasibility of using iron nanoparticles for gene delivery in the eye (6,7). These studies describe the use of DNA tethered nanoparticles to deliver genetic biosensors to retinal endothelial cells in vitro. Oxidative stress was evaluated, because the core of these nanoparticles is composed of iron. One possibility would be that the nanoparticles would degrade and expose the iron core. This free iron could then be involved in Fenton cycling, generating oxidative stress. Therefore, different concentrations of magnetic nanoparticles were incubated with cultured endothelial cells. Oxidative stress was monitored by fluorescence of CM-H2DCFDA by flow cytometry. Ultimately there was no detectible increase in oxidative stress with any treatment group. These nanoparticles were also tested in vivo, with very little toxicity observed. The magnetic nanoparticles were given in vivo through intravitreal and sub-retinal injection. Intravitreal injection resulted in transfection of mostly hyalocytes, dendritic cells of vitreous. Subretinal injection resulted in transfection of several cell types in retina but RPE were the most prominent cell type transfected. There was little to no signs of inflammation, retinal degeneration, and minor changes in RPE (8).

Chen and associates have used another metallic nanoparticle, cerium oxide (termed nanoceria particles), as a therapeutic agent itself (9). They found that nanoceria particles protected cultures of rat retinal neuronal cells from H_2O_2-induced cell death. Furthermore, nanoceria particles also protected against photoreceptor death in vivo if injected intravitreally before the rats were exposed to intense light, which causes a form of retinal degeneration. Not only was cell death prevented but visual function was preserved after administration of nanoceria nanoparticles (9).

Condensed DNA Nanoparticles

The Naash laboratory at the University of Oklahoma Health Sciences Center has been developing a unique nanoparticle for gene delivery to the sensory retina (10). This DNA compacted nanoparticle has been an effective gene delivery agent for plasmids up to 20 Kb. The nanoparticle is composed of a neutrally-charged complex with a single plasmid compacted with PEG-substituted lysine peptides. The resulting nanoparticles are reported to be quite stable in a variety of biological fluids and conditions. Sub-retinal injections into mice did not lead to an inflammatory response as determined by histological analysis. Electroretinography results demonstrated that the injection of these nanoparticles had no deleterious effect on the function of the photoreceptors at 30 days post injection. Overall these nanoparticles achieved a physiologically significant level of gene transduction and did not show any signs of toxicity (10).

PLGA

Poly(D,L-lactide-co-glycolide (PLGA) has been used in the eye frequently. It has been evaluated for topical drug delivery by Vega and associates (11). They found that PLGA NP loaded with fluripofen were nontoxic when delivered to cornea and it controlled inflammation of cornea. Bejjani et al. investigated the route of uptake of Texas red dye loaded PLGA NP by RPE cells in vitro and found that it was through absorptive endocytosis (12). These NP were judged non-toxic to RPE in vitro based on trypan blue exclusion.

PLGA has recently been investigated for gene therapy in the eye as well. In the study by Bejjani et al, green fluorescent protein (GFP) and red nuclear fluorescent protein plasmids (RNFP) were incorporated in PLGA NP (12). Bovine and human RPE cells were exposed to the NP for up to six hours and then toxicity and gene expression were evaluated. Fourteen percent of the cells expressed the GFP gene with no toxicity. These NP were also injected intravitreally and preferential RNFP expression was observed in RPE cells with no apparent toxicity. A potential therapeutic construct was incorporated in PLGA NP by Aukunuru et al. and the effects on RPE viability and vascular endothelial growth factor (VEGF) gene expression were evaluated in vitro (13). VEGF is an angiogenic growth factor produced by RPE and other cells during hypoxia (14). It has been implicated in stimulating angiogenesis in several ischemic retinopathies and in age-related macular degeneration, when neovascularization grows from the choroid into the sub-retinal space (15). In their study, Aukunuru et al. incorporated antisense VEGF nucleotides into PLGA and exposed human RPE cells in vitro to the NP (13). The antisense PLGA NP inhibited VEGF mRNA production and protein secretion. No toxicity was observed.

PLA

Poly (lactic acid) (PLA) has been evaluated for drug and gene delivery in the eye. Bourges et al. encapsulated dyes in PLA nanoparticles and injected them intravitreally (16). They found that NP settled on the internal limiting membrane of retina (Fig. 3A) but were not toxic. However, there was an inflammatory response between 18 and 24 hours after injection that subsided with time. They observed fluorescence of the dyes in RPE up to four months later. Sakai et al. incorporated betamethasone phosphate in PLA nanoparticles in hopes of using them as a therapy for experimental autoimmune uveoretinitis (EAU) induced by injection of S-antigen (17). Intravitreal injection of these NP was nontoxic and effective against EAU but systemic delivery of the NP was superior therapeutically. Giannavola et al. incorporated acyclovir into PLA NP and applied the NP topically to the cornea (18). Using a modified Draize test they found these NP were nontoxic. This has potential for treating viral conjunctivitis.

PLA NP were also used for gene delivery by Bejjani et al (12). The details of transfection efficiency and the toxicity from intravitreal injection are not clearly stated in the manuscript, but it is implied that PLA NP were nontoxic.

PEI

Polyethylenimine (PEI) is a chemical that has been investigated for over three decades and has since been reported in about 1300 publications. PEI is a very popular molecule for drug and gene delivery and has previously been used in the eye. One study used PEI to deliver anti-TGF-β2 oligonucleotides (ODN) to improve the outcome of glaucoma surgery (19). The surgery creates a drainage canal for excess intra-ocular fluid and pressure, but scarring, which is stimulated by TGF-β, can close the drainage canal. This nanomaterial was tested in vitro for ODN release and then in vivo. The PEI-ODN was evaluated after subconjunctival administration to rabbits. This nanomaterial was able to achieve a sustained release of the ODN, thus inhibiting scarring. No toxicity was seen at the injection site, up to seven days after injection (19).

Chitosan

Chitosan is a deacetylated form of chitin, which is the second most abundant polymer in nature after cellulose. It is a desirable polymer for drug delivery and gene therapy because of its mucoadhesiveness and its bio-degradability (20). Maria Alonso's laboratory in Santiago de Compostela, Spain, has done extensive work with drug delivery from chitosan NP applied topically to the eye. The positively charged groups on chitosan bind to the negatively charged groups in mucin prolonging the residence of chitosan in extraocular fluids and on surfaces, assuring slow release of drugs and prolonged half-life of chitosan on the ocular surface (20). The toxicity was assessed on a human conjunctival cell line by determining cell survival and viability (21). No toxicity was observed in vitro and in vivo application demonstrated that these NP penetrated into the corneal and conjunctival epithelia. The prolonged release of drug from the chitosan NP on the surface of the eye was demonstrated using cyclosporin (22). Their most recent study demonstrated that the uptake of the chitosan NP by conjunctival and corneal epithelial cells was by active transport mechanisms that did not compromise cell viability (23). Kao et al evaluated chitosan nanoparticles for delivery of pilocarpine, a commonly used drug for management of glaucoma (24). They found that Carbopol contributed to the stabilization of the pilocarpine/chitosan NP and the Carbopol/chitosan/ pilocarpine NP had good biocompatibility, biodegradability and low toxicity.

Chitosan has also been used for gene delivery. One of the first applications was oral delivery in a murine model of peanut allergy (25). We have investigated the use of chitosan as an intraocular gene therapy vehicle in rabbit (8). In this study, plasmid DNA containing a Cytomegalovirus (CMV) promoter driven enhanced green fluorescent protein (EGFP) reporter was complexed with chitosan and injected via an intravitreal route. The animals were kept for seven days. The eyes were evaluated for toxicity by gross and histological analysis (Fig. 3). The gross analysis revealed strong signs of inflammation that the histological analysis confirmed (Fig. 3, Panel D). This molecule has been used successfully on the surface of the retina, but injecting it into the eye led to massive inflammation. This illustrates the need for tissue specific, in vivo toxicity assays for all nanomaterials that are to be used in humans.

PCEP

In 2004, a novel biodegradable polyphosphoester, poly[[(cholesteryl oxocarbonylamido ethyl) methyl bis(ethylene) ammonium iodide] ethyl phosphate] (PCEP), was introduced as a gene delivery tool by Wen et al. (26). This biodegradable polymer was promising because of its low toxicity and ability to be formed into nanoparticles, films, or shaped as needed. We tested PCEP for toxicity and gene delivery in the rabbit eye. PCEP was complexed with plasmid DNA containing a CMV promoter driven EGFP reporter. The eyes were injected via two routes: intravitreal and sub-retinal. After injection, the animals were maintained for seven days. After seven days, the eyes were evaluated grossly and by histological means for toxicity and for EGFP reporter expression. PCEP did not induce inflammation although there was some retinal degeneration. The retinal degeneration was thought to come from residual solvents from the preparation of the PCEP (Fig. 3, Panel B). However, this was never proven. Ultimately, in subsequent preparations, PCEP appeared to be non-toxic, but there was essentially no transfection of retinal cells (8).

Polycarboxylic Acid Nanoparticles

De et al. evaluated two types of polycarboxylic acid NP for controlled release of Brimonidine on the surface of the cornea (27). Brimonidine is an alpha2 agonist used to control intraocular pressure in glaucoma, so slow topical release is desirable. Their toxicity was evaluated in vitro with human corneal epithelial cells. Polyacrylic acid NP seemed to not be toxic for corneal epithelial cells while polyitanconic acid NP were toxic to these cells. Neither of these NP was evaluated in vivo.

Eudragit Nanoparticles

The inert polymer resins Eudragit RS100 and RL100 were made into nanoparticles and evaluated topically on the eye (28). A modified Draize test was used to evaluate toxicity of these NP 24 hours after application and no toxicity was observed. Topical non-steroidal anti-inflammatory drugs are the most commonly used drugs after ocular trauma. Ibuprofen was loaded in Eudragit RS100 NP and evaluated topically after ocular trauma, in this case paracentesis, a penetrating wound resulting in leakage of aqueous humor (28). These NP were nontoxic and a reasonable level of drug was observed in aqueous and in the conjunctival sac. Cloricromene, a coumarin that was evaluated for control of uveitis, was loaded in Eudragit RL100 NP and the NP delivered topically (29,30). The NP were non-toxic and said to have potential as an anti-inflammatory agent for uveitis.

Albumen Nanoparticles

CMV infection affects neural retina, optic nerve, and blood vessels of retina resulting in uveitis. Gancyclovir is an effective therapy if delivered into vitreous but its half- life is short. Merodia and associates incorporated this drug into albumen nanoparticles (31). Two weeks after intravitreal injection, there was neither any inflammatory reaction nor toxicity. The albumin nanoparticles remained mostly at the vitreous/retina interface. They also appeared to improve the antiviral activity of gancyclovir and, in subsequent experiments, another antiviral reagent formivirisin (32).

CONCLUSIONS

No study to date, in the eye, has applied rigorous toxicological analysis to the effects of NP to any ocular tissue. However, the Draize test has been used for corneal toxicity from topical NP and traditional histological evaluation used for intraocular toxicity. The logical progression for the evaluation of toxicity is to test the NP on the target cells in vitro using standard toxicity analysis. If nontoxic in vitro, NP must then be evaluated in vivo where the immune system is present and all cells in target tissue are present in the correct association. This is the standard procedure for topical drugs in the US; in vitro analysis must be done before Draize test evaluation of topical substances. Chitosan is a good example of the need for both in vivo and in vitro testing. Chitosan also demonstrates the need to evaluate NP in different compartments of the eye as well, since it was nontoxic when applied topically but toxic when injected into the eye.

REFERENCES

1. Ambati J, Canakis C, Miller JW, et al. Diffusion of high molecular weight compounds through sclera. Invest Ophthalmol Vis Sci 2000; 41:1181–5.
2. Ambati J, Gragoudas E, Miller JW, et al. Transscleral delivery of bioactive protein to the choroid and retina. Invest Ophthalmol Vis Sci 2000; 41:1186–91.

3. Thorek DL, Chen AK, Czupryna J, et al. Superparamagnetic iron oxide nanoparticle probes for molecular imaging. Ann Biomed Eng 2006; 34:23–38.
4. Krause M, Kwong KK, Xiong J, et al. MRI of blood volume and cellular uptake of superparamagnetic iron in an animal model of choroidal melanoma. Ophthalmic Res 2002; 34:241–50.
5. Krause MH, Kwong KK, Gragoudas E, et al. MRI of blood volume with superparamagnetic iron in choroidal melanoma treated with thermotherapy. Magn Reson Imaging 2004; 22:779–87.
6. Prow T, Grebe R, Merges C, et al. Nanoparticle tethered antioxidant response element as a biosensor for oxygen induced toxicity in retinal endothelial cells. Mol Vis 2006; 12:616–25.
7. Prow T, Smith JN, Grebe R, et al. Construction, gene delivery, and expression of DNA tethered nanoparticles. Mol Vis 2006; 12:606–15.
8. Prow T, Bhutto I, Kim SY, et al. Nanoparticle toxicity and transfection of the retina. Nanoletters, 2007.
9. Chen J, Patil S, Seal S, et al. Rare earth nanoparticles prevent retinal degeneration induced by intracellular peroxides. Nat Nanotechnol 2006; 1:142–150.
10. Farjo R, Skaggs J, Quiambao AB, et al. Efficient non-viral ocular gene transfer with compacted DNA nanoparticles. PLoS ONE 2006 Dec 20; 1:e38.
11. Vega E, Egea M, Valls O, et al. Flurbiprofen loaded biodegradable nanoparticles for ophthalmic administration. J Pharm Sci 2006; 95:2393–405.
12. Bejjani RA, Benezra D, Cohen H, et al. Nanoparticles for gene delivery to retinal pigment epithelial cells. Mol Vis 2005; 11:124–32.
13. Aukunuru J, Ayalasomayajula S, and Kompella U. Nanoparticle formulation enhances the delivery and activity of a vascular endothelial growth factor antisense oligonucleotide in human retinal pigment epithelial cells. J Pharm Pharmacol 2003; 55:1199–206.
14. Adamis AP, Shima DT, Yeo KT, et al. Synthesis and secretion of vascular permeability factor/vascular endothelial growth factor by human retinal pigment epithelial cells. Biochem Biophys Res Commun 1993; 193:631–8.
15. D'amore PA. Mechanisms of retinal and choroidal neovascularization. Invest Ophthalmol Vis Sci 1994; 35:3974–79.
16. Bourges J, Gautier S, Delie F, et al. Ocular drug delivery targeting the retina and retinal pigment epithelium using polylactide nanoparticles. Invest Ophthalmol Vis Sci 2003; 44:3562–9.
17. Sakai T, Kohno H, Ishihara T, et al. Treatment of experimental autoimmune uveoretinitis with poly(lactic acid) nanoparticles encapsulating betamethasone phosphate. Exp Eye Res 2006; 82:657–63.
18. Giannavola C, Bucolo C, Maltese A, et al. Influence of preparation conditions on acyclovir-loaded poly-d,l-lactic acid nanospheres and effect of PEG coating on ocular drug bioavailability. Pharm Res 2003; 20:584–90.
19. Gomes dos Santos AL, Bochot A, Doyle N. et al. Sustained release of nanosized complexes of polyethylenimine and anti-TGF-beta 2 oligonucleotide improves the outcome of glaucoma surgery. J Control Release 2006; 112: 369–81.
20. Alonso MJ and Sanchez A. The potential of chitosan in ocular drug delivery. J Pharm Pharmacol 2003; 55:1451–63.

21. De Campos AM, Diebold Y, Carvalho E, et al. Chitosan nanoparticles as new ocular drug delivery systems: in vitro stability, in vivo fate, and cellular toxicity. Pharm Res 2004; 21:803–10.
22. De Campos AM, Sanchez A, Alonso MJ. Chitosan nanoparticles: a new vehicle for the improvement of the delivery of drugs to the ocular surface. Application to cyclosporin A. Int J Pharm 2001; 224:159–68.
23. Enriquez De Salamanca A, Diebold Y, et al. Chitosan nanoparticles as a potential drug delivery system for the ocular surface: toxicity, uptake mechanism and in vivo tolerance. Invest Ophthalmol Vis Sci 2006; 47:1416–25.
24. Kao H, Lin H, Lo Y, et al. Characterization of pilocarpine-loaded chitosan/ Carbopol nanoparticles. J Pharm Pharmacol 2006; 58:179–86.
25. Roy K, Mao H-Q, Huang S-K, et al. Oral gene delivery with chitosan-DNA nanoparticles generates immunologic protection in a murine model of peanut allergy. Nat Med 1999; 5:387–91.
26. Wen J, Mao H-Q, Li W, et al. Biodegradable polyphosphoester micelles for gene delivery. J Pharm Sci 2004; 93:2142–57.
27. De T, Bergey E, Chung S, et al. Polycarboxylic acid nanoparticles for ophthalmic drug delivery: an ex vivo evaluation with human cornea. J Microencapsul 2004; 21:841–55.
28. Pignatello R, Bucolo C, Puglisi G. Ocular tolerability of Eudragit RS100 and RL100 nanosuspensions as carriers for ophthalmic controlled drug delivery. J Pharm Sci 2002; 91:2636–41.
29. Bucolo C, Maltese A, Maugeri F, et al. Eudragit RL100 nanoparticle system for the ophthalmic delivery of cloricromene. J Pharm Pharmacol 2004; 56: 841–6.
30. Bucolo C, Maltese A, Puglisi G, et al. Enhanced ocular anti-inflammatory activity of ibuprofen carried by an Eudragit RS100 nanoparticle suspension. Ophthalmic Res 2002; 34:319–23.
31. Merodio M, Irache JM, Valamanesh F, et al. Ocular disposition and tolerance of ganciclovir- loaded albumin nanoparticles after intravitreal injection in rats. Biomaterials 2002; 23:1587–94.
32. Irache J, Merodio M, Arnedo A, et al. Albumin nanoparticles for the intravitreal delivery of anticytomegaloviral drugs. Mini Rev Med Chem 2005; 5:293–305.

21

Nanoparticle Interactions with Biological Systems and Subsequent Activation of Intracellular Signaling Mechanisms

Vicki Stone

Centre for Health and the Environment, School of Life Sciences, Napier University, Edinburgh, U.K.

Ian Kinloch

School of Materials, University of Manchester, Manchester, U.K.

INTRODUCTION

This chapter aims to describe some of the intracellular signaling pathways that have been studied in relation to the control of inflammation for pathogenic particles, and in particular for nanoparticles. In addition, this article will highlight some of the methods that are most appropriate for such studies, and those in which the use of particles provide specific problems that need to be controlled in order to allow appropriate interpretation of the data.

Inflammation is considered to play a key role in driving diseases induced by a number of pathogenic particles that enter the body via inhalation. The field of nanotechnology opens some interesting new avenues of research in relation to particle toxicology, due to the potential for uptake via a wide variety of routes into the body. For example, the use of nanoparticles in cosmetics and suntan lotions increases the likelihood for absorption via the skin (1), while the inclusion of nanoparticles in foods and medicines suggests that uptake via the gastrointestinal tract will be a significant route of entry for some types of nanoparticles, and of course some nanoparticles will be injected directly into the body for medicinal (2) or diagnostic purposes (3). The nanotechnology area therefore provides challenges to the field of particle toxicology, to first examine the current literature relating to respirable particles, and then to use this literature to apply to other types of particles administered alternative exposure routes and to design new studies. Much of the following chapter will describe studies that were originally conducted in relation to respirable particle toxicology, but due to their in vitro nature, and similarity between the cell types found in different organs, could easily apply to other exposure scenarios including injection, ingestion or dermal absorption.

INFLAMMATION

The pathogenic effects of many types of particles (α-quartz, asbestos and PM_{10} air pollution particles) have all been demonstrated to involve the induction or promotion of inflammation (4–6). Inflammation involves a number of cell types, including epithelial cells, macrophages and neutrophils, whose activation results in the initiation, progression or prolongation of the signaling mechanisms that control inflammation. These signaling can be divided into extracellular (outside or between cells) and intracellular (inside cells) mechanisms. In the extracellular environment, inflammation is activated and controlled by a wide range of molecules such as cytokine proteins (7), leukotrienes (8) and prostaglandins (9). Much of the pro-inflammatory effects of pathogenic particles have focused on the impact of these particles on pro-inflammatory cytokine expression (10). In the coming years it will interesting to investigate whether any of the additional extracellular signaling pathways play a significant role in the potential toxic effects of nanoparticles. With respect to the intracellular signaling pathways, these generally control the production of the extracellular pro-inflammatory mediators described above. This article will focus on the ability of a variety of nanoparticles to impact on these intracellular signaling pathways.

FACTORS AFFECTING NANOPARTICLE SURFACE AREA AND SURFACE REACTIVITY

Many pathogenic particles, including carbon (11), polystyrene (12), TiO_2, cobalt and nickel (13) nanoparticles have also been demonstrated to generate reactive oxygen species (ROS) including hydroxyl radicals in a cell free environment (e.g., cell culture medium), possibly due to their surface functional groups. A number of these studies have compared particles of different sizes, suggesting that particles of smaller size are more potent at generating ROS per mass of particles (11,12). The surface area per unit mass is much larger for nanoparticles than larger particles, and thus the ROS production has been proposed to be related to the particle surface area.

The surface of particles is often used in chemistry as a catalytic surface, and it has been suggested that for smaller particles, in addition to the surface area being greater, the surface catalytic reactivity per unit area is also greater, (14). A relatively simple explanation for this size effect is previously described (15). This hypothesis suggests that biological molecules can only react with the atoms in the particle to which they have access. This means that the extent of the reaction between a nanoparticle and the surrounding fluid depends on the area of interface between the two, which is equal to the total surface area of the particle dose. (Note: In the case of ultrafine porous particulates, not all of the pores and hence surface area will be accessible to large biomolecules.) As the particle radius decreases the surface area to volume ratio increases, resulting in a greater proportion of the atoms at the surface of the particle compared to the bulk (Fig. 1).

Many toxicological studies use aggregated or agglomerated particles, which consequently influence the available surface area. In some preparations and manufacturing methods, the primary particles sinter together to form relatively stable aggregates which are held together by covalent or ionic bonding (e.g., fumed silica). In the case of these aggregated particles the specific surface area available for interaction with biological molecules is much less than for monodispersed particles, but remains greater than for a

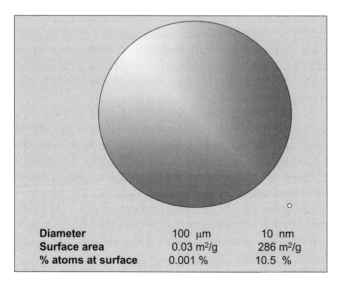

Diameter	100 μm	10 nm
Surface area	0.03 m²/g	286 m²/g
% atoms at surface	0.001 %	10.5 %

Figure 1   A comparison of the size, surface area, and percentage of atoms at the surface for two carbon particles four orders of magnitude different in diameter. (Particles not drawn to scale.)

single particle of equal mass. This stable aggregation status also impacts upon how these particles interact with biological systems. For example, the aggregated particle has an overall particle size that is an amalgamation of the individual particles and which phagocytic cells would need to fully engulf to allow phagocytosis. For those particles made of soluble materials the shape of the stable aggregate would also effect the dissolution rate in biological media and hence their biopersistence (16).

Non-aggregated nanoparticles can however still agglomerate via weaker electrostatic forces or van der Waal forces (e.g., single-walled nanotubes in bundles). The degree to which this agglomeration will occur depends on the degree of favorable interaction between the solvent and the particle's surface chemistry. Upon entering a biological system the interaction can be modified by either the binding of biomolecules such as endogenous proteins or surfactants or, in the case of the electrostatically dispersed particles, the concentration of ions in the surrounding media. While the impact of such agglomeration forces may be sufficient to affect available surface area, this is much more difficult to quantify due to the propensity for agglomeration status to change depending upon mechanical agitation, the chemical composition of the media and interaction with cells. It is currently unclear as to whether a phagocytic cell would engulf an agglomeration of particles as one particle, or whether agglomerated particles would be dissociated by the cell and engulfed singularly or in smaller agglomerates. Preliminary data from the author's laboratory in Edinburgh using live imaging combined with confocal microscopy of macrophages ingesting carboxylated polystyrene nanoparticles (20 nm primary particle diameter) suggests that large agglomerates (2–5 μm diameter) are not taken in as a single entity, but instead the cell appears to take 'bites' in order to internalize single particles or small agglomerates. This work requires further study to verify such observations and the dependence of the effect on the strength of the interparticulate forces.

It is important to note that a majority of the in vivo and in vitro studies that have been published over the last decade using a variety of nanoparticles, have used particles that are aggregated and/or agglomerated. In studies that have compared the same mass dose of particles of different primary particle size, those of smaller dimensions are almost always found to be more reactive in terms of generating inflammation (12,17), cytokine expression (10,18), intracellular signaling (19) and cytotoxicity (11). In many of these studies, despite the full surface area not being completely exposed, their remains a clear relationship between particle surface area and biological effect (12,20,21).

In addition to size, the chemistry of the surface is also important in determining a material's behavior within a biological system. For many engineered nanoparticles, the chemistry of the particle surface is purposefully different to that within its centre. In particular, much work has been conducted to engineer particles with a surface chemistry that influences or controls dispersion and interaction with other materials. Typical approaches include using surfactants, substituting ligands or functionalising the surface. All these modifications will either charge the surface to give Coulomb forces (forces associated with the relative charge of the particles, for example like charges repel, opposite charges attract), introduce long molecular chains to increase steric forces or improve the solvent-material interaction (e.g., make the surface hydrophilic for aqueous dispersions).

For particles in the micrometer range and larger, the electronic properties of the particle are independent of particle size. At the nanometer range the size is sufficiently small to confine the electrons, which subsequently impacts upon the physicochemical properties of the particle. Electron confinement within such a material generates discrete (*quantized*) energies which become increasingly apparent as one, or more, of the dimensions of the particle decreases below 10 nm (22). Through control of the particle composition and production process, these quantized energy levels can be tuned to generate specific particle characteristics. The particles generated by such processes include quantum wells, wires and dots with electron confinement in one, two or three dimensions respectively (23). Also, for very small particles, below a diameter of approximately 5 nm, there can be increased strain in the bonds between the atoms, leading to increased reactivity or change in the crystal structure (16).

A range of in vivo and in vitro toxicology studies of particles within the nanometer size range have been published over the last decade that address the relationship between particle size, surface area and inflammation. Such particles include TiO_2, carbon black and polystyrene beads, with the particles referred to as 'ultrafine' rather than 'nano'. All of these particles are generated by industrial processes and most are made in bulk quantities. However, many of these studies were conducted to test the hypothesis that smaller particles have a greater capacity to induce inflammation in the lung after inhalation, and that these pro-inflammatory properties are responsible for driving the adverse health effects induced by particulate air pollution (24,25). The wording and focus of these articles is therefore dominated by air pollution and respiratory toxicology, and while these observations are important, it is now essential to re-evaluate these results in order to investigate whether the lessons learnt also apply to newly engineered nanoparticles (26). This chapter will review some of these studies and put them into the context of nanotoxicology in general.

Many of the studies published over the last decade suggest that as particle size decreases, potential to induce oxidative stress and inflammation increases (11,27,28). A number of studies from different research groups have demonstrated a linear relationship between the surface area dose of the particle delivered into the rat lung via instillation and the ability to induce inflammation, as indicated by neutrophil influx 18 to 24 hours after exposure. These studies include a variety of low solubility, low toxicity materials including polystyrene beads (12), carbon black (21), and TiO_2 (20). Stoeger et al., 2006 recently identified a link between surface area and the ability of six different carbon particles to induce inflammation in the mouse lung (21). Such models may provide in the future useful benchmarking tools to compare the relative toxicity of different nanoparticles, especially if an in vitro alternative can be identified. In vitro systems have proved to be useful when comparing the ability of particles to enhance signaling responsible for driving inflammation, and as such these endpoints may provide the in vitro tools for alternative testing. However, at this time in vitro models have not been validated as alternatives to inhalation, instillation, injection, ingestion or dermal absorption studies to determine the ability of nanoparticles to induce inflammation. This work will form the basis of important research in the near future.

NANOPARTICLE CYTOTOXICITY

Before the ability of nanoparticles to induce cell signaling and inflammation can be determined, the cytotoxicity must be assessed in order to ensure appropriate interpretation of the responses observed. There are a wide variety of assay techniques to assess cell viability, a review of which would be beyond the scope of this article. Instead, we will focus on tests that have been used for particle treated cells, while pointing out some of their advantages and pitfalls.

Many studies have measured release of the cytoplasmic protein lactate dehydrogenase (LDH). This protein leaks into the extracellular media either as a consequence of direct membrane insult leading to death, or due to cell death resulting in membrane breakdown. Therefore the enzyme activity of LDH measurable within the cell culture medium of exposed cells should be directly proportional to the level of cell death. However, we (12) and others (29) have observed that micro and nanoparticles have a large capacity to either bind proteins or to induce their degradation (30, See Monteiro-Riviere Chapter 19), which could lead to an underestimation of that protein content in the cell culture supernatant. Our own recent data clearly shows that LDH mixed with nanoparticles results in an underestimation of the LDH content of media (15). It is interesting to note that activated carbons are used as medical absorbents and filters. They are commonly used to remove poisons and toxins and have been proposed to remove inflammatory markers in blood (31).

The MTT (3-(4,5-dimethylthiazol-2-yl)-2,5-diphenyltetrazolium bromide) assay is also widely published as a useful tool to measure cell viability (32). The MTT molecule is converted to a blue formazan product by the mitochondrial enzyme succinate dehyrogenase, and so a decrease in metabolic competence of the cells is used as an indicator of viability. However the colored formazan product is actually a combined measure of the amount of functional succinate dehydrogenase per cell and the number of cells per culture well. While a decrease in MTT absorbance can clearly be used as an indicator of toxicity, it is not clear whether this is due to decreased cell function or decreased cell number, although in fact for many purposes it may not be necessary to distinguish between the two. Interpretation of an increase in MTT absorbance, or in fact of no change, is also confused by these issues and may need to be considered carefully. The production of the colored formazan involves an oxidative reaction. In phagocytic cells generating an oxidative burst on exposure to nanoparticles, this additional oxidative effect could lead to an underestimation of cytotoxicity and again requires careful control. Since measurement of the formazan product is via absorbance, the light absorbing properties of any particles also needs to considered, monitored and controlled for. For example, black carbon particles will generate a significant background absorbance over many wavelengths.

Annexin V combined with propidium iodide staining is proving to be a reliable and relatively easy technique to quantify viability, but also to distinguish between cell death via apoptosis and necrosis (33). The technique involves staining the cells using immunofluorescence techniques followed by subsequent quantification by flow cytometery or flourimetry. It is also possible to image the cells by fluorescence or confocal microscopy to observe changes in individual cells within a culture.

The Live/Dead assay has also been used in some studies (34). This assay involves treating the cells with calcein acetoxymethylester (AM) which diffuses into cells due to the lipophillic nature of AM. Once inside viable cells, cytoplasmic esterase enzymes will cleave the dye to release fluorescent calcein. In addition, the cells are treated with ethidium homodimer that can only enter cells if the cell membrane is compromised and hence the cell is dead. Once inside the cell the ethidium binds to DNA to generate a fluorescent signal which can be quantified or imaged alongside the calcein signal.

With any of the assays using fluorescence as an endpoint, the ability of the particles to interfere with fluorescence quantification must be taken into consideration, for instance, TiO_2 can reflect UV light, while carbon black absorbs light and can alter the background fluorescence.

THE LINK BETWEEN OXIDATIVE STRESS, CALCIUM SIGNALING, AND INFLAMMATION

Oxidative stress-responsive signaling pathways are known to exist and to control the expression of genes that are involved in the recruitment and activation of neutrophils and macrophages leading to inflammation (35,36).

Many studies using non-particle oxidant sources provide evidence that ROS and oxidative stress impact upon calcium signaling in cells. This is important since calcium is a key intracellular signaling molecule that controls a variety of cellular processes including exocytosis, the cytoskeleton and enzymes that regulate transcription factor activity (37). Concentrations of calcium within the cytoplasm are maintained at low levels, in the nM range by a combination of Ca^{2+} ATPase pumps in the plasma membrane that actively extrude calcium from the cell, Ca^{2+} ATPase pumps in the endoplasmic reticulum (ER) that actively sequester calcium, and calcium binding proteins; this allows relatively small changes in calcium to generate very effective signals (38). The nM intracellular calcium concentration is in contrast to the mM concentrations of the extracellular medium, resulting in a constant concentration gradient for the entry of calcium into the cell. Activation of a wide variety of cell signaling events can stimulate calcium release from the ER and entry via calcium channels in the plasma membrane, generating a very effective intracellular calcium signal that can be quickly recovered by the Ca^{2+} ATPase pumps. Oxidants, including ROS, appear to affect calcium signaling by oxidation of thiol groups in the Ca^{2+} ATPase pumps of the plasma membrane and ER (37,39), leading to decreased extrusion and sequestration. It has also been suggested that ROS can affect the activity and function of membrane calcium channels and calcium binding proteins (40). This would suggest, that during exposure to ROS the leak of calcium into the cytoplasm down its concentration gradient is not counteracted, allowing the intracellular calcium concentration to increase. There is also substantial evidence from the literature that calcium signaling can control inflammation, as has been demonstrated during sepsis (41). Taken together this evidence indicates that ROS modulate calcium signaling leading to the activation of an intracellular signaling cascade involving transcription factor activation and culminating in the production of pro-inflammatory cytokines. Brown et al. recently demonstrated that the lipophilic oxidant *tert*-butyl hydroperoxide (tBHP) activates calcium influx in macrophages and the production TNFα, a pro-inflammatory cytokine (42). Calcium signaling inhibitors, including verapamil a calcium channel blocker and BAPTA-AM a calcium chelator were able to prevent the tBHP induced TNFα production by macrophages in culture. This data indicates that calcium plays a key role in oxidant induced pro-inflammatory cytokine production by macrophages.

Transcription of the genes that regulate inflammation is controlled by transcription factors including nuclear factor kappa B (NFκB) and activator protein 1 (AP1), both of which are redox sensitive (43). In many cell types, the transcription factor NFκB takes the form of a heterodimer of the proteins p50 (NF-κB1) and p65 (RelA) (44), although this can vary to include other proteins. When this signaling pathway is inactive NFκB is retained within the cytoplasm by binding to an inhibitor subunit (IκB).

Activation of the enzyme IκB kinase results in phosphorylation of IκB and dissociation of the inactive IκB-NFκB complex (45), revealing a nuclear localization sequence on the NFκB subunits. Translocation of NFκB to the nucleus follows, where the transcription factor binds the specific promoter motifs of pro-inflammatory genes resulting in their transcription. Oxidants possess the ability to both enhance and inhibit NFκB mediated gene transcription, leading to confusion with respect to this pathway. For example, in HeLa cells, Byun *et al* have demonstrated that exposure to H_2O_2 leads to inhibition of acute IκB kinase mediated NFκB activation, while chronic exposure results in NFκB activation via an IκB kinase independent pathway (46).

In fact, the signaling pathways of calcium and NFκB are linked. Activation of intracellular calcium signaling initiates a number of signaling cascades, for example, calcium binds to calmodulin and activates Ca^{2+}/ calmodulin-dependent kinase (CaMK) enzymes. Brown demonstrated that inhibition of calmodulin by the antagonist W-7 was able to prevent tBHP induced NFκB activation and TNFα protein production by macrophages in culture (42).

In response to LPS stimulation, CaMK II enzymes have been shown to activate intracellular signaling via NFκB leading to TNFα production (47). Inhibition of CaMK in this study also increased IL10 production. IL10 is a cytokine associated with an anti-inflammatory effect (48), and so pathways other than calcium may be working to induce an effect that dampens or modulates the pro-inflammatory effects of stimuli such as LPS and may discriminate pro-inflammatory from non-inflammatory particles. In fact, calmodulin activity is altered by ROS through methionine oxidation (49), thereby linking calcium and ROS signaling at a molecule level. The oxidized calmodulin is still able to bind its target proteins, but once bound stabilizes them in an inactive state, preventing further activation, potentially providing a protective mechanism against oxidative induced inflammation (49).

Cyclic AMP (cAMP) also plays a key role in controling inflammation by promoting an anti-inflammatory signaling environment. A number of phosphodiesterase (PDE) enzymes are responsible for regulating the break down and hence concentration of cAMP in cells, relieving its anti-inflammatory effects and allowing pro-inflammatory cell signaling to dominate (50). The calcium/calmodulin complex stimulates the PDE1 family of enzymes (42,51) provided evidence that addition of PDE 1 and 4 inhibitors to macrophages in culture prevented oxidant (tBHP) induced TNFα production. The PDE inhibitors were also found to inhibit the tBHP induced calcium increase in the macrophage cell line, suggesting that cAMP may play a role in regulating calcium signaling in these cells.

Calcium plays an important role in apoptotic and necrotic cell death (52), it is therefore important in any study of calcium signaling to differentiate between cellular responses to stress, versus signaling related to cell death.

LINKING ROS, NANOPARTICLES AND INFLAMMATION

Carbon black nanoparticles (14 nm primary diameter) have been demonstrated to induce glutathione depletion, indicative of oxidative stress in a lung epithelial cell line (11). The same particles also induce a calcium influx in a human monocytic cell line (Monomac 6) (19) and in primary rat alveolar macrophages (53). This effect is not limited to carbon nanoparticles, polystyrene nanoparticles also have the ability to induce calcium signaling in macrophages (12). The ability of carbon black nanoparticles to induce an increase in cytosolic calcium concentration in the macrophages was inhibited by antioxidants, clearly showing a link between the ability of the particles to induce ROS and their ability to induce calcium signaling (19,53).

Brown et al. also investigated the impact of carbon black on NF-κB and AP-1 in human monocyte derived macrophages (10). Nanoparticulate carbon black (agglomerations made from 14nm primary particles) induced nuclear translocation of NF-κB subunits p50 and p65, as well as increasing DNA binding of AP-1, suggesting that these particles activated these transcription factors. In contrast, larger carbon black particles (260 nm diameter) had no impact on either of the transcription factors. Addition of lipophilic (trolox) and hydrophilic (Nacystelyn) antioxidants prevented the nuclear translocation of NF-κB and DNA binding of AP-1 supporting a role for ROS in the carbon nanoparticle mediated activation of these transcription factors. Furthermore, inhibition of calcium signaling via the inclusion of verapamil, BAPTA-AM and W7 also completely prevented the activation of these transcription factors. This was also reflected in the ability of the nanoparticles to induce production of TNFα protein, which was significantly inhibited by the antioxidants and calcium signaling antagonists (10). The pro-inflammatory effects of nanoparticle carbon black were not due to endotoxin contamination, since baking the particles at 180°C overnight did not alter the potency of the particles to induce the calcium signaling response.

A number of studies using environmentally relevant particulate samples, such as diesel exhaust particles (DEP), which consists of elemental and organic carbon nanoparticles, have also investigated their ability to induce inflammation via signaling pathways including oxidative stress. For example, DEP activates the antioxidant response element (ARE) (54), a nucleotide sequence found in the promoter of many genes. This sequence controls the expression of antioxidant defence pathways including the enzymes heme-oxygenase-1 (HO-1) and glutathione S-transferase (GST) (55,56). Treatment of macrophages with either organic or inorganic extracts of diesel exhaust particulates has been demonstrated to induce HO-1 and GST expression in via a transcription factor Nrf-2 (57). The ARE also contain a binding sequence for AP-1, a redox sensitive transcription factor, which (58) demonstrated lead to inhibition of ARE preventing the up-regulation of antioxidant defences. This therefore demonstrates that pro-oxidant treatments such as DEP have the ability to up-regulate antioxidant defence mechanisms via ARE, HO-1 and GST. The ability of engineered nanoparticles to activate such defence mechanisms could be advantageous but has not yet been investigated. The ability to activate such defence mechanisms may depend upon the chemical and physical nature of the particulate, the dose and the route of exposure.

Both PM_{10} and 14 nm carbon black particles can activate the expression of heat shock protein 70 (HSP70) by the A549 lung epithelial cell line (59). HSP70 is a molecular chaperone, the intracellular expression of which is up-regulated by ROS and during inflammation can protect the cell from damage (59). However, extracellular HSP70 secretion also increases in response to pathogenic particles such as asbestos (60), PM_{10} and nano-particle carbon black (59). Addition of antioxidants prevented the PM_{10} and carbon black stimulated increase in HSP70 secretion by epithelial cells, suggesting a role for ROS (59). The role of the released HSP70 is not fully understood, but extracellular HSP70 has been shown to activate macro-phages leading to calcium influx, NFκB activation and TNFα production (61) and to be elevated during cardiovascular disease (62).

HIGH-ASPECT RATIO NANOPARTICLES AND CELL SIGNALING

High-aspect ratio nanoparticles include carbon nanotubes (63), nanorods (64), nanofibers (65) and nanowires (64). Much attention has been given to the apparent similarity between such nanoparticles and asbestos due to their fiber-like dimensions and the known pathogenic effects of asbestos (66). However, it is worth noting that for asbestos fibers, the pathogenicity is highly dependent on the fiber length, with short fibers being less toxic than longer fibers (approximately greater than 10–20 µm) (67,68). Length is important because this determines the ability of macrophages (diameter 10–20 mm) to completely phagocytose the fibers, allowing their transport and clearance from the lung surface. Longer fibers result in frustrated phagocytosis, reduced clearance and hence the potential to persist in the body to cause disease. Many of the high aspect ratio nanoparticles currently engineered are only a few µm in length, and so if the same rules apply to these particles, their length would be unlikely to play a role in their toxicity. However, many of the applications requiring high aspect ratio nanoparticles enhance their characteristics positively if the particles are longer, and so industry and scientists are working hard to enhance the production processes to generate longer particles. Therefore in the future, length may become more of an issue.

The molecular and cellular mechanism of asbestos fiber induced inflammation and toxicity is well studied (69,70). With evidence that fibers generate reactive oxygen species (71) induce antioxidant depletion in lung lining fluid, indicative of oxidative stress (72) and lipid peroxidation in macrophages (73). In addition fibers have been shown to activate cell signaling pathways including mitogen activated protein kinase (74,75), calcium (76,77), activation of the NFκB and NF-IL6 like transcription factors (78,79) and the production of cytokines (80), with oxidative stress playing a key role in many of these pathways. Since asbestos is known to be carcinogenic, a number of studies have also looked at the ability of fibers to activate proto-oncogenes such as c-*fos* and c-*jun* (81), which are in fact the genes that code for the subunits of the transcription factor AP-1. Activation of c-*fos* and c-*jun* was subsequently found be directly related to the ability of asbestos to induce proliferation and transformation of primarily hamster tracheal epithelial cells (82).

To date, many of the studies investigating high aspect ratio nanoparticles have focused on carbon nanotubes, with some evidence in vivo that these particles are able to induce inflammation and granuloma formation in mice (83,84). However, these studies administered large doses of the particles via instillation, and so future studies will be of interest to verify whether inhalation exposure to more realistic doses confirm the potential for the pathogenicity of these particles. Our own in vitro studies, used multiwalled carbon nanotubes of 60 μm in length with few relatively defects, that formed large aggregates of long straight nanotubes with a small number of flakes. Administration of such nanotubes resulted in incomplete uptake by some macrophages, superoxide production and TNFα release. This was in contrast to shorter nanotubes, and curved nanotubes that were aggregated into "*balls*" or complex bundles, which were more easily ingested by macrophages and resulted in less superoxide and TNFα production (85). The relationship between the activity of these nanotubes in vitro and in vivo is yet to be investigated.

CONCLUSION

Much work is required to improve our understanding of the factors responsible for determining the potential for engineered nanoparticles to induce toxicity and disease. Studies using environmental particulate air pollution, model nanoparticles (published as ultrafine particles), and asbestos provide some useful guides as to techniques that can be employed to study nanoparticles, but also the endpoints that might be most relevant. However, it is also anticipated that due to the diversity of nanoparticle composition and form, that their may be special properties that have not yet been identified in relation to biological interaction. Some of these properties may enable improved biocompatibility, while others may be related to as yet disease. An improvement of understanding of such factors will enable a safer development of nanotechnology in the future. For the safe development of nanotechnology it is essential that we develop predictive models of toxicity as well as toxicity screening models, both in vitro and in vivo. With respect to other particle types, oxidative stress and inflammation, the in vitro effects are often indicative of the in vivo response. However, validation of such tests have not been rigorously conducted. Nanotechnology provides the incentive to invest in developing such tests. If the in vitro effects turn out to be representative of the in vivo response then these assays coupled with those measuring signaling responses may prove to be useful in vitro alternatives to predict toxicity and reduce the requirement for in vivo testing as well as telling us more about the mechanism of toxicity.

REFERENCES

1. Monteiro-Riviere NA. Dermal Effects of Nanomaterials. In:Monteiro-Riviere NA, Tran, CL, eds. Chapter 19, Nanotoxicology: Characterization, Dosing, and Health, Informa, 2007 (311–331).
2. Vicent MJ, Duncan R. Polymer conjugates: nanosized medicines for treating cancer. Trends Biotechnol 2006; 24(1):39–47.
3. Dudeck O, Bogusiewicz K, Pinkernelle J, et al. Local arterial infusion of superparamagnetic iron oxide particles in hepatocellular carcinoma: a feasibility and 3.0 T MRI study. Invest Radiol 2006; 41(6):527–35.
4. Albrecht C, Schins RP, Hohr D, et al. Inflammatory time course after quartz instillation: role of tumor necrosis factor-alpha and particle surface. Am J Respir Cell Mol Biol 2004; 31(3):292–301.
5. Warheit DB, Driscoll KE, Oberdoerster G, Walker C, Kuschner M, Hesterberg TW. Contemporary issues in fiber toxicology. Fundam Appl Toxicol 1995; 25(2):171–83.
6. Li XY, Gilmour PS, Donaldson K, MacNee W. In vivo and in vitro proinflammatory effects of particulate air pollution (PM10). Environ Health Perspect 1997; 105(Suppl 5):1279–83.
7. Kelley J. Cytokines of the lung. Am Rev Respir Dis 1990; 141(3):765–88.
8. Grayson MH, Korenblat PE. The emerging role of leukotriene modifiers in allergic rhinitis. Am J Respir Med 2003; 2(6):441–50.
9. Park GY, Christman JW. Involvement of cyclooxygenase-2 and prostaglandins in the molecular pathogenesis of inflammatory lung diseases. Am J Physiol Lung Cell Mol Physiol 2006; 290(5):L797–805.
10. Brown DM, Donaldson K, Borm PJ, et al. Calcium and reactive oxygen species-mediated activation of transcription factors and TNFa cytokine gene expression in macrophages exposed to ultrafine particles. Am J Physiol Lung Cell Mol Physiol 2004; 286:L344–53.

11. Stone V, Shaw J, Brown DM, MacNee W, Faux SP, Donaldson K. The role of oxidative stress in the prolonged inhibitory effect of ultrafine carbon black on epithelial cell function. Toxicol. In Vitro 1998; 12:649–59.

12. Brown DM, Wilson MR, MacNee W, Stone V, Donaldson K. Size-dependent proinflammatory effects of ultrafine polystyrene particles: a role for surface area and oxidative stress in the enhanced activity of ultrafines. Toxicol Appl Pharmacol 2001; 175(3):191–9.

13. Dick CA, Brown DM, Donaldson K, Stone V. The role of free radicals in the toxic and inflammatory effects of four different ultrafine particle types. Inhal Toxicol 2003; 15(1):39–52.

14. Zhou WP, Lewera A, Larsen R, Masel RI, Bagus PS, Wieckowski A. Size effects in electronic and catalytic properties of unsupported palladium nanoparticles in electrooxidation of formic acid. J Phys Chem B Condens Matter Mater Surf Interfaces Biophys 2006; 110(27):13393–8.

15. Stone V, Kinloch I, Clift M, et al. Nanoparticle toxicology and ecotoxicology; the role of oxidative stress. In: Nalwa HS, Zhao YL, eds. Nanotoxicology. American Scientific Publishers, 2007.

16. Borm P, Klaessig FC, Landry TD, et al. Research strategies for safety evaluation of nanomaterials, part V: role of dissolution in biological fate and effects of nanoscale particles. Toxicol Sci 2006; 90(1):23–32.

17. Oberdoerster G, Ferin J, Finkelstein J, Wade P, Corson N. Increased pulmonary toxicity of ultrafine particles? II. Lung lavage studies. J Aerosol Sci 1990; 21:384–7.

18. Hohr D, Steinfartz Y, Schins RP, et al. The surface area rather than the surface coating determines the acute inflammatory response after instillation of fine and ultrafine TiO2 in the rat. Int J Hyg Environ Health 2002; 205(3): 239–44.

19. Stone V, Tuinman M, Vamvakopoulos JE, et al. Increased calcium influx in a monocytic cell line on exposure to ultrafine carbon black. Eur Respir J 2000; 15(2):297–303.

20. Duffin R, Tran CL, Clouter A, et al. The importance of surface area and specific reactivity in the acute pulmonary inflammatory response to particles. Ann. Occup. Hyg 2002; 46(Suppl. 1):242–45.

21. Stoeger T, Reinhard C, Takenaka S, et al. Instillation of six different ultrafine carbon particles indicates a surface area threshold dose for acute lung inflammation in mice. Environ Health Perspect 2006; 114(3):328–33.

22. Edelstein AS. In: Edelstein AS, Cammarata RC, eds. Nanomaterials: Synthesis, Properties and Applications. Bristol, UK: Institute of Physics Publishing, 2002.

23. In: Poole CP, Owens. FJ, eds. Introduction to Nanomaterials. NJ, USA: Wiley and Sons, 2003.

24. Donaldson K, Stone V, Gilmour PS, Brown DM, MacNee W. Ultrafine particles: mechanisms of lung injury. Phil Trans R Soc Lond 2000; 358: 2741–49.

25. Seaton A, MacNee W, Donaldson K, Godden D. Particulate air pollution and acute health effects. Lancet 1995; 345(8943):176–8.

26. Donaldson K, Tran CL, Jimenez LA, et al. Combustion-derived nano-particles: A critical review of their toxicology following inhalation exposure. Particle Fiber Toxicol 2005; 2(10):1–14.

27. Oberdorster G, Ferin J, Lehnert BE. Correlation between particle size, in vivo particle persistence, and lung injury. Environ Health Perspect 1994; 102 (Suppl 5):173–9.

28. Li XY, Brown D, Smith S, MacNee W, Donaldson K. Short-term inflammatory responses following intratracheal instillation of fine and ultrafine carbon black in rats. Inhal Toxicol 1999; 11(8):709–31.

29. Thiele L, Diederichs JE, Reszka R, Merkle HP, Walter E. Competitive adsorption of serum proteins at microparticles affects phagocytosis by dendritic cells. Biomaterials 2003; 24(8):1409–18.

30. Zhang W-S. Nanoscale iron particles for environmental remediation: an overview. J Nanoparticle Res 2003; 5:323–32.

31. Yushin G, Hoffman EN, Barsoum MW, et al. Mesoporous carbide-derived carbon with porosity tuned for efficient adsorption of cytokines. Biomaterials 2006; 27(34):5755–62.

32. Mossman T. Rapid colorimetric assay for cellular growth and survival: Application to proliferation and cytotoxicity assays. J Immunol Meth 1983; 65:55–63.

33. Huang YC, Li Z, Harder SD, Soukup JM. Apoptotic and inflammatory effects induced by different particles in human alveolar macrophages. Inhal Toxicol 2004; 16(14):863–78.

34. Sayes CM, Liang F, Hudson JL, et al. Functionalization density dependence of single-walled carbon nanotubes cytotoxicity in vitro. Toxicol Lett 2006; 161(2):135–42.

35. Barnes PJ. Reactive oxygen species and airway inflammation. Free Radic Biol Med 1990; 9(3):235–43.

36. Rahman I. Oxidative stress, chromatin remodeling and gene transcription in inflammation and chronic lung diseases. J Biochem Mol Biol 2003; 36(1): 95–109.

37. Berridge MJ. Calcium signal transduction and cellular control mechanisms. Biochim Biophys Acta 2004; 1742(1–3):3–7.

38. Orrenius S, Burkitt MJ, Kass GE, Dypbukt JM, Nicotera P. Calcium ions and oxidative cell injury. Ann Neurol 1992; 32(Suppl):S33–42.

39. Barnes KA, Samson SE, Grover AK. Sarco/endoplasmic reticulum Ca^{2+}-pump isoform SERCA3a is more resistant to superoxide damage than SERCA2b. Mol Cell Biochem 2000; 203(1–2):17–21.

40. Kourie JI. Interaction of reactive oxygen species with ion transport mechanisms. Am J Physiol 1998; 275(1 Pt 1):C1–24.

41. Deaciuc IV, Spitzer JA. Calcium content in liver and heart and its intracellular distribution in liver during endotoxicosis and sepsis in rats. Cell Calcium 1987; 8(5):365–76.

42. Brown DM, Hutchison L, Donaldson K, MacKenzie J, Dick CAJ, Stone V. The effect of oxidative stress on macrophages and lung epithelial cells: the role of phosphodiesterases 1 and 4. Am J Physiol Lung Cell Mol Physiol 2006; Submitted.

43. Sen CK, Packer L. Antioxidant and redox regulation of gene transcription. FASEB J 1996; 10(7):709–20.

44. Blackwell TS, Christman JW. The role of nuclear factor-kappa B in cytokine gene regulation. Am J Respir Cell Mol Biol 1997; 17(1):3–9.

45. DiDonato JA, Hayakawa M, Rothwarf DM, Zandi E, Karin M. A cytokine-responsive Ikappa B kinase that activates the transcription factor NF-kappa B. Nature 1997; 388(6642):548–54.

46. Byun MS, Jeon KI, Choi JW, Shim JY, Jue DM. Dual effect of oxidative stress on NF-kappak B activation in HeLa cells. Exp Mol Med 2002; 34(5): 332–9.

47. Cuschieri J, Bulger E, Garcia I, Jelacic S, Maier RV. Calcium/calmodulin-dependent kinase II is required for platelet-activating factor priming. Shock 2005; 23(2):99–106.

48. Hamilton TA, Ohmori Y, Tebo J. Regulation of chemokine expression by antiinflammatory cytokines. Immunol Res 2002; 25(3):229–45.

49. Bigelow DJ, Squier TC. Redox modulation of cellular signalling and metabolism through reversible oxidation of methionine sensors in calcium regulatory proteins. Biochim Biophys Acta 2005; 1703(2):121–34.

50. Hoffmann R, Baillie GS, MacKenzie SJ, Yarwood SJ, Houslay MD. The MAP kinase ERK2 inhibits the cyclic AMP-specific phosphodiesterase HSPDE4D3 by phosphorylating it at Ser579. EMBO J 1999; 18(4): 893–903.

51. Yan C. Determination of Ca2+/calmodulin-stimulated phosphodiesterase activity in intact cells. Methods Mol Biol 2005; 307:85–92.

52. Orrenius S, Ankarcrona M, Nicotera P. Mechanisms of calcium-related cell death. Adv Neurol 1996; 71:137–49.

53. Stone V, Brown DM, Watt N, et al. Ultrafine particle-mediated activation of macrophages: Intracellular calcium signalling and oxidative stress. Inhal Toxicol 2000; 12(Suppl. 3):345–51.

54. Baulig A, Garlatti M, Bonvallot V, et al. Involvement of reactive oxygen species in the metabolic pathways triggered by diesel exhaust particles in human airway epithelial cells. Am J Physiol Lung Cell Mol Physiol 2003; 285(3):L671–9.

55. Ishii T, Itoh K, Ruiz E, et al. Role of Nrf2 in the regulation of CD36 and stress protein expression in murine macrophages: activation by oxidatively modified LDL and 4-hydroxynonenal. Circ Res 2004; 94(5):609–16.

56. Ishii T, Itoh K, Sato H, Bannai S. Oxidative stress-inducible proteins in macrophages. Free Radic Res 1999; 31(4):351–5.

57. Li N, Alam J, Venkatesan MI, et al. Nrf2 is a key transcription factor that regulates antioxidant defense in macrophages and epithelial cells: protecting against the proinflammatory and oxidizing effects of diesel exhaust chemicals. J Immunol 2004; 173(5):3467–81.

58. Ng D, Kokot N, Hiura T, Faris M, Saxon A, Nel A. Macrophage activation by polycyclic aromatic hydrocarbons: evidence for the involvement of stress-activated protein kinases, activator protein-1, and antioxidant response elements. J Immunol 1998; 161(2):942–51.

59. Ramage L, Guy K. Expression of C-reactive protein and heat-shock protein-70 in the lung epithelial cell line A549, in response to PM10 exposure. Inhal Toxicol 2004; 16(6–7):447–52.

60. Timblin CR, Janssen YM, Goldberg JL, Mossman BT. GRP78, HSP72/73, and cJun stress protein levels in lung epithelial cells exposed to asbestos, cadmium, or H2O2. Free Radic Biol Med 1998; 24(4):632–42.

61. Asea A, Kraeft SK, Kurt-Jones EA, et al. HSP70 stimulates cytokine production through a CD14-dependant pathway, demonstrating its dual role as a chaperone and cytokine. Nat Med 2000; 6(4):435–42.

62. Pockley AG, Georgiades A, Thulin T, de FU, Frostegard J. Serum heat shock protein 70 levels predict the development of atherosclerosis in subjects with established hypertension. Hypertension 2003; 42(3):235–8.

63. Donaldson K, Aitken R, Tran CL, et al. Carbon Nanotubes: A review of their properties in relation to pulmonary toxicology and workplace safety. Toxicol Sci 2006; Epub.

64. Chen J, Xiong Y, Yin Y, Xia Y. Pt Nanoparticles Surfactant-Directed Assembled into Colloidal Spheres and used as Substrates in Forming Pt Nanorods and Nanowires. Small 2006; 2(12):1399.

65. Melaiye A, Sun Z, Hindi K, et al. Silver(I)-imidazole cyclophane gem-diol complexes encapsulated by electrospun tecophilic nanofibers: formation of nano-silver particles and antimicrobial activity. J Am Chem Soc 2005; 127(7):2285–91.

66. Donaldson K, Aitken R, Tran L, et al. Carbon nanotubes: a review of their properties in relation to pulmonary toxicology and workplace safety. Toxicol Sci 2006; 92(1):5–22.

67. Donaldson K, Li XY, Dogra S, Miller BG, Brown GM. Asbestos-stimulated tumour necrosis factor release from alveolar macrophages depends on fiber length and opsonization. J Pathol 1992; 168(2):243–8.

68. Donaldson K, Brown GM, Brown DM, Bolton RE, Davis JM. Inflammation generating potential of long and short fiber amosite asbestos samples. Br J Ind Med 1989; 46(4):271–6.

69. Mossman BT, Faux S, Janssen Y et al. Cell signalling pathways elicited by asbestos. Environ Health Perspect 1997; 105(Suppl. 5):1121–5.

70. Mossman BT, Lounsbury KM, Reddy SP. Oxidants and signalling by mitogen-activated protein kinases in lung epithelium. Am J Respir Cell Mol Biol 2006; 34(6):666–9.

71. Gilmour PS, Brown DM, Beswick PH, MacNee W, Rahman I, Donaldson K. Free radical activity of industrial fibers: role of iron in oxidative stress and activation of transcription factors. Environ Health Perspect 1997; 105 (Suppl. 5):1313–17.

72. Brown DM, Beswick PH, Bell KS, Donaldson K. Depletion of glutathione and ascorbate in lung lining fluid by respirable fibers. Ann Occup Hyg 2000; 44(2):101–8.

73. Goodglick LA, Pietras LA, Kane AB. Evaluation of the causal relationship between crocidolite asbestos-induced lipid peroxidation and toxicity to macrophages. Am Rev Respir Dis 1989; 139(5):1265–73.

74. Swain WA, O'Byrne KJ, Faux SP. Activation of p38 MAP kinase by asbestos in rat mesothelial cells is mediated by oxidative stress. Am J Physiol Lung Cell Mol Physiol 2004; 286(4):L859–65.

75. Mossman BT, Lounsbury KM, Reddy SP. Oxidants and signalling by mitogen-activated protein kinases in lung epithelium. Am J Respir Cell Mol Biol 2006; 34(6):666–9.

76. Tuomala M, Hirvonen MR, Savolainen KM. Changes in free intracellular calcium and production of reactive oxygen metabolites in human leukocytes by soluble and particulate stimuli. Toxicology 1993; 80(1):71–82.

77. Faux SP, Michelangeli F, Levy LS. Calcium chelator Quin-2 prevents crocidolite-induced DNA strand breakage in human white blood cells. Mutat Res 1994; 311(2):209–15.

78. Janssen YM, Barchowsky A, Treadwell M, Driscoll KE, Mossman BT. Asbestos induces nuclear factor kappa B (NF-kappa B) DNA-binding activity and NF-kappa B-dependent gene expression in tracheal epithelial cells. Proc Natl Acad Sci USA 1995; 92(18):8458–62.

79. Simeonova PP, Luster MI. Asbestos induction of nuclear transcription factors and interleukin 8 gene regulation. Am J Respir Cell Mol Biol 1996; 15(6): 787–95.

80. Drumm K, Messner C, Kienast K. Reactive oxygen intermediate-release of fiber-exposed monocytes increases inflammatory cytokine-mRNA level, protein tyrosine kinase and NF-kappaB activity in co-cultured bronchial epithelial cells (BEAS-2B). Eur J Med Res 1999; 4(7):257–63.

81. Janssen YM, Heintz NH, Marsh JP, Borm PJ, Mossman BT. Induction of c-fos and c-jun proto-oncogenes in target cells of the lung and pleura by carcinogenic fibers. Am J Respir Cell Mol Biol 1994; 11(5):522–30.

82. Timblin CR, Janssen YW, Mossman BT. Transcriptional activation of the proto-oncogene c-jun by asbestos and H2O2 is directly related to increased proliferation and transformation of tracheal epithelial cells. Cancer Res 1995; 55(13):2723–6.

83. Shvedova AA, Kisin ER, Mercer R, et al. Unusual inflammatory and fibrogenic pulmonary responses to single-walled carbon nanotubes in mice. Am J Physiol Lung Cell Mol Physiol 2005; 289(5):L698–708.

84. Lam CW, James JT, McCluskey R, Hunter RL. Pulmonary toxicity of single-wall carbon nanotubes in mice 7 and 90 days after intratracheal instillation. Toxicol Sci 2004; 77(1):126–34.

85. Brown DM, Kinloch IA, Windle AH, et al. Inflammogenic Potential of Carbon Nanotubes and Nanofibers in vitro. Carbon 2006; Accepted.

22

Environmental Considerations: Occurrences, Fate, and Characterization of Nanoparticles in the Environment

Gregory V. Lowry

Department of Civil and Environmental Engineering, Carnegie Mellon University, Pittsburgh, Pennsylvania, U.S.A.

Mark R. Wiesner

Department of Civil and Environmental Engineering, Duke University, Durham, North Carolina, U.S.A.

INTRODUCTION

Nanomaterials are rapidly finding their way into an increasing number of industrial products (e.g., automotive, biomedical, environmental remediation, catalysis) (1–3) and in an ever-increasing number of consumer products (e.g., clothing, cosmetics, sun screens) (4–6). The ability to manipulate nanomaterials at the atomic scale offers the potential to greatly improve their properties and to improve the quality and efficiency of many processes. In the environmental technology industry alone, nanomaterials will enable new means of reducing the production of wastes, using resources more sparingly, cleaning-up industrial contamination, providing potable water, and improving the efficiency of energy production and use. However, as increasing quantities of nanomaterials are produced, used, and disposed of, it becomes increasing likely that these materials will find their way into the environment. The challenge of a growing nanomaterials industry is therefore to ensure that nanotechnologies evolve as tools that enable sustainability rather than environmental liabilities.

Recent investigations of the toxicity of nanomaterials have demonstrated or indicated the potential for these materials to be cytotoxic and bactericidal (7–9), or neurotoxic (10) and have demonstrated their ability to enter biological systems and food cycles (11). For nanomaterials to pose a risk they need to present both a hazard and a potential for exposure. Given the potential hazards based on work to date, responsible uses of manufactured nanomaterials in commercial products and environmental applications, as well as prudent management of the associated risks, require a better understanding of the sources, types and distributions of nanomaterials in the environment. In addition, the fate processes (e.g., aggregation and transformation) affecting the mobility and lifetime of nanomaterials in the environment must be understood, and methods to detect and characterize nanomaterials in the environment must be determined to properly assess the potential for exposure and the likely exposure concentrations to a wide variety of organisms. Here we discuss the types and distributions of nanomaterials in the environment, the fate of those materials, and methods to detect and characterize them in the environment.

TYPES AND DISTRIBUTIONS OF NANO-SCALE MATERIALS IN THE ENVIRONMENT

Nano-scale materials may come from either natural sources or they may be manufactured. It is important to understand the potential sources and types of nanomaterials that currently exist or that may be released into the environment. Based on the production and use of nanomaterials in high volume products such as tires or sunscreens it may also be possible to estimate the potential concentrations of these materials in the environment.

SOURCES AND TYPES OF NANO-SCALE MATERIALS

Naturally Occurring Nano-scale Materials

There are myriad nano-scale materials present in the environment of natural origin. Products from natural combustion (e.g., forest fires), bacterial products and exudates, mineral precipitates and aerosols are just a few examples. The fact that these materials may be either carbonaceous or mineral (12,13), and are produced by widely differing processes is indicative of the wide range of properties that these material may exhibit. Moreover, some manufactured nanomaterials may also have natural sources. The C_{60} fullerene is one such example of a newly discovered nanomaterial that has been detected in geologic deposits and may be readily produced by some combustion processes. Naturally formed atmospheric aerosols known as ultrafines are formed from sulfuric and nitric acids or from organic gases and are ubiquitous in the atmosphere. These ultrafine nanoparticles have a relatively short lifetime in the atmosphere, however, and typically coalesce into larger particles. Nanoparticulate iron oxides such as goethite and hematite are constituents of soils and sediments.

Their high surface area and sorption capacity for heavy metals and anionic contaminants make them important constituents controlling the fate and cycling of many environmental contaminants (14). Biological systems virtually bathe in nano-scale materials, and it is reasonable to assume that mechanisms have been developed at the cellular and organism levels to co-exist with many materials in the nanometer size range.

Manufactured and Other Anthropogenic Sources of Nanomaterials

The degree to which manufactured nanomaterials may present new challenges for environmental systems is unknown. In some cases, manufactured nano-materials such as quantum dots, and the heavy metals they contain, may differ from naturally occurring nano-scale materials in terms of composition. In other cases, composition may be similar but the structure maybe drastically different (e.g., carbon nanotubes vs. diamonds). Human activities may also lead to the unintentional production of nano-scale materials in air or water. Internal combustion engines, grinding operations, and welding are among the many possible sources of inadvertently produced nano-scale materials that may find their way into the environment. While the focus of most current risk assessment activities has been on quantifying exposure and hazards associated with manufactured nanomaterials alone, the relative exposures to other anthropogenic sources of nano-scale materials, exposure to naturally occurring materials, and the interactions between these materials, are pertinent factors in quantifying the risks posed by manufactured nanomaterials.

The production, use, and disposal of nanomaterials will inevitably lead to their appearance in air, water, soils, or organisms. The relevant format in which these materials are introduced to the environment must be considered. In some cases, manufactured nanomaterials may be used in products that suggest introduction to the environment as relatively distinct particles. For example, it may be reasonable to consider the transport and fate of individual nanoparticles introduced to the environment through the production and use of products such as silica nanoparticles used as solid lubricants; fullerene cage molecules added to cosmetics; metal and metal oxide nanoparticles injected for groundwater remediation; and protein-based nanomaterials in soaps, shampoos, and detergents. In other cases, manufactured nanomaterials may be incorporated into consumer products as composites or mixtures that may drastically alter the properties of the nanomaterials used in these products. For example, titania particles may be used in sunscreens and paints and fullerene nanotube composites may be used to make tires, tennis rackets, and video screens. The form of the released nanomaterials is unclear at this point and many questions remain, i.e., will they be individual particles or agglomerates of particles, will they be encapsulated in the matrix that they are used in or will the encapsulation wear away.

Accidental releases to the environment may come from point sources such as factories manufacturing the nanomaterials or facilities using nanomaterials in their products. As the use of products containing nano-materials increases, these products will inevitably be disposed of in landfills which may serve as point sources of nanomaterials into the environment. Nanomaterials used for targeted drug delivery will be excreted and sent to wastewater treatment plants which may ultimately serve as point sources of nanomaterials. With due diligence releases of nanomaterials from these point sources should be minimal provided adequate controls are in place, but accidental releases may be possible.

As with many environmental contaminants, nonpoint sources of nanomaterials are more difficult to control and will likely represent the majority of nanomaterial releases to the environment. Nonpoint sources such as wet deposition of particles from the atmosphere are possible. Attrition from products containing nanomaterials will be an ever increasing nonpoint source of nanomaterials in the environment as nanomaterials find their way into consumer products. Storm-water runoff from manufacturing sites or city roads and highways also represents a significant nonpoint source. As nanotubes find their way into automobile tires and brake pads, attrition from these products will constitute a large source of nanomaterials into the environment.

FATE OF NANOMATERIALS IN THE ENVIRONMENT

The risks posed by nanomaterials released to the environment are a function of their toxicity and the exposure. It is therefore important to understand the fate and transport of nanomaterials in the environment in order to assess exposure pathways and estimate the expected exposure concentrations. Once released into the environment, nanomaterials may be subjected to a variety of transport mechanisms and undergo physical and chemical changes as a result of biogeochemical weathering (Fig. 1). These changes can dram-atically affect their distribution and persistence in the environment, and their ability to be removed in conventional water treatment processes. Aggregation, biotic and abiotic transformations, and specific adsorption of constituents in natural waters (e.g., natural organic matter) can affect the mobility and fate of nanomaterials in the environment and in treatment systems. Each of these processes is discussed here.

TRANSFORMATIONS OF NANOMATERIALS IN THE ENVIRONMENT

Aggregation, sedimentation, and deposition of nanoparticles are likely to play an important role in determining the exposure and persistence of these materials in air or water. There is a large body of literature addressing

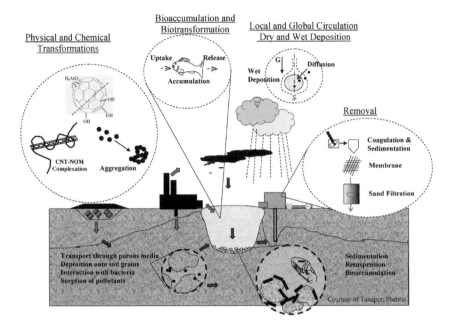

Figure 1 Nanomaterial releases to the environment may come from point sources such as factories where they are synthesized or used as feedstocks, or landfills where products containing nanomaterials are disposed. Releases from non-point sources include wet deposition from the atmosphere, stormwater runoff, or attrition from products containing nanomaterials. Physical and chemical transformations may include photochemical reactions in the atmosphere, aggregation, or uptake, accumulation, transformation, and degradation in organisms. Long-range atmospheric transport, as well as transport in saturated and unsaturated regions in the subsurface are possible. Nanomaterials in groundwater and surface water used for drinking water will be subject to conventional treatment methods such as flocculation/sedimentation and sand or membrane filtration. Human exposure to nanomaterials will most likely be during nanomaterial manufacturing, but inhalation of nanomaterials released to the atmosphere and ingestion of drinking water or food (e.g., fish) that have accumulated NPs can also be speculated. Bioaccumulation of hydrophobic nanomaterials such as nanotubes may occur in sediment benthic organisms and tropic transfer to higher organisms is also possible.

colloidal and aerosol transport and aggregation that is relevant to understanding nanoparticles. Similarly, mineral weathering has been studied extensively. However, the specifics of transformations of given classes of manufactured nanoparticles as the result of biogeochemical weathering are largely unknown. Other processes such as redox transformations, mediated abiotically or biologically, will undoubtedly alter the chemistry of particles in the environment, however, the rate of these processes and the ultimate effect on the chemistry and toxicity of engineered nanomaterials are not known.

Aggregation/Sedimentation

Although many nanomaterials are often produced as distinct particles with diameters of 1 to 100 nm, these particles are frequently observed to form much larger, colloidal aggregates in water. For example, 20-nm anatase particles form aggregates with a narrow size distribution and stable diameter of ~200 nm. Hydroxylated C_{60} (fullerols) forms aggregates ~20 nm in diameter in pure water. These aggregates may be highly stable, showing little propensity to aggregate over periods of several months or more (15). The basis for this stability is not clear. Fullernenes are reported to have high Hamaker constants that may favor aggregation. Hamaker constants of 50–60 × 10^{-20} J are reported for carbon nanotubes which is similar to that the value of 47 × 10^{-20} J reported for graphite. Hydrophobicity or chemical bonding between nanoparticles can also promote aggregation in water. These effects may be exacerbated in the presence of specifically adsorbing counterions that bridge between particles or for the smallest nanoparticles that tend to have high surface energies. Magnetic attractive forces between Fe^0 nanoparticles used for groundwater remediation cause them to aggregate more rapidly than less magnetic iron oxide nanoparticles with similar dimensions (16).

Nanoparticles can be stabilized in water due to electrostatic repulsive forces between particles, or due to steric repulsions. For electrostatically stabilized particles, when even small amounts of salts (e.g., Na^+, Mg^{2+}) are added, nanomaterials that are electrostatically stabilized will readily form large settleable aggregates, and this has been observed in the case of colloidal aggregates of fullerenes (15). Most natural fresh surface waters and groundwaters contain mM or greater levels of monovalent and divalent cations that may promote the aggregation of nanoparticles in water. Aggregation is particularly evident in biological fluids. For example, Degussa P25 TiO_2 nanoparticles (~30 nm) rapidly aggregate into micrometer sized aggregates in physiological buffer that is 155 mM ionic strength and contains high concentrations of divalent cations Ca^{2+} and Mg^{2+} (10). Some evidence suggests that the deleterious effects on bacterial populations are greater for smaller aggregates of C_{60} than for larger ones. Thus, aggregation of nanoparticles may mitigate both exposure and toxicity in some cases.

Agglomeration and aggregation can affect the fate of nanomaterials in natural water an in treatment systems. Nanoparticles and colloids up to a few microns in size that are present as individual particles do not readily settle from solution. This is because the particles are small enough such that the gravity force acting on these particles is small compared to the buoyancy force, and the drag force acting to keep them suspended in solution, or for very small particles the thermal diffusivity of the particles. Nanoparticles can agglomerate or aggregate into larger micron sized aggregates to a critical size where the gravity force dominates the other forces and allowing them to settle from suspension. Aggregates or agglomerates of nanoparticles that settle can be expected to accumulate in sediments of lakes or rivers in the absence of nanoparticle degradation. The tendency to aggregate will typically be higher as the ionic strength of a solution increases and as the concentration of divalent cations such as Ca^{2+} and Mg^{2+} increases. Thus nanoparticles will tend to aggregate more in seawater (high ionic strength) than in fresh water. Aggregation is a particularly vexing problem when evaluating the toxicology of nanoparticles as many of these studies require the use of physiological buffers of high ionic strength that promote aggregation and sedimentation of nanoparticles. Thus, it is difficult for example in vitro studies, to evaluate the effects of single nanoparticles and distinguish the effects of single nanoparticles versus nanoparticle aggregates. Since physiological buffers cause rapid aggregation the nanoparticles sediment from solution onto cells cultured on the bottom of the plates, even at low exposure concentrations of a 5 mg/L (10).

Redox Transformations

Reduction and oxidation (redox) reactions are very important in the environment. Redox reactions can occur abiotically or biologically, and are the basis of transformations of organic chemicals in the environment and of various precipitation and dissolution reactions that influence the sequestration and mobility of inorganic metals. Redox reactions can alter the surface chemistry of nanoparticles and thus can potentially affect the toxicity, mobility, and ultimate fate of these particles in the environment.

Abiotic transformations of nanoparticles may include the binding of water (17) which was shown to significantly modify the structure of ~3 nm ZnS nanoparticles, and chemical oxidation or reduction. For example, zero-valent iron nanoparticles used for groundwater remediation are designed for rapid oxidation upon release to the environment. The Fe^0 in the particles oxidizes to Fe-oxides while the target contaminant (e.g., trichloroethylene) is reduced (1,18). Upon oxidation the surface properties of the particle change; the pH of the isoelectric point of the particles is lowered from 6.5 to 4, the N_2-BET specific surface area of the particles decreases by ½, and the chemical composition of the particles changes from predominantly Fe^0 to Fe-oxides (magnetite and maghemite). The changes in the particle properties can affect their aggregation potential and mobility, and hence fate in the environment, and may also change their inherent toxicity since particle size, surface area, and surface charge can all affect the toxicity of a nanoparticle (10). The oxidation and hydroxylation of fullerenes has been demonstrated in laboratory studies (19). The hydroxylation of fullerenes in water was rapid at elevated temperatures (85–90°C), or under strongly basic conditions (aqueous sodium hydroxide solutions). Based on these studies, it is therefore unclear if these reactions would occur in the environment. More recently, Brant et al. (15) demonstrated that fullerenes, which are very hydrophobic will in fact become soluble after several months in aqueous solution (15), indicating that the hydroxylation reaction is probably slow but is occurring under typical environmental conditions. Despite the limited studies of redox transformations of engineered nanoparticles, most nanoparticles (either carbonaceous, metals, or metal oxides) should be expected to weather slowly over time analogous to chemical weathering of minerals in the environment. Future investigations of the environmental factors (e.g., pH, temperature, salinity) influencing the rates of weathering and the weathering products formed will provide insight into the significance of these transformations on the fate nanomaterials in the environment.

Biologically mediated oxidations and reductions of nanoparticles released to the environment may substantially increase the rate of weathering of these particles relative to chemical weathering, and may lead to different weathering products. Despite the limited amount of direct observations of biologically-mediated redox transformations of nano- particles, there is evidence that suggests these types of transformations will occur. For example, the oxidation of C_{60} fullerene in a cytochrome P450 (P450) chemical model system resulted in several oxidation products. Fenton's chemistry, as $H_2O_2 + Fe(II)$ generating hydroxyl radicals, was the model system (20). Cytochrome P450 as well as peroxidases and laccases should be able to catalyze these oxidations and thus is proof of principle that these types of oxidations are possible.

Adsorption of Organic Matter, Oxoanions, and Proteins

The surface chemistry of nanoparticles will ultimately control their fate in the environment and their toxicity. Engineered nanomaterials are typically highly surface active, either through specific chemical architecture or simply because they have such a high surface to volume ratio and hence high surface energy. Because of their exceptionally high surface reactivity, it is likely that they will tend to adsorb dissolved species present in natural waters. Species such as dissolved organic matter or heavy metal-containing cations and anions are common in the environment. Dissolved organic matter (DOM) (also referred to as aquatic humic substances) derived from algae or higher plants is ubiquitous in the environment. It is comprised of agglomerated organic molecules such as humic acids, fulvic acids, and polysaccharides. Typically they are highly functionalized (e.g., carboxylic acid groups, phenolic groups, etc.) and negatively charged at neutral pH, and may also contains groups (chromophores) that absorb sunlight. Absorption of light by chromophoric groups can lead to formation of short-lived reactive products such as singlet oxygen ($^1O_2$) (21) which may increase the toxicity of a particle, or transform it. The adsorption of DOM onto nanoparticles can alter the surface charge, and inhibit aggregation and attachment to surfaces thereby enhancing their mobility in the environment. For example, alginate which is a common polysaccharide found in natural waters was shown to readily adsorb to hematite (Fe_3O_4) nanoparticles, lowering its surface charge, and significantly enhanced the aggregation kinetics of hematite particles relative to unmodified particles (22). The increase in aggregation was attributed to the increase in the collision radii of the particles due to the alginate coating.

The adsorption of oxoanions (e.g., AsO_4^{3-} or CrO_4^{2-}) to nanoparticles is also common. For example, Fe^0 or Fe-oxide nanoparticles can be used to remove AsO_4^{3-} from water (23). The AsO_4^{3-} oxoanion strongly adsorbs to the Fe-oxide surfaces and is sequestered. Hexavalent chromium (CrO_4^{2-}), a common environmental pollutant, is reduced and strongly adsorbs to the Fe-oxide surface of a Fe^0/Fe-oxide core shell particle (24). The sequestration of potentially toxic heavy metals such as As(III)/As(IV) and Cr(VI) implies that nanomaterials have the potential to enhance transport of the pollutants in the environment (assuming the nanoparticles ware mobile), enhance the uptake of these toxic metals into biological organisms, or to affect the toxicity of nanoparticles that are taken up by organisms. Protein adsorption onto carbon nanotubes (25) and onto gold nanoparticles (26) has been demonstrated, and strong protein binding onto metal-oxides (27) is well documented so adsorption onto metal oxide nanoparticles is likely. As with adsorbed oxoanions, adsorbed proteins can affect the mobility and fate of nanoparticles in the environment as well as their toxicological properties.

MOBILITY AND FATE OF NANOMATERIALS IN THE ENVIRONMENT

A higher mobility of nanomaterials in the environment implies a greater potential for exposure as nanomaterials are dispersed over greater distances and their effective persistence in the environment increases. One phenomenon that may reduce nanomaterial exposure is a propensity to attach to surfaces (deposition) as well as to each other (aggregation). Aggregation (particle-particle attachment) and deposition (particle-media grain attachment) are related phenomena and the magnitude of these two phenomena depend on similar geochemical parameters. For example, particles that are water soluble and highly mobile in the atmosphere or in surface water may be less mobile in porous media such as ground water aquifers if the particles readily attach to mineral surfaces. Particle attachment is common, particularly for highly surface active particles. Controls such as filters used in potable water treatment or respirators rely on particle attachment to retain nanoparticles. Intuitively, the assumption is often made that nanoparticles will be more mobile in porous media due to their small size. However, all other factors being equal (ionic strength and composition, filter media grain size, and hydrodynamics), smaller particles should be less mobile due to their relatively large diffusivity that produces more frequent contacts with the surfaces of the porous media. Similar considerations lead to a high deposition rate of ultrafine air-borne particles in the lungs. We now discuss the factors controlling deposition and methods currently used to control the rate and extent of deposition for certain types of nano-materials. The environmental compartments where we would expect to find nanomaterials released to the environment is postulated based on the known common properties of many nanomaterials.

Deposition

Particle deposition and aggregation are closely-related phenomena and factors that favor particle removal by deposition, frequently tend to favor particle aggregation and subsequent removal by settling or deposition. Both deposition and aggregation can be described as a two-step process of particle transport followed by attachment. For example, particle deposition in an aquifer can be described as a sequence of particle transport to the immobile surface or aquifer material "collector" followed by attachment to the collector (28). Particles are transported to the collector surface when fluid streamlines, as described for example by the Happel model (29), pass sufficiently close to the collector surface such that particles make contact with the surface. Particles entrained by the fluid flow may also contact collectors if they cross streamlines within a critical region due to the effects of gravity or Brownian diffusion. Transport of engineered nanoparticles and nano-scale particles will be dominated by Brownian diffusion. Particle trajectory calculations have been combined with the analytical solution for Brownian transport to yield closed-form solutions for the transport of particles to the surface of spherical collectors (30,31) expressed as the theoretical single collector efficiency, η_0. Data for particle deposition have been found to be adequately represented by this model for particle transport in the absence of a repulsive energy barrier when near-field conditions therefore favor particle attachment (32–36). However, when particle attachment is not favorable, only a fraction of the collisions with the collector surface will result in particle deposition.

Forces such as attractive London-van der Waals and attractive or repulsive electrical double-layer forces (e.g., the classic Derjaguin, Landau, Verwey and Overbeek or DLVO forces, (37,38) are known to influence particle attachment. The ratio of the rate of particle deposition on a collector to the rate of collisions with that collector is referred to as the attachment efficiency factor, α. Attachment efficiency is a function of near-field phenomena that, in addition to those accounted for in the classical form of the DLVO model, may include steric interactions, hydration forces, and solvation forces. When the sum of all near-field phenomena is attractive, particle attachment is favorable and $\alpha \geq 1$. The value of α is unity when there are no near-field barriers to particle deposition and is less than unity when energy barriers are present and attachment is not favored. Particle transport and attachment can be represented as the product of the collector efficiency and the attachment efficiency:

$$\eta_r = \alpha\eta_0$$

The attachment efficiency may be treated as an empirical parameter that captures all aspects of particle deposition not described by the more extensively validated particle transport models. Particle transport to the vicinity of the collector surface is described by expressions that consider forces on particles in a fluid flowing past collectors where the fluid is treated as a continuum. These expressions for particle transport to collectors account for factors such as flow rate, fluid viscosity, particle density, and collector geometry. The empirically determined attachment efficiency will vary as a function of factors such as ionic strength, pH, the nature of ions in the solution, the nature of the nanoparticles and the characteristics of the collector surfaces.

A mass balance of particles over a differential volume of porous medium can be integrated over distance within a homogenous medium to yield an expression for the attachment efficiency factor, α, as a function of the observed removals, the characteristics of the porous medium and the flow:

$$\alpha = -\frac{4r_c}{3(1-\varepsilon)\eta_0 L}\ln(C/C_{in})$$

where r_C is the radius of a collector (assumed to be spherical) in the porous medium, L is the length of the porous medium, C and C_{in} are respectively the particle concentrations present at distance L (effluent) and the influent concentration at $L = 0$, and η_0 is the single collector efficiency which describes the particle transport to an individual collector and can be calculated as function of the Darcy velocity, porous medium grain size, porosity and temperature among other variables. Using experimental C/C_{in} values (fraction of influent particles remaining) and theoretical η_o values, experimental values for α can be calculated for a given particle suspension. Such experimental values can be used to express nanoparticle stability in these aqueous systems and calculate a mobility index useful for comparing the relative mobilities of different nanoparticle types. Deposition and aggregation differ in the sense that particle deposition involves attachment to an immobile site (e.g., aquifer grain), while particle aggregation involves attachment between mobile sites (nanoparticles).

Initial work on nanomaterial mobility in formations resembling groundwater aquifers or sand filters has shown that while one type of nanomaterial may be very mobile, a second may stay put (3,39). Differences in nanoparticle mobility in porous media appear to be a function of both surface chemistry and particle size and the size of the aggregates that are formed. Under the conditions investigated to date, low ionic strength and formations of relatively high hydraulic conductivity, the mobility of most nanoparticles in the porous media is limited, with log α values ranging from 10^{-2} to 10^{-4}. While these results underscore the need to avoid general-izations of nanoparticle risks based on differences in potential exposure, they also suggest that even the most mobile of the nanomaterials evaluated to date are likely to be removed in filters during water treatment. Con-ditions such as high ionic strength and the presence of divalent ions in even small quantities tend to increase retention of nanoparticles by porous media (15). Since ground water aquifers and surface waters typically have ionic strengths in excess of 10^{-4} M and frequently have significant (0.5–1.0 mM) concentrations of calcium or magnesium, conditions should tend to favor nanomaterial deposition and limited mobility. There are possible exceptions such as transport in fractured bedrock which can be more like channel flow than flow in porous media, but in general nanomaterial mobility in porous media such as groundwater aquifers should be limited (40).

Coatings to Minimize Deposition

The surface properties of nanoparticles largely control their aggregation and deposition characteristics. In general, particles with minimal aggregation and deposition onto surfaces will be more mobile in the environment than particles that do aggregate and deposit. Many novel nanoparticles with unique reactivity and functions have been synthesized and characterized, however engineering applications employing these novel nanomaterials have lagged their development because they are difficult to process. For example, they may not be readily dispersible in either aqueous or organic solvents or otherwise rapidly aggregate in suspension. To combat the ill behavior of nanoparticles in solution and to improve their functionality, the surfaces of most particles are functionalized, e.g., functionalized particles can provide the targeted delivery of drugs to specific receptors (41) or form stable colloidal suspensions in both organic and aqueous solvents (42). There are as many novel surface coatings as there are nanoparticles. For example, peptides have been used to label quantum dots used for imaging tumors (43).

The use of low molecular weight surfactants or high molecular weight polymeric coatings to protect nanoparticles from rapid flocculation is a well established technique (2,44). Sodium dodecylbenzene sulfonate or alkyl polyglucosides are commonly used surfactants. Uncharged polymers such as polyethylene glycols or carboxymethyl cellulose and charged polyelectrolytes such as polystyrene sulfonate or poly(aspartic acid) are also common stabilizers for nanoparticles. Both natural and synthetic varieties of each type of stabilizer are available. For example, polystyrene sulfonate is a synthetic polyelectrolyte where as poly(aspartic acid) is a biopolymer. In general, high molecular weight polymers (synthetic or natural) provide steric repulsions. Polyelectrolytes are large polymers containing charged functional groups (anionic or cationic) and provide both steric and electrostatic (electrosteric) repulsions. Surfactants can provide electrostatic repulsive or attractive forces (depending on their charge), but are less effective than polymers or polyelectrolytes because their small size is unsuitable for steric repulsions. The coatings provide strong electrostatic and/or electrosteric repulsions that dominate over attractive van der Waals forces between particles or between particles and collector grains and thereby limit both aggregation and deposition in the environment (45). Coatings may also affect the toxicity of nanoparticles, either by inhibiting contact between the particles and the organisms or by altering the surface chemistry, thereby affecting the mode of toxicity. The ability to reduce or eliminate the toxicity of a nanoparticle through surface coatings is an attractive proposition worthy of future study.

There are many open questions regarding the ability of surface coatings to alter the fate and toxicity of nanoparticles in the environment. Evidence suggests that surface coatings affect nanoparticle toxicity found that gold nanoparticles with positively charged side chains were toxic to *Escherichia coli*, but negatively charged particles were not (46), however the mechanisms by which toxicity reduction occurs are uncertain. The fate of the surface coatings upon release to the environment is uncertain. Surfactant adsorption is readily reversible and would be expected to desorb upon release to the environment where free-surfactant in absent, whereas adsorption for high molecular weight polymers is essentially an irreversible process (47,48). Despite this, biodegradation of polymeric coatings may occur, especially for biopolymers such as poly(aspartic acid). Since the fate of nanomaterials in the environment is highly dependent on their surface coatings, it is imperative to understand the fate of these coatings as well as the fate of the particles.

Environmental Compartments as Sinks (Water, Air, Soil/Sediment)

Knowing the sources, sinks, and transformations of nanoparticles will help to identify the most likely environmental compartments for nanomaterials released in the environment. Such knowledge will help direct efforts in determining the relevant exposure concentrations for organisms and humans, can be used to design nanomaterials that are benign in the environment, and used to implement regulatory policies based on scientific knowledge rather than ignorance.

The environment is a complex and dynamic system that is difficult if not impossible to model accurately. As such, it is typically represented by a simple box model with partitioning between water, air, and solids (sediment and/or soil) compartments. An understanding of the mass transport between the compartments allows for more complex kinetic models to be developed, however in the absence of kinetic data we typically rely on simple equilibrium partitioning modeling between the compartments. Based on our current understanding of the science and technology of nanoparticles, their transport and transformation in the environment, and some preliminary information on the interaction of nanoparticles with biota we can infer that most nanoparticles will have low mobility in porous media and that aggregates or agglomerates of nanoparticles will sediment from solution and are likely to be found in soils and sediments rather than remaining in suspension or in the atmosphere. Thus, the highest concentrations of nanomaterials in the environment should be at or near their source for those released into water of soils.

The potential biotransformation of nanomaterials has not been widely studied, however some initial data (e.g., nanotube interactions with benthic copepods) has been collected (11). The persistence of nanomaterials in the environment will depend highly on their ability to be biotransformed as biotransformation will probably turn out to be an important destructive and/or transformation mechanism. For nanomaterials that are hydrophobic (e.g., nanotubes or fullerenes) and not readily biodegradable, their fate upon release into the environment may end up being analogous to polychlorinated biphenyls and other types of persistent organic pollutants (POPs). POPs are highly persistent and tend to be associated with particles in the environment. More research is needed to determine the ultimate fate of nanomaterials in the environment.

TREATMENT TECHNOLOGIES FOR NANOMATERIALS

If nanoparticles are found to have negative consequences (e.g., toxicity) and must themselves be removed from water drinking water, it is important to determine their potential for removal by standard processes used in water treatment systems such as coagulation and sedimentation or sand filters and membranes. The fate of nanoparticles in these treatment systems and the potential for these treatment systems to be effective is discusses here.

Flocculation/Sedimentation

Surface water and groundwater used for drinking water supply contains fine particles such as clays and silts, natural organic matter, oxides of iron and manganese, and microorganisms. Flocculation is a water treatment processes used to combine or coagulate these small particles into larger particles, which settle (sediment) from solution in a clarifier and are removed. Alum and iron salts or synthetic organic polymers (used alone or in combination with metal salts) are generally used to promote coagulation. Alum and iron increase the ionic strength and precipitate a high concentration of particles of $Al(OH)_3$ or $Fe(OH)_3$ that agglomerate with other particles (e.g., clay particles or engineered nanoparticles) and then settle from solution. Nanoparticles that are most susceptible to aggregation and deposition should be the most effectively removed using these standard treatment technologies designed to remove naturally occurring fine particles.

Filtration

Many water treatment facilities use filtration to remove all particles from the water. Filtration is used alone or after coagulation/sedimentation to remove nonsettlable particles. The most common type of filter used granular media such as anthracite coal underlain by sand. Sand filters rely on particle deposition to remove particles, so the same properties (e.g., ionic strength and composition) that affect the mobility of nanomaterials through aquifers also affects the ability of granular media filters to remove particles. Engineered nanomaterials evaluated thus far (e.g., nanotubes, TiO_2, nanoscale Fe^0 and Fe-oxides) have aggregation and deposition characteristics that suggest these materials will be readily removed during aggregation and sedimentation (3,15,16,39). Thus, there is not yet evidence to support the scenario of a new nano-particulate contaminant that our current water treatment infrastructure is ill-suited to handle.

CHARACTERIZING AND DETECTING NANOMATERIALS IN THE ENVIRONMENT

The increased use of engineered nanomaterials will ultimately lead to their appearance in soil, sediment, and waterways. Methods to detect and characterize nanomaterials present in environmental matrices such as soil or sediment are limited. It is difficult enough to fully characterize the chemical composition and morphology of relatively pure suspensions of nanomaterials in the laboratory, let alone in a complex matrix containing a mixture of engineered as well as natural nanomaterials. Relevant properties include particle size or size distribution, shape (e.g., aspect ration), structure, chemical composition, surface charge (zeta potential), surface area, and the presence/absence and characteristics of surface coatings on the particles. There are a variety of techniques available to measure these parameters, but no single technique can be employed to determine all of these properties so reliable characterization requires the use of multiple techniques (49). The common tools used to measure each of these parameters are provided in Table 1 along with the benefits and primary shortcomings and difficulties applying them to nanomaterials present in the environment.

Challenges in Characterizing Nanomaterials in "Natural" Systems

Characterizing relatively pure dispersions of nanomaterials under laboratory conditions using the tools in Table 1 is common. Many of the tools are straightforward and easy to apply, although the equipment needed is costly (e.g., TEM's range from $250,000 to several million U.S. dollars). There are several challenges to characterizing nanomaterials in the environment which is not a well controlled system. First, the concentration of nanomaterials in the environment will typically be low. Further, engineered nanomaterials which will likely be present at a lower concentration than a variety of natural nanomaterials. Methods to separate nanomaterials from their matrix such as a water sample are unsophisticated (e.g., centrifugation) and there are no reliable methods to distinguish between natural nanomaterials and engineered nanomaterials in a sample unless those nanomaterials should have specific features built into them to make them stand out, e.g., fluorescent tags or specific rare earth metals. Separating nanomaterials from soils and sediments is even more challenging. Near-term research is needed to identify methods to isolate and characterize nanomaterials in natural samples. Many of the characterization techniques require that the sample be dried and analyzed under vacuum (e.g., TEM, N_2-BET) which can alter the sample from its form in solution. At the very least, aggregation of the samples will occur upon drying and information regarding particle size or particle (or aggregate) size distribution may contain artifacts. These measurements can also be strongly biased due to sampling inhomogeneity. Surface area measurements of aggregated samples may be biased due to mesopore structures formed during agglomeration. Complete and reliable characterization of nanomaterials will require the application and multiple techniques and a good understanding of the biases resulting from sampling artifacts.

Table 1 Characterization Methods for Nanoparticles

Method	Advantages	Disadvantages
Particle Size and Size Distribution		
Dynamic Light Scattering (DLS)	Measures particle size distribution (PSD) in situ. Applicable to a size range of 0.6 nm to 6 μm.	Polydisperse samples make data interpretation difficult. Cannot distinguish particle types and provides no information on shape. Measured sizes can be concentration and time dependent. No chemical information.
Atomic Force Microscopy (AFM)	Determines particle size and shape.	No chemical information. Particles must be adhered to a surface.
Transmission Electron Microscopy (TEM)	Direct imaging of particle size and shape. Can provide chemical information with proper detectors.	Requires dried samples, which aggregates samples and introduces other sample preparation artifacts.
Differential Mobility Analyzer	Measure particles in gas phase. Simple and inexpensive.	Requires low particle concentrations ($< 10^8$ particles/m^3). Provides no chemical or structure information.
Shape		
TEM	Direct image of particle shape.	Requires dried samples, which aggregates samples and introduces other artifacts.
AFM	Indirect image of shape.	
Chemical Composition		
TEM with Energy Dispersive X-Ray Detection (EDS)	Provides chemical information at specific locations on a particle.	Only semi-quantitative in most cases.
ICP-MS or AES	Provides chemical composition for a particle.	Bulk measurement and reveals no information on structure. Destructive technique.
XPS	Provides surface chemical composition and oxidation state.	Vacuum technique and usually semi quantitative. No shape or size information.

(Continued)

Table 1 Characterization Methods for Nanoparticles (*Continued*)

Method	Advantages	Disadvantages
XRD	Determines crystalline phases present. Can be an indirect measure of crystal size in a particle.	Low sensitivity. Overlapping peaks in a complex sample make positive identification difficult.
Surface Charge Electrophoretic Mobility	Allows calculation of surface (zeta) potential.	Zeta potential value depends on model applied to convert EM to zeta potential. No size or shape information or chemical information.
Specific Surface Area N_2-BET	Easy measurement that provides a specific surface area accessible to N_2.	No size or shape information or chemical information. Requires dried samples which may not be representative of the surface area in situ in water or biological systems.

Abbreviation: TK. AES, atomic emission spectrometry; ICP-MS, inductively coupled plasma mass spectrometry; XPS, X-ray photo electron spectroscopy; XRD, X-ray diffraction.

REFERENCES

1. Liu YQ, Lowry GV. Effect of particle age (Fe-o content) and solution pH on NZVI reactivity: H-2 evolution and TCE dechlorination. Environ Sci Technol 2006; 40(19):6085–90.
2. Saleh N, Phenrat T, Sirk K, et al. Adsorbed triblock copolymers deliver reactive iron nanoparticles to the oil/water interface. Nano Lett 2005; 5(12): 2489–94.
3. Saleh N, Sirk K, Liu Y, et al. Surface modifications enhance nanoiron transport and DNAPL targeting in saturated porous media. Environ Eng Sci 2007; 24(1):45–57.
4. Biswas P, Wu CY. Critical review: nanoparticles and the environment. J Air Waste Manage Assoc 2005; 55(6):708–46.
5. Maynard AD, Aitken RJ, Butz T, et al. Safe handling of nanotechnology. Nature 2006; 444(7117):267–9.
6. Maynard AD, Michelson E. The Nanotechnology Consumer Products Inventory. Washington D.C.; Woodrow Wilson International Center for Scholars, 2006:1–8.
7. Auffan M, Decome L, Rose J, et al. In vitro interactions between DMSA-coated maghemite nanoparticles and human fibroblasts: a physicochemical and cyto-genotoxical study. Environ Sci Technol 2006; 40(14):4367–73.

8. Thill A, Zeyons O, Spalla O, et al. Cytotoxicity of CeO2 nanoparticles for Escherichia coli. Physico-chemical insight of the cytotoxicity mechanism. Environ Sci Technol 2006; 40(19):6151–6.

9. Wiesner MR, Lowry GV, Alvarez P, et al. Progress and research needs towards assessing the risks of manufactured nanomaterials. Environ Sci Technol 2006; 40(14):4336–45.

10. Long T, Saleh N, Tilton R, et al. Titanium dioxide (P25) produces oxidative stress in immortalized brain microglia (BV2): implication of nanoparticle neurotoxicity. Environ Sci Technol 2006; 40(14):4346–52.

11. Templeton RC, Ferguson PL, Washburn KM, et al. Life-cycle effects of single-walled carbon nanotubes (SWNTs) on an Estuarine Meiobenthic Copepod. Environ Sci Technol 2006; 40(23):7387–93.

12. Banfield JF, Zhang HZ. Nanoparticles in the environment, In: Nanoparticles and the Environment. 2001:1–58.

13. Poulton SW, Raiswell R. Chemical and physical characteristics of iron oxides in riverine and glacial meltwater sediments. Chem Geol 2005; 218(3–4):203–21.

14. Waychunas GA, Kim CS, Banfield JF. Nanoparticulate iron oxide minerals in soils and sediments: unique properties and contaminant scavenging mechanisms. J Nanoparticle Res 2005; 7(4–5):409–33.

15. Brant J, Lecoanet H, Wiesner MR. Aggregation and deposition characteristics of fullerene nanoparticles in aqueous systems. J Nanoparticle Res 2005; 7(4–5):545–53.

16. Phenrat T, Saleh N, Sirk K, et al. Aggregation and sedimentation of aqueous nanoiron dispersions. Environ Sci Technol 2007; 41(1):284–290.

17. Zhang HZ, Gilbert B, Huang F, et al. Water-driven structure transformation in nanoparticles at room temperature. Nature 2003; 424(6952):1025–9.

18. Liu YQ, Majetich SA, Tilton RD, et al., TCE dechlorination rates, pathways, and efficiency of nanoscale iron particles with different properties. Environ Sci Technol 2005; 39(5):1338–45.

19. Chiang LY, Wang LY, Swirczewski JW, et al. Efficient synthesis of polyhydroxylated fullerene derivatives via hydrolysis of polycyclosulfated precursors. J Organ Chem 1994; 59(14):3960–8.

20. Hamano T, Mashino T, Hirobe M. Oxidation of (60)fullerene by cytochrome-P450 chemical-models. J Chem Soc—Chem Commun 1995; 15:1537–8.

21. Goldstone JV, Del Vecchio R, Blough NV, et al. A multicomponent model of chromophoric dissolved organic matter photobleaching. Photochem Photobiol 2004; 80(1):52–60.

22. Chen KL, Mylon SE, Elimelech M. Aggregation kinetics of alginate-coated hematite nanoparticles in monovalent and divalent electrolytes. Environ Sci Technol 2006; 40(5):1516–23.

23. Kanel SR, Manning B, Charlet L, et al, Removal of arsenic(III) from groundwater by nanoscale zero-valent iron. Environ Sci Technol 2005; 39(5):1291–8.

24. Cao HS, Zhang WX. Stabilization of chromium ore processing residue (COPR) with nanoscale iron particles. J Hazardous Mater 2006; 132(2–3): 213–19.

25. Bradley K, Briman M, Star A, et al. Charge transfer from adsorbed proteins. Nano Lett 2004; 4(2):253–6.

26. Chithrani BD, Ghazani AA, Chan WCW. Determining the size and shape dependence of gold nanoparticle uptake into mammalian cells. Nano Lett 2006; 6(4):662–8.

27. Kenausis GL, Voros J, Elbert DL, et al. Poly(L-lysine)-g-poly(ethylene glycol) layers on metal oxide surfaces: Attachment mechanism and effects of polymer architecture on resistance to protein adsorption. J Phys Chem B 2000; 104(14): 3298–309.

28. Omelia CR. Aquasols—the behavior of small particles in aquatic systems. Environ Sci Technol 1980; 14(9):1052–60.

29. Happel J, Viscous flow in multiparticle systems: slow motion of fluids relative to beds of spherical particles. A.I.Ch.E J 1958; 4(2):197–201.

30. Rajagopalan R.Tien C.Trajectory analysis of deep-bed filtration with sphere-in-cell porous-media model. Aiche J 1976; 22(3):523–33.

31. Tufenkji N, Elimelech M. Correlation equation for predicting single-collector efficiency in physicochemical filtration in saturated porous media. Environ Sci Technol 2004; 38(2):529–36.

32. Adamczyk Z. Particle deposition from flowing suspensions. Colloids Surfaces 1989; 39(1–3):1–37.

33. Elimelech M. Effect of particle-size on the kinetics of particle deposition under attractive double-layer interactions. J Colloid Interface Sci 1994; 164(1):190–9.

34. Elimelech M, Omelia CR. Kinetics of deposition of colloidal particles in porous-media. Environ Sci Technol 1990; 24(10):1528–36.

35. Veerapaneni S, Wiesner MR. Role of suspension polydispersivity in granular media filtration. J Environ Eng 1993; 119(1):172–90.

36. Yao KM, Habibian MM, Omelia CR. Water and waste water filtration—concepts and applications. Environ Sci Technol 1971; 5(11):1105–1112.

37. Derjaguin BV, Landau LD. Theory of the stability of strongly charged lyophobic sols and of the adhesion of strongly charged particles in solutions of electrolytes. Acta Physicochim URSS 1941; 14:733–62.

38. Verwey EJW, Overbeek JTG. Theory of the Stability of Lyophobic Colloids. Amsterdam: Elsevier, 1948.

39. Lecoanet HF, Bottero JY, Wiesner MR, Laboratory assessment of the mobility of nanomaterials in porous media. Environ Sci Technol 2004; 38(19): 5164–9.

40. Schrick B, Hydutsky BW, Blough JL, et al. Delivery vehicles for zerovalent metal nanoparticles in soil and groundwater. Chem Mater 2004; 16(11): 2187–93.

41. Chen CC, Dormidontova EE. Architectural and structural optimization of the protective polymer layer for enhanced targeting. Langmuir 2005; 21(12): 5605–15.

42. Duan HW, Kuang M, Wang DY, et al. Colloidally stable amphibious nanocrystals derived from poly (2-(dimethylamino)ethyl) methaerylatel capping. Angewandte Chemie—Int Edn 2005; 44(11):1717–20.

43. Cai WB, Shin DW, Chen K, et al. Peptide-labeled near-infrared quantum dots for imaging tumor vasculature in living subjects. Nano Lett 2006; 6(4):669–76.

44. Rosen MJ. Surfactants and Interfacial Phenomena. 3rd ed. New York: Wiley-Interscience, 2002.

45. Romet-Lemonne G, Daillant J, Guenoun P, et al. Thickness and density profiles of polyelectrolyte brushes: dependence on grafting density and salt concentration. Phys Rev Lett 2004; 93(14):148301-1–148301-4.

46. Goodman, CM, McCusker CD, Yilmaz T, et al. Toxicity of gold nanoparticles functionalized with cationic and anionic side chains. Bioconjugate Chem 2004; 15(4):897–900.

47. Braem AD, Prieve DC, Tilton RD. Electrostatically tunable coadsorption of sodium dodecyl sulfate and poly(ethylene oxide)-b-poly(propylene oxide)-b-poly(ethylene oxide) triblock copolymer to silica. Langmuir 2001; 17(3): 883–90.

48. Holmberg K, Jönsson B, Kronberg B, et al. Surfactants and Polymers in Aqueous Solution. 2nd ed. West Sussex: John Wiley & Sons, 2003.

49. Burleson DJ, Driessen MD, Penn RL. On the characterization of environmental nanoparticles. J Environ Sci Health Part A—Toxic/Hazardous Substances Environ Eng 2004; 39(10):2707–53.

23

Impact of Nanoparticles on Aquatic Organisms

Patricia D. McClellan-Green

Department of Environmental and Molecular Toxicology and Center for Marine Sciences and Technology, North Carolina State University, Raleigh, North Carolina, U.S.A.

Eva Oberdörster

Department of Biology, Southern Methodist University, Dallas, Texas, U.S.A.

Shiqian Zhu

Environmental Toxicology Research Program, National Center for Natural Products Research and Department of Pharmacology, School of Pharmacy, The University of Mississippi, University, Mississippi, U.S.A.

T. Michelle Blickley

Integrated Toxicology Program and Division of Coastal Systems Science and Policy, Duke University Marine Laboratory, Beaufort, North Carolina, U.S.A.

Mary L. Haasch

USEPA Mid-Continent Ecology Division, Molecular and Cellular Mechanisms Research Branch, Duluth, Minnesota, U.S.A.

INTRODUCTION

When the first nano-sized materials were being investigated, they were considered to have limited environmental or health consequences. The techniques for synthesizing these materials were costly and extremely inefficient. Today, however, technological advancements in the manufacturing of nanomaterials have made them a commercially viable product. The applications being proposed that will use nanoparticles are phenomenal. Nanoparticles have been suggested and tested for use in tumor ablation cancer treatments, as a surface for bone re-growth, a construction material for the space elevator, a source for alternative energy, even as remediation material for negating decades of environmental damage to groundwater. The nanotechnology market is projected to be valued at $1 trillion by 2012 (1). The underlying concern with a dramatic increase in production and use of nanomaterials is that they will be intentionally or unintentionally released into the environment in large quantities posing a potential risk to humans and ecosystems. The National Nanotechnology Initiative (USA) as well as the governments of other nations and technology entrepreneurs have directed huge amounts of funding exclusively into nanoparticle research. Forming the basis of this technology are four major types of nanomaterials that are commercially manufactured. These include: (1) carbon-based materials such as fullerenes and nanotubes, (2) metal-based materials such as quantum dots and metal oxides (titanium dioxide), (3) dendrimers, which are multi-branched chains and (4) composites, which are a combination of nanomaterials or a mixture of nanoparticles and other materials (2).

Manufactured nanoparticles, ranging in size from 1 to 100 nm, are unique in that they bridge the divide between being a bulk material and being an atomic or molecular structure (3). Because of their small size, these particles have a large surface area to mass ratio that contributes to their unique properties. The chemical composition of the particle, its surface charge, shape and reactivity all influence the potential application(s) of these materials. These traits also influence their potential to move through the environment, accumulate in tissues and elicit biological and physiological responses in exposed organisms. The purpose of this review is to highlight some of the problems and obstacles encountered when working with nanomaterials, especially when trying to assess their effects on aquatic species. We will present some of our findings as well as discuss the results of other investigators involved in research on the effects of nanomaterial exposure in aquatic organisms.

PROBLEMS OF SOLUTION

The solubility of nanomaterials in aqueous media is one of the limiting factors when working with these materials. Most nanoparticles are coated, conjugated or otherwise have their surface structures modified to increase their solubility in aqueous media. This process allows the creation of many "designer" particles that are being developed for medicinal applications or as electronic components. Degraded and unadulterated nanoparticles, such as fullerenes, are largely insoluble and require the use of organic solvents to prepare workable solutions. In 1993, Ruoff et al. (4) examined the solubility of fullerenes in a variety of solvents. They discovered that the material, while easily dissolved in some solvents, e.g., naphthalenes (33–51 mg/ml), was intermediately soluble in other solvents, e.g., benzenes (0.4–8.5 mg/ml), and practically insoluble in polar solvents, such as methanol, ethanol, acetone or water (0.00–0.002 mg/ml).

This variation in solubility, which is due to the surface charge and structure of the parent material, has been one of the hardest obstacles to overcome when working with nanomaterials. The preparation of working suspensions of nanoparticles has only been possible when the interaction of the particle surface with an appropriate solvent was strong enough to overcome differences in the density of the material (5). Unfortunately, in many instances the solvents are highly toxic and potential adverse effects due to the nanoparticle can be masked by the adverse effects of the solvent. To overcome this problem, several methodologies that remove or decrease the use of organic solvents have been employed for solubilizing nanomaterials. One of the first methods used in the solubilization of fullerenes involved the sequential dissolution of the nanomaterial into benzene, followed by dilution into tetrahydrofuran (THF), then into acetone, and finally into water. The aqueous dispersion was finally obtained following distillation to remove the organic solvents (6). Other investigators have prepared their material by sonicating a mixture of fullerene, toluene and water for several hours until the organic solvent was removed and only the aqueous suspension remained (7).

Still others have attempted to dissolve fullerenes without the use of highly toxic solvents. Deguchi et al. (8) and Fortner et al. (9) both described procedures for the preparation of stable dispersions of fullerenes in water using the solvent THF. They prepared their solutions by stirring the fullerenes in THF under an argon atmosphere for 24 hours followed by dilution into water and purging with nitrogen to remove the THF. Unfortunately, all of these described methods including the THF methods, contained trace amounts of solvent within the matrix of the nanoparticle solution that altered the characteristics and toxicity of the suspensions (5). In an effort to alleviate this problem, Brant et al. (5) prepared suspensions of C_{60} aggregates in water by extended mixing of the fullerene in water alone for up to two months. This method avoids introducing any solvent into the preparations and can be used to obtain a reasonable concentration of material with particle sizes < 200 nm. However, other factors such as temperature, mixing speed and the presence of light can all influence the dissolution of fullerenes by this process. For example, as shown in Fig. 1, 200 mg/L of a fullerene powder (99.9+%, Alfa Aesar, Ward Hill, MA) prepared according to the method of Brant et al. (5) in the presence of light (fluorescent room lights plus filtered sunlight) for 30 days was twice as concentrated as an identical preparation that was prepared in the dark with identical temperature and stirring rates (McClellan-Green laboratory). In this case, it appears that light affects the charge transfer or hydrolysis reactions of the parent compound to increase the solubility of the fullerene (5). The ability of the material to be solubilized or suspended in aqueous media portends the potential risk these nanomaterials may pose to aquatic species.

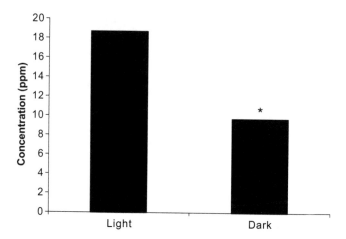

Figure 1 Comparison of the effects of light on the preparation of an aqueous suspension of C_{60} ($p \leq 0.05$). *Note*: * indicates statistical significance.

ENVIRONMENTAL FATE AND UPTAKE

Many investigators have previously demonstrated that the effects of environmental contaminants on an ecosystem and its resident organisms are not based on the total concentration of the chemical but rather on the sub-fraction of the contaminant that is biologically available (10). It has been generally assumed that only desorbed contaminants are biologically available to an organism (i.e., the compound must be desorbed from the sediment particles into the pore water or into an organism's digestive fluids) (11). Thus, sorption and de-sorption of a compound from water and sediment particles are very important factors that determine the accumulation potential of nanomaterials.

The strength of the adsorption of manufactured nanomaterials to organic particles is most likely dependent on its size and chemistry, whether it has a modified surface structure and the environmental conditions under which it is exposed. Lecoanet and Wiesner (12) recently modeled the mobility of a variety of nanomaterials through a sandy aquifer. Their results indicate that single wall carbon nanotubes (SWCNT) were significantly (100×) more mobile in sandy soil than C_{60} aggregates. In addition, they demonstrated that fullerol, C_{60} hydroxide, had a mobility range of 40 feet while C_{60} aggregates, ferroxane (nano-size iron), and anatase (nano-size titanium) had a mobile range of less than one foot. In each case the mobility of the materials was independent of the velocity of the solution through the medium. In a similar study, Zhang (13) demonstrated that nano-size iron particles formed aggregates which strongly adhered to the surface of soil particles and did not undergo leaching to any appreciable extent.

While Lecoanet and Weisner (12) and Zhang (13) demonstrated the ability of nanomaterials to bind to the organic fraction of sediments, Oberdörster et al. (14) demonstrated that nanomaterials could be taken up by aquatic organisms. In separate studies, it was shown that daphnids take up significant amounts of both nC_{60} and nano-iron from the aqueous media (2,14). Tissue levels of >2 ppm were achieved when they were exposed to 30 ppm of water-stirred nC_{60} for 72 hours. Lethality toxicity testing revealed that 48 hour or 96 hour LC_{50} levels could not be achieved in this species using water-stirred C_{60} and no mortality was observed until after five to six days of exposure. Mortality was observed at concentrations of 1, 2.5 and 5 ppm with the highest mortality (40%) achieved at 2.5 ppm. Exposure of daphnids to nano-iron did result in significant levels of mortality with a 50% level achieved in 24 hours using 62.5 mg/L, which is considered a very large dose in environmental toxicology terms (2). In addition, these organisms (Fig. 2a) exhibited significant binding of the nano-iron particles to their exoskeleton surface and antennae as well as significant ingestion of the particles. Fullerenes which were ingested did not visibly bind to the daphnid exoskeleton or antennae. In contrast, harpacticoid copepods not only ingest the material but bind clusters of fullerene aggregates to their exo-skeleton and setae (Fig. 2b) similar to that observed with nano-iron in the daphnia.

A majority of aquatic organisms eat particulate foods. These particles may be consumed by engulfing the material, ingesting through suspension feeding processes (sieving via mucus traps or the use of setae and setule bearing appendages), through filter feeding or through deposit feeding where sediment containing food particles are ingested (15). Daphnids are suspension feeders that selectively feed on phytoplankton within a specific size range. In addition, they utilize unique setae structures to facilitate this feeding process. Thus, their uptake of nanomaterials is largely based on the size of the aggregates. The attraction of the nano-iron particles to the setae and to the exoskeleton of the daphnid is likely due to the surface charge of the exoskeleton surface. Although there are no detailed descriptions of daphnid exoskeleton composition, most crustacean exoskeleton consists of at least four distinct layers, the epicuticle, the exocuticle, the endocuticle and the membranous layer. The epicuticle consists of acidic proteins, lipids and calcium salts. The exocuticle and endocuticle layers consist of calcified matrices of chitin and protein containing a high number of acidic amino acids. The membranous layer, which is the inner-most component of the exoskeleton, is rich in neutral amino acids. The exact composition of the membranous layer amino acids and proteins varies depending on the species and is highly influenced by environmental factors such as salinity, temperature or the presence of metals (16). It would not be unreasonable to assume that the surface of the exoskeleton of some species of crustaceans would be reactive with charged structures such as nanomaterials, while other

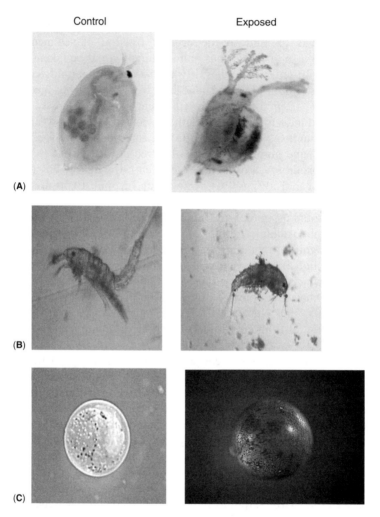

Figure 2 Adsorption and binding of nanomaterials to external surface of aquatic organisms (A) Daphnia exposed to 6.5 mg/L nano-iron (B) Harpacticoid copepods exposed to 15 ppm aqua-C_{60} for 4 days. (C) *Funchilus heteroclitus* embroys exposed to 10 ppm aqua-C_{60} for 6 days. The C_{60} colors the chorion amber.

species would not be reactive. It has also been demonstrated by Conova (17) that wettability of molecules affects their interaction with the surface structures of many invertebrate setae. The results showed that particle capture increased as wettability decreased, indicating that hydrophobic particles were more likely to adhere to the setae. It should be reiterated that not all nanomaterials will bind to all surfaces. This was clearly illustrated with the interaction of the nano-iron and lack of interaction of fullerenes to the daphnid exoskeleton.

Harpacticoid copepods feed on detritus and other material in the sediments and serve as the major food source for many fish and other aquatic organisms. These organisms are bathed in a complex mixture of polysaccharides, lipids, humic acids and other benthic sediment components, many of which have the potential to interact with nanomaterials. Uptake of nanomaterials by microscopic invertebrates would facilitate movement of the compounds through the food-chain and with concomitant reproductive or behavioral adverse effects or toxicity could result in population-level changes. It was demonstrated by Templeton et al. (18) that exposure of the meiobenthic copepod *Amphiascus tenuiremis* to the fluorescent nanocarbon byproduct of single-walled carbon nanotubes (SWNCT) resulted in a significant reduction in life-cycle molting success and reduced the predicted population sizes of future generations. In addition, binding of the nanomaterials to the external surfaces of daphnids, copepods or other microscopic invertebrates could potentially hinder the ability of the invertebrates to escape predators thereby further decreasing the overall populations.

This sorption phenomenon is not limited to invertebrates. Fish embryos (*Fundulus heteroclitus*) exposed to water stirred-C_{60} adsorb a great deal of this material to their chorion (Fig. 2c). Embryos exposed to 0, 2, 5, or 10 ppm for six days bind an increasing level of C_{60} to their chorion surface (Fig. 3). Depending upon the configuration of the nanomaterial on the surface, this binding could have an effect on the hatching ability of the organisms and would definitely make them more visible to predators in the environment.

In a recent paper, Kashiwada (19) demonstrated that nanoparticles, in this case fluorescent polystyrene beads, not only bound to the exterior of the chorion in Japanese medaka, *Oryzias latipes*, but were able to pass through the pores and enter the embryo. Target tissues were largely dependent on the size of the particle and the stage of development of the organism. It was observed that smaller sized particles (39.4 nm) readily partitioned into the yolk and gall bladder of the embryo during development. In the adult fish exposed to the 39.4 nm particles, a significant level of absorption was observed in the gill and intestines with detectable levels present in other tissues such as liver and blood.

PHYSIOLOGICAL EFFECTS

After nanoparticle uptake, their effects, if present, are manifested through various biochemical and molecular perturbations that result in developmental pathologies, endocrine disruption, physiological stress or

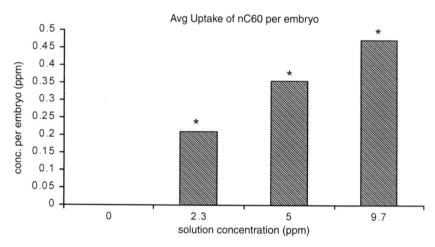

Figure 3 C_{60} adsorption to the chorion of *Fundulus heteroclitus* embryos following a 6-day exposure to increasing concentration of aqueous fullerenes. ($p \leq 0.05$). *Note*: *indicates statistical significance.

ecosystem level dysfunction (2). In 2004, Oberdörster first reported that THF-solubilized nC_{60} was taken up by juvenile large mouth bass (LMB). This uptake most likely occurred via the normal routes of ingestion or by diffusion across the membrane of the gills. In addition, it has been shown that nanoparticles have the ability to be retro-grade transported *via* olfactory neurons (and other neurons of the upper respiratory tract) of mammals into the brain (2,20,21). Interaction of nanomaterial with the chemoreceptors present in the nares of fish could facilitate this transport in teleosts and result in metabolic effects. Therefore, increased lipid peroxidation (LPO) (10–17-fold higher than control fish) in the brain of LMB treated with THF-solubilized nC_{60} was not unexpected. Oberdörster (22) also reported that LPO was reduced in both gill and liver tissue of the exposed animals. It was likely that repair enzymes or anti-oxidants in these latter tissues were induced by exposure to the compound. But in any case, the increased lipid damage observed in these fish indicated that C_{60} partitioned into lipid-rich areas such as the brain and plasma membranes.

This hypothesis was verified using suppressive subtractive hybridization of liver mRNA, which demonstrated that proteins related to metabolism (e.g., oxidoreductases), tissue repair (e.g., hepatocyte growth factor activator) and inflammation (e.g., macrophage stimulating factor) were up-regulated, while proteins related to maintaining homeostasis and acclimation (e.g., proteins involved in glucose metabolism, organic solute transporters) were suppressed (14).

Since the publication of this early study (22), it has been determined that the presence of THF within the C_{60} cluster may be responsible for many of the toxic effects. This supposition was strongly supported in subsequent investigations. Comparison of the LPO data from the LMB study to that of fathead minnows (FHM) exposed to water-stirred C_{60} (Fig. 4) demonstrated that LPO in brain while elevated in water-stirred nC_{60} FHM was not statistically different from levels observed in control fish. Haasch et al. (2005) compared the LC_{50} for THF-nC_{60} and water-stirred nC_{60} in FHM (*Pimephales promelas*). The THF-nC_{60} exhibited an acute toxicity with 100% mortality at 0.5 ppm within 16 hours whereas the water-stirred nC_{60} elicited no mortality at any concentration up to 7 ppm.

In addition, Haasch et al. (23) and Zhu et al. (24) examined the liver for changes in cytochrome P450 expression and PMP70 protein levels. From the earlier studies in bass using THF-nC_{60}, it had been observed that several oxidoreductases and specifically CYP2K4 were up-regulated following exposure. To determine whether this change in P450 expression was conserved between species, they investigated whether P450 isozymes in the CYP2 family were altered in FHM and medaka (*Oryzias latipes*) but this time they employed water-stirred C_{60}. Their results were surprising in that they indicated that CYP2 and many other enzymes were not up-regulated. They did however observe a reduction in PMP70 expression. PMP70 (also known as ABCD3 and PXMP1) is a peroxisomal membrane protein that functions as an ATP-binding half-transporter whose function is the import of very-long-chain fatty acids for peroxisomal β-oxidation (25). Decreased

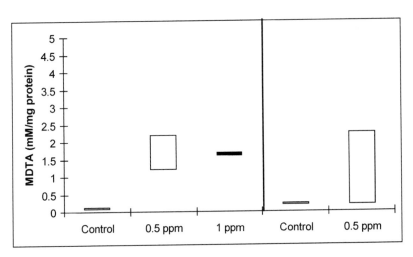

Figure 4 Brain LPO in large mouth-bass and fathead minnows. (provided by Dr. Eva Oberdörster). *Abbreviation*: FHM, fathead nunnows; LMB, large-mouth bass; LPO, lipid peroxidation; THF, tetrahydrofuran. *Source*: Dr. Eva Oberdörster.

expression of this protein could indicate an alteration in the number or size of peroxisomes, an inhibition of the membrane repair process or a reduction in the lipid transport into peroxisomes. Similar results were reported by Henry et al. (26) in zebra fish exposed to fullerenes prepared by the two methods. They reported a 3–7 fold increase in expression of genes involved with the oxidative response. However, this increase was attributable to the presence of THF oxidation products γ-butyrolactone and tetrahydro-2-furanol rather than the presence of C_{60}. They did not examine the expression of PMP70 in their assays.

REPRODUCTIVE AND OTHER EFFECTS

Aside from the ROS response observed by many investigators, the potential for nanoparticle exposure to affect reproduction and development raises the most concern. Oberdörster et al. (14) noted significant decreases in the number of offspring over a 21-day life cycle for daphnia exposed to water-stirred nC_{60}. The number of cumulative offspring dropped from ~80 for control organisms to ~15–30 for daphnids exposed to 5.0 and 2.5 ppm respectively. Likewise, Templeton et al. (18) reported significant reduction in fertilization rates and molting success in the estuarine copepod, *Amphascus tenuiremis*, following exposure to unpurified single walled carbon nanotubes (SWNT). Only one female copepod exposed to 10 mg/L reached adulthood compared to >90% of the females in the control group. Interestingly, this study showed that these toxic effects were not elicited by the purified SWNT but rather by the manufacturing by-products, fluorescent nanocarbon particles. Projections by this group on the environmental significance of exposure to the waste material indicated significant reductions in the population growth rates. This portends serious environmental consequences unless proper oversight is maintained during the production process.

SUMMARY AND CONCLUSIONS

The design and construction of new and useful nanotechnology products is limited only by our imagination. Nanotechnology holds the promise of creating new products and treatments for disease, for enhancing and improving our environment and for the development of new "gee-whiz" technologies. The usefulness and versatility of manufactured nanoparticles is based on their unique electrical, structural and thermal properties. The redox active properties of nanomaterials while extremely useful under controlled conditions may pose a risk to non-target species through unintentional environmental release.

Based on the results of our studies as well as that by other investigators, we do know that nanomaterials, especially those with carbon-based structures such as fullerenes and nanotubes, can elicit toxic responses. This has been documented in cell culture systems, in invertebrate species, and with various vertebrate organisms including mammals and fish. These materials as well as the quantum dots and the metal oxides discussed in this book can readily enter the tissues of exposed organisms and be transported throughout the body. Thus, the critical question; "Are they taken up and are they biologically available to organisms in the environment?" has partially been answered. We know that organisms can take-up these materials and we know that these materials have the potential to enter and move within the environment. The remainder of that question, "Are nanoparticles entering the environment?" has not been totally addressed. Based on current and historical literature many lipophilic environmental contaminants, such as dioxins and PCBs, readily enter the environment through accidental or intentional release. These contaminants are then tend to bioaccumulate in tissues and are extremely mobile within the food web/food chain. Using a precautionary approach, it is likely that nanoparticles will behave in a similar fashion.

Another question that has arisen regarding the manufacture and use of nanomaterials is; "How persistent are the effects of nanomaterial exposure and do they pose a risk to successive generations?" The study by Templeton et al. (18) clearly indicates that population levels of organisms can be affected by exposure to nanoparticles. However, there are still many unanswered questions regarding nanoparticles and the environment. Because of the diverse nature of the nanomaterials being developed and the multiple ways these materials can be modified and manipulated, this will not be a simple question to answer. The establishment of guidelines using approved testing protocols will be a great benefit. In addition, cooperative efforts between industrial, regulatory and private interests should assist in streamlining this process and avoid repeating mistakes of the past.

BIBLIOGRAPHY

Colvin, V. The potential environmental impacts of engineered nanomaterials. Nature Biotech 2003; 21(10):1166–70.

Ringwood AH, Khambhammettu S, Santiago P, Bealer E, Stogner M, Collins J, Gonsalves KE. Characterization, imaging and degradation studies of quantum dots in aquatic organisms. In: Stella P, Vasilis F, eds. Life-Cycle Analysis Tools for "Green" Materials and Process Selection, Mater Res Soc Symp Proc 895, Warrendale, PA, 2006:0895-G04-06-S04-06.

REFERENCES

1. Service RF. Nanotechnology grows up. Science 2004; 304:1732–4.
2. Oberdörster G, Oberdörster E, Oberdörster J. Nanotoxicology: An emerging discipline evolving from studies of ultrafine particles. Environ Health Perspect 2005; 113:823–39.

3. Hoet PHM, Brüske-HohlfeldI Salata OV. Nanoparticles: known and unknown health risks. J Nanobiotechnol 2004; 2:12(doi:10.1186/1477-3155-2-12).

4. Ruoff RS, Tse DS, Malhotra R, Lorents DC. Solubility of C60 in a variety of solvents. J Phys Chem 1993; 97:3379–83.

5. Brant J, Lecoanet H, Hotze M, Wiesner M. Comparison of electrokinetic properties of colloidal fullerenes (nC60) formed using two procedures. Environ Sci Technol 2005; 39:6343–51.

6. Scrivens WA, Tour JM, Creek KE, Pirisi L. Synthesis of 14C-labeled C60, Its suspension in water and its uptake by human keratinocytes. J Am Chem Soc 1994; 116:4517–18.

7. Andrievsky GV, Kosevich MV, Vovk OM, Shelkovsky VS, Vashchenko, LA. On the production of an aqueous colloidal solution of fullerenes. J Chem Soc Chem Commun 1995; 12:1281–82.

8. Deguchi S, Alargova RG, Tsujii K. Stable dispersions of fullerenes, C_{60} and C_{70}, in water. Preparation and characterization. Langmuir 2001; 17:6013–17.

9. Fortner JD, Lyon DY, Sayes CM, Boyd AM, Falkner JC, Hotze EM, Alemany LB, Tao YJ, Guo W, Ausman KD, Colvin VL, Hughes JB. C_{60} in water: Nanocrystal formation and microbial response. Environ Sci Technol 2005; 39:4307–16.

10. Haung W, Peng P, Yu Z, Fu, J. Effects of organic matter heterogeneity on sorption and desorption of organic contaminants by soils and sediments. Appl Geochem 2003; 18:955–72.

11. Lu X, Reible DD, Fleeger JW. Bioavailability and assimilation of sediment-associated benzo(a)pyrene by *Ilyodrilus templetoni* (Oligochaeta). Environ Toxicol Chem 2004; 23:57–64.

12. Lecoanet HE, Wiesner MR. Velocity effects on fullerene and oxide nano-particle deposition in porous media. Environ Sci Technol 2004; 38:4377–82.

13. Zhang W. Nanoscale iron particles for environmental remediation: an overview. J Nanoparticle Res 2003; 5:323–32.

14. Oberdörster E, McClellan-Green P,. Haasch M. Ecotoxicology of engineer-ednanomaterials. Nanomaterials-Toxicity, Health and Environmental Issues. Xhalla S, Kumar SR, eds. Weinheim: Wiley-VCH Verlag GmbH & Co, KGaA, 2006:35–49.

15. Valiela I. Marine Ecological Processes, 2nd ed. New York: Springer-Verlag, Inc. 1995:686.

16. O'Brien J, Kumari S, Skinner D. Proteins of crustacean exoskeletons: I. Similarities and differences among proteins of the four exoskeletal layers of four brachyurans. Biol Bull 1991; 181:427–41.

17. Conova S. Role of particle wettability in capture by suspension-feeding crab (*Emerita talpoida*). Mar Biol 1999; 133:419–28.

18. Templeton RC, Ferguson PL, Washburn KM, Scrivens WA, Chandler GT. Life-cycle effects of single-walled carbon nanotubes (SWNTs) on an estuarine meiobenthic copepod. Environ. Sci. Technol . 2006; 40:7387–93.

19. Kashiwada S. Distribution of nanoparticles in the see-through medaka (*Oryzias latipes*). Environ Heallth Perspect 2006; 114:1697–02.

20. Tjälve H, Mejare C, Borg-Neczak K. Uptake and transport of manganese in primary and secondary olfactory neurones in pike. Pharmacol Toxicol 1995; 77(1):23–31.
21. Tjälve H, Henriksson J. Uptake of metals in the brain *via* olfactory pathways. Neurotoxicology 1999; 20(2–3):181–96.
22. Oberdörster E. Manufactured nanomaterials (fullerenes, C60) induce oxidative stress in brain of Juvenile Largemouth Bass. EnvironHealth Perspect 2004; 112(10):1058–62.
23. Haasch ML, Patricia M-G, Oberdörster E. Consideration of the toxicity of manufactured nanoparticles. In: Kuzmany H, Fink J, Mehring M, Roth S, eds. XIX International Winterschool/Euroconference on Electronic Properties of Novel Materials, Vol. 786. Tirol, Austria: American Institute of Physics (AIP), Kirchberg, 2005:586–9.
24. Zhu S, Oberdörster E, Haasch ML. Toxicity of an engineered nanoparticle (fullerene, C_{60}) in two aquatic species, *Daphnia* and fathead minnow. Mar Environ Res 2006; 62:S5–9.
25. Kim J-H, Yamaguchi K, Lee S-H, Tithof PK, Sayler GS, Yoon J-H, Baek, SJ. Evaluation of polycyclic aromatic hydrocarbons in the activation of early growth response-1 and peroxisome proliferator activated receptors. Toxicol Sci 2005; 85:585–93.
26. Henry TB, Menn F-M, Fleming JT, Wilgus J, Compton RN, Sayler GS. Attributing the toxicity of aqueous C_{60} nano-aggregates to tetrahydrofuran decomposition products in larval zebrafish by assessment of gene expression. Cambridge, MA: TFI Learning Nanotoxicology Conference, April 24–25, 2006.

24

The Environmental Implications of Nanomaterials

Theresa F. Fernandes, Nic. Christofi, and Vicki Stone

*Centre for Health and the Environment, School of Life Sciences,
Napier University, Edinburgh, U.K.*

INTRODUCTION

There is general lack of information regarding the environmental implications of engineered nanomaterials. Results from human toxicology indicate that the toxicity of these materials is related to their ability to induce oxidative stress and inflammation in the lung leading to impacts on respiratory and cardiovascular health. Studies which investigate the ability of nanoparticles (NP) made from low toxicity materials to generate oxidative stress and inflammation suggest that potency is dependent upon their surface area. Furthermore, studies that compare low toxicity materials and particles made from more noxious substances, such as nickel or alpha-quartz, demonstrate that biological reactivity is a function of both surface reactivity and surface area.

There is now a widespread use of nanomaterials in a variety of consumer products. Some of those uses involve the deliberate release of nanomaterials (e.g., removal of pollutants from contaminated water or soil, water treatment filters and control of algal growth). It is also possible that the increased use of nanomaterials will lead into an increase in the release of NP into the environment, although little is known about this process and its significance. Once organisms are exposed to NP, immediate or long-term toxic effects may be observed. Results from environmental studies indicate rapid uptake and translocation from the gut to other parts of the body of the test species. Recently, deleterious effects on crustacean and fish exposed to

C_{60}, TiO_2 and carbon black NPs have been published. Although these studies have not yet addressed NP uptake, bioaccumulation or biomagnification, they suggest some short term effects (e.g., oxidative stress) and some behavioural and reproductive effects. It is possible that these effects may be reflected at population level and potentially also at food web level, including bioacumulation and biomagnification effects. It is therefore important that overall impacts and risks of newly engineered NP released into the environment are addressed.

Nanotechnology involves the development and manufacture of materials in the nanometer size range and includes the production and use of nanoparticles (NP; defined as particles with lengths in two or three dimensions greater than 1 nm and smaller than 100 nm, and which may or may not exhibit a size-related intensive property1). Due to their small size a relatively large proportion of the atoms and molecules making up the particles are exposed at the particle surface compared to larger particles. This structural difference, coupled with the relatively large surface area per unit mass of NP, allows such materials to exhibit properties that differ from bulk chemicals, making them useful in a wide variety of applications including electronics, paints, cosmetics, medicines, foods, textiles and environmental remediation (2,3). This means that the potential for human and environmental exposure to NP is large.

NANOPARTICLE TOXICOLOGY

In general, there is still lack of information regarding the human health and environmental implications of engineered NP (4). Some toxicological studies have been conducted in relation to the inhalation of NP made from low toxicity materials such as carbon black (5), TiO_2 (6) and polystyrene (7). Such studies demonstrate that the toxicity of these materials is related to their ability to induce oxidative stress and inflammation in the lung leading to impacts on lung and cardiovascular health. The cells of the body contain a number of antioxidant defense molecules (e.g., glutathione and vitamin E) that protect cells against reactive oxygen species (ROS) and free radicals that due to their electrophillic properties damage proteins, lipids and DNA. Such ROS and free radicals include superoxide anion radicals ($O_2^{-\bullet}$) and hydroxyl radicals ($OH^\bullet$) and are generated at the surface of NP (8,9). Depletion of antioxidant defense molecules by these ROS and production of free radicals lead to oxidative stress and damage to cells. NP causing oxidative stress may also lead to the production of reactive nitrogen, sulphur and other species (i.e., RNS, RSS and others) stressing the body in a similar manner to the effect of ROS. In the case of RSS (10), reactive sulphur substances such as thiyl radicals and disulphides can oxidize and ultimately inhibit thiol proteins and enzymes.

Oxidative stress and cell damage can also activate inflammation. This involves activation of various white blood cells within the immune system. Such cells include macrophages that migrate to the site of particle deposition and then engulf the particles by phagocytosis. The macrophages then remove the particles from the lung surface by either moving out of the airways along with mucus, or by migrating into the body's lymph nodes. Successful particle clearance allows the inflammation to subside and any tissue damage to be repaired.

Unsuccessful particle clearance leads to persistent inflammation and oxidative stress that causes cellular damage leading to a variety of disease effects (11,12). Acute effects associated with particulate air pollution result in increased hospitalization and deaths from both respiratory and cardiovascular diseases. Such effects have been attributed to airborne NP (13). Acute effects tend to affect people who are susceptible due to pre-existing inflammatory diseases.

Chronic effects associated with other respirable particles, such as environmental particulate air pollution, crystalline silica (alpha-quartz) and asbestos fibres, include fibrosis (scarring of lung tissue making breathing difficult) and cancer. The long term health effects of respirable NP as yet have not been elucidated. Epidemiological evidence from industrial processes, such as the manufacture of carbon black, where workers may potentially be exposed to NP, is not clear-cut.

Studies which investigate the ability of NP made from low toxicity materials to generate oxidative stress and inflammation suggest that potency is dependent upon their surface area (7,14). Furthermore, studies that compare low toxicity materials and particles made from more noxious substances, such as nickel or alpha-quartz, demonstrate that biological reactivity is a function of both surface reactivity and surface area (14).

For non-spherical particles such as fibres, it is well recognized that dimensions (long and thin particles) and durability are important factors in determining their ability to induce fibrosis and cancer (15,16). It is conceivable that these properties will also be relevant to NP such as nanotubes, nanowhiskers and nanofibres. For new, more novel forms of engineered NP it is likely that a combination of the factors described above will be important in determining their ability to induce adverse effects in human and wider environmental systems. To summarize, such factors will include small size, large surface area per surface reactivity (determined by chemistry), dimensions (spherical versus fibre) and durability (biopersistence).

ECOTOXICOLOGY OF NP

Many of the current and intended uses of NP are 'environmental' including remediation (removal of pollutants from contaminated water or soil where large quantities are used in e.g., permeable reactive barriers, PRB), water treatment filters and control of algal growth in water systems (3). The rapid growth of nanotechnologies will also lead to increased accidental and purposeful release of NP into the environment. It is, therefore, important that overall impacts and risks of newly engineered NP released into the environment are addressed (4,17,18).

As yet very little work has been conducted to determine the fate of NP in the aquatic and terrestrial habitats and their effects on the biota within these environments. Even less work has been conducted on the mechanism of this potential ecotoxicity. However, the environmental impact of NP is a key area of research since many NP will enter the environment via wastewater from both domestic and industrial use of NP (4,17,18). Input through numerous diffuse sources will be possible as many of the current and intended uses of NP are environmental.

Such applications include remediation to remove pollutants from contaminated water and soil, water treatment filters and the control of algal growth in water systems (3). It has also been advocated that silicon and rubber NP be used as reinforcements in rubber tires with implications for environment released through rubber wear. There are a number of recommendations, both in Europe and in the United States, for enacting caution in the development of nanosciences and nanotechnology, especially concerning the use of free NP.

NP are released into the environment via air, water or soil will which means that they have access to a wide range of species from microorganisms such as bacteria and algae, through to more complex organisms including terrestrial and aquatic vertebrates. Obviously, deleterious effects on any organism within the ecosystem can lead to significant consequences for the remainder of the ecosystem in a number of ways, including impacting upon food chains and altering interactions between different species. For these reasons it is important to assess the fate and distribution of NP that are released into the environment to determine which environments and species are most exposed, and what the consequences may be. NP have enhanced structural, chemical, magnetic, optical and electrical properties. The fate and distribution of NP within the environment are highly dependent upon these properties including their hydrophobicity and surface charge.

Very little information is available in relation to the tracking and behavior of engineered NP in the environment, although there are a number of studies on colloidal particles which have tried to address such issues (19,20). A more detailed analysis of this area of research is outside the scope of this chapter, but is warranted since this information is likely to be relevant to engineered NP. For example, in studies using TEM to characterize nanoparticle colloids in environmental water samples, the substances most studied include humic substances, polysaccharide fibrils, hydrous iron oxides, viruses, clay minerals and heavy metal agglomerates

(20), suggesting that the technology to track such particles in the environment is now available.

In addition to determining the fate and distribution of NP in the environment, it is also essential to assess their potential toxicity to a wide range of species. A handful of studies have begun to emerge in this area (21–23).

Microorganisms

The effects of NP on microorganisms has been more extensively studied than other areas of ecotoxicology. There is currently an effort to develop a range of metal oxide and silver NP as antibacterials to reduce the dependency on antibiotics to which many microorganisms are becoming resistant. A problem may be the release and effect of these 'nanobiotics' to non-target microorganisms involved in biogeochemical cycling in the environment. Currently it is not known whether NP as sole toxicants are toxic to cells in the environment, as in real systems they undergo modification including aggregation with other NP (agglomeration) due to dissolved salts and adsorption of a range of organics and inorganic constituents of the matrix in which they are distributed. Williams et al., examined the effects of various NP on the growth and activity of *Escherichia coli* (24). They found that with silica, gold and composite silica/iron oxide NP, at concentrations from 1.1×10^{-4} g ml^{-1} to 4.4×10^{-2} g ml^{-1}, there was little or no effect on microbial growth. This study did not attempt to determine more subtle physiological and genetic functional changes in the bacterium. Of course the NP tested represent only a small fraction of available nanomaterials and it has been shown, for example, that C_{60} fullerenes inhibit prokaryotes at low concentrations (0.4 mg l^{-1}) and affect their respiration at 4 mg l^{-1} (25).

NP such as those made from silver are widely used in a range of projects as antimicrobial agents, for example in wound dressings. From available studies it is not clear whether the antimicrobial effects are simply due to the silver rather than the nanoparticulate form. Some studies suggest that silver NP can accumulate in the membrane of *E. coli* bacteria causing the cell walls to pit, so that cell permeability is altered and death ensues (26). The large surface area of NP makes them ideal for use as absorbents and so a number of products are being developed for the destruction or removal from the environment of bacteria, including biological warfare agents (27).

Composite materials containing different nanomaterials are also being developed for antimicrobial applications. For example, Lee et al. investigated the ability of TiO$_2$-coated multi-walled nanotubes to kill bacterial endospores (28). They found that the composite irradiated with UV light was more effective than either UV light alone or UV irradiated TiO_2 particles. However, the composite of nanotubes and TiO_2 appeared to cause endospore aggregation so that some of the spores were protected and survived. Magnetic NP have also been developed to remove bacteria from aquatic environments (29).

In addition to effects on bacteria, TiO_2-coated hollow glass beads have been shown to inhibit the photosynthetic activity of cyanobacteria, and diatoms, suggesting potential useful applications in preventing excessive algal growth (30).

The enhanced structural, chemical, magnetic, optical and electrical properties of NP can be utilized in environmental remediation/waste treatment. Zero valent iron is used in the remediation of trichloroethylene in groundwaters with trials taking place to affect better remediation using nanoscale zero valent iron (NZVI). As with many metallic NP agglomeration is a common feature in the environment and efforts are directed at reducing agglomeration in the field to retain nanoparticle effectiveness. There should be consideration of the potential hazard from NZVI particles.

These studies would suggest that intended or accidental release of NP in the environment may affect natural ecosystem microorganism populations and microorganisms involved in waste degradation (e.g., soil and waste-water).

Plants

Very little work has been done in relation to the effects of NP on plants. Yang and Watts investigated the phytotoxicity of 13 nm aluminium NP (Al-NPs) on root growth by the seeds of five different plant species (31). The Al-NPs inhibited root growth at high concentrations ($2 \, mg \, ml^{-1}$), while larger aluminium particles (size of 200–300 nm) had no effect supporting suggestions that the size of NP is important in the study of their toxicity. Interestingly, when Yang and Watts loaded Al-NPs with the polycyclic aromatic hydrocarbon phenanthrene, the inhibiting effects on root growth were reduced (31). The authors suggest the reason for the reduced inhibition to be due to the disappearance of free hydroxyl groups and a consequential change in particle surface characteristics. This suggestion was supported by loading Al-NPs with DMSO (a known free hydroxyl group scavenger) and observing similar results. Murashov, however, suggested that some of the effects noted in this study may have resulted from increased solubility of nanoscale alumina which was likely to have lead to increased concentrations of alumina species (32). This may have contributed to the observed phytotoxicity, as opposed to nanoscale properties of the alumina.

Invertebrates and Vertebrates

One of the main problems encountered in the animal testing of nanoparticle ecotoxicology, has been the protocol used to prepare the NP. Many NP tend to form large aggregates, and it is not currently clear whether the NP in the aggregates possess the same toxic potential and bioavailability as single NP. What is important to consider, however, is the form of nanoparticle that is found in the environment, and this is likely to depend upon the formulation of the released nanoparticle along with the substances with which the nanoparticle interacts with once released. For example, release of NP via waste water suggests that NP will be mixed with significant quantities of household and industrial detergents that could help to disaggregate the particles. Furthermore, naturally occurring surfactants, such as humic acids may help to disaggregate particles.

A number of the ecotoxicology studies that have been published have used the organic solvent tetrahydrofuran (THF) to disaggregate NP such as C_{60} prior to treatment of organisms. However, THF is not representative of materials widely found naturally or via pollution in the environment. Brant et al. (33) have demonstrated that even after filtration and evaporation that THF remains trapped between the aggregated C_{60} particles, suggesting that the studies described below by Oberdorster and by Lovern and Klaper (21,34), outlined below, have investigated the effects of C_{60} combined with THF rather than the effects of C_{60} per se. THF is classified by many regulatory bodies as a neurotoxin and so could in part explain some of the effects observed in the fish. For these reasons it is worth considering some of the following information with caution. No evidence could be found in the literature that THF per se is able to induce oxidative stress.

Lovern and Klaper exposed *Daphnia magna* to C_{60} or TiO_2 (Degussa P25, 25 nm diameter) (34). The particles were treated to break up the aggregates by either sonicating in medium for 30 minutes, or by solubilization in the organic solvent THF. The TiO_2 and the C_{60} particles were both more potent at killing the organisms when prepared in THF than when prepared by sonication, and the C_{60} was more potent than the TiO_2. The question remains as to whether the particles prepared in THF were more toxic because they were better dispersed or because of THF induced toxicity. Similar results were obtained by Zhu et al. (35). These authors compared the effects of THF-treated with water-stirred fullerenes on *D. magna* and on adult male fathead minnow (*Pimephales promelas*). When lethal tests were conducted, THF-treated fullerenes proved to be more toxic than water-stirred to both *Daphnia* and minnow. Zhu et al. suggest that even sonication can enhance toxicity and therefore stress the need to use environmentally-relevant doses and preparation techniques (35).

Oberdorster et al. tried to overcome the preparation-linked problems by stirring the fullerenes in water (23). They exposed the aquatic crustaceans

D. magna and *Hyalella azteca,* and marine harpacticoid copepods to a range of fullerene concentrations. These could not be prepared at high enough concentration levels to cause 50% mortality of the invertebrate species tested (LC_{50}) at 48 or 96 hours. The maximum concentrations tested were 35 ppm for freshwater and 22.5 ppm for full-strength (35 ppt) seawater, since at higher concentrations the fullerene precipitated out of solution. *D. magna* exposures for 21 days to 2.5 and 5 ppm concentrations, respectively resulted in a significant delay in moulting and significantly reduced offspring production, which could have negative impacts at the population level (23).

Recent work (35) has studied the effects of exposing a range of aquatic crustaceans *(D. magna, Artemia salina* and Gammarids) exposed to several NP (TiO_2, ultra-fine carbon black, C_{60}). Preliminary results indicate that particles are ingested, resulting in accumulation in the gastrointestinal tract (Fig. 1). The particles also adhere to the exoskeleton surfaces of the exposed organisms, suggesting multiple routes of exposure and absorption. In the *D. magna* fluorescent polystyrene NP were found to be rapidly taken up by neonate *D. magna* into their fat storing droplets (Fig. 1). In addition, LC_{50} (48 hours) results ranged between 5–20 ppm. Subtoxic doses of carbon black and TiO_2 NP were also found to be associated with increased moulting of the carapace by neonates (35). In these studies, the methodology employed involved sonication but not the use of a solvent such as THF.

The results so far obtained from the acute tests conducted on *D. magna* indicate that the lethality of the NP tested is relatively low, but that they may still be cause for concern (22,23,34,35). Preliminary results indicate increased oxidative stress in *D. magna* with increased ultrafine carbon black concentrations. Therefore, although there is still much ongoing work in this area, the indication of accumulation within body compartments suggests that such research is essential. In addition, published studies on the effects of any NP on other invertebrates have been limited, with only Oberdorster and

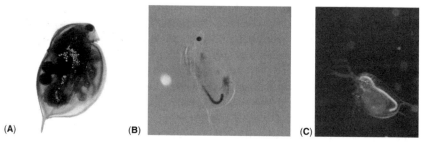

(A)   **(B)**   **(C)**

Figure 1 *Daphnia magna* exposed to (**A**) 20 nm fluorescent carboxylated polystyrene beads (2.6 g/L for 1 hour); (**B**) 14 nm carbon black (1 mg/L for 48 hours); (**C**) 25 nm TiO_2 particles (1 mg/L for 48 hours).

colleagues focussing additionally on the freshwater amphipod *H. azteca* and on marine benthic harpacticoid copepods (23).

A publication by Oberdorster using juvenile largemouth bass is the first non-human, non-rodent vertebrate study on nanoparticle toxicity to be published (21). As in the studies described above the C_{60} was pre-treated with THF to aid dispersion of the NP. The fish were exposed to 0.5 and 1ppm C_{60} for 48 hours and were found to exhibit signs of lipid peroxidation in the brain. Selective transport of NP to the brain of rodents has been observed in rodent studies (the authors suggest that this, along with the lack of neural antioxidant defense mechanisms, could explain the enhanced brain lipid peroxidation. However, THF is classified as a neurotoxin, and so it will be important to repeat such studies using alternative procedures. In a subsequent study Zhu et al. demonstrated that THF prepared C_{60} induced 100% mortality within 6 to 18 hours of exposure in adult fat head minnow (*P. promelas*) (34). Conversely, C_{60} generated by water stirring had no impact on lethality over the same time period, although lipid peroxidation was observed in the gill, suggestive of oxidative damage, as well as a significantly increased expression of CYP2 family isoenzymes in the liver as compared to control fish. This study again suggests that the method of preparation can increase toxicity (34).

As described, Oberdorster et al. tried to overcome the preparation-linked problems by stirring the fullerenes in water (36). The effects of this preparation were assessed on fish species, fathead minnow and japanese medaka (*Oryzias latipes*) at 0.5 ppm concentration for 72 hours. Results indicated no change in mRNA or protein-expression levels of cytochrome P450 isoenzymes CYP1A, CYP2K1 and CYP2M1. The peroxisomal lipid transport protein PMP70 was found to be significantly reduced in fathead minnow but not medaka which the authors attribute to potential changes in acyl-CoA pathways (36).

A recent study by Oberdorster et al. explores the potential application of microarray technology to ecotoxicity screening of NP (36). Specifically, their work focussed on the development and application of a genomic-based, ecotoxitity screening method to nano-scale iron particles being used for environmental remediation.

Smith et al. studied the toxicity of single walled carbon nanotubes (SWCNT) to rainbow trout (37). SWCNT exposure caused a dose-dependent rise in ventilation rate, gill pathologies (oedema, altered mucocytes, hyperplasia), and mucus secretion with SWCNT precipitation on the gill mucus. SWCNT exposure caused statistically significant increases in Na^+ K^+-ATPase activity in the gills and intestine, but not in the brain. Thiobarbituric acid reactive substances (TBARS) showed dose-dependent and statistically significant decreases especially in the gill, brain and liver during SWCNT exposure compared to controls. SWCNT exposure caused statistically significant increases in the total glutathione levels in the gills

(28%) and livers (18%), compared to the solvent control. Pathologies in the brain included possible aneurisms or swellings on the ventral surface of the cerebellum. Liver cells exposed to SWCNT showed condensed nuclear bodies (apoptotic bodies) and cells in abnormal nuclear division. Fish ingested water containing SWCNT during exposure (presumably stress-induced drinking) which resulted in precipitated SWCNT in the gut lumen and intestinal pathology. Aggressive behavior and fin nipping caused some mortalities at the end of the experiment, which may be associated with the gill irritation and brain injury, although the solvent may also partly contribute to aggression. Overall the authors concluded that SWCNTs are a respiratory toxicant in trout, and that observed cellular pathologies suggest cell cycle defects, neurotoxicity, and blood borne factors that possibly mediate systemic pathologies.

The Way Forward

The little data that are available on the ecotoxicology of NP on a variety of organisms, coupled with the scale of nanoparticle use and potential release into the environment, suggests that this is an area of research that is important to pursue. It is worth using the literature relating to the toxicology of NP as a guide when conducting such studies, especially in determining the role of oxidative stress in driving any adverse effects identified. An understanding of the mechanism of toxicity would help in determining safe limits of release for new NP as well as the design of safer NP in the future.

NANOPARTICLE PREPARATION PRIOR TO EXPERIMENTATION

The THF used in some of the studies described above is not necessarily representative of materials widely found naturally or via pollution in the environment, as this has marred the debate regarding the validity of such studies. Brant et al. have demonstrated that even after filtration and evaporation that THF remains trapped between the aggregated C_{60} particles suggesting that the studies by Oberdorster and by Lovern and Klaper have investigated the effects of C_{60} combined with THF rather than the effects of C_{60} per se (22,33). THF is classified by many regulatory bodies as a neurotoxin and so could in part explain some of the effects observed in the fish. For these reasons, Brant et al. suggest that the studies published so far need to be reinterpreted (33). Recent studies have employed different approaches.

It is clear that more work is required to address the development of an optimal procedure for the study of the effects of nanomaterials on aquatic species. As described, many nanomaterials are insoluble and do not tend to stay in suspension when in liquid media. A variety of methods, including stirring, probe sonication and bath sonication for a differing amount of time, have been proposed and it is as yet unclear how realistic they may be and how they may affect the results of whole organism toxicity assessments. There are a number of surfactants found naturally and as pollutants (e.g., detergents) that may be useful tools to study the effects of particle dispersion on their subsequent toxicity. However, the question regarding the behavior of NP in the environment has not yet been addressed and so the relevance of generating a stable homogenous suspension of NP is not yet know.

For all organism types, it is also important to consider that transformations and interactions between different compounds and pollutants do take place in the natural environment. For example, microparticles have been demonstrated to serve as a transport medium for toxic chemicals (e.g., PCBs, DDE, nonylphenols) (38). In addition, an indication of particles synergisms between nanomaterials and metals or organic compounds has also been put forward (39).

STRATEGIC PRIORITIES FOR ECOTOXICOLOGY

Considering the rapid expansion of nanotechnologies, and the potential for nanoparticulates to be released into the environment, it is essential that regulatory authorities and ecotoxicologists prioritize their research. It is beyond the scope of this paper to list fully the studies required, however, a development of such a strategy will require the establishment of a panel of well-characterized NP that vary in size, shape, durability, composition and surface reactivity, as well as varying the presence of potential contaminants such as metals. In addition, tests should also include natural materials, such as humic acids, which may act as dispersants. This panel can then be used in multiple laboratories and models in order to generate a data set amongst which comparisons, and hence conclusions, can be made. However, these should also take into account the extent of current and near-future NP discharged into the environment. The toxicity tests conducted will require both acute and chronic exposures preferably using standard laboratory models. It is important that the models employed cover a wide range of trophic levels and encompass a variety of organisms which different modes of feeding/respiration (e.g., filter, detritus feeders, carnivores) and will consider bioaccumulation/biomagnification, as well as food web effects. It might be appropriate to use endpoints that have been identified as relevant in mammalian and human toxicological studies using NP, for example, oxidative stress appears to be an important process driving particle toxicity. Finally, it will be necessary to develop standard methodologies for the assessment of nanomaterial toxicity or hazard that are relevant to the full lifecycle of NP.

CONCLUSIONS

To date very little is known regarding the ecotoxicology of NP, and many of those studies that have been conducted may require careful consideration and interpretation due to the protocols employed. Future studies will need to address a range of species from different guilds (levels of complexity) and from different environments (air, water, and soil). The route of exposure will need to be carefully considered in order to generate a system that resembles scenarios that are feasible in the environment. The endpoints that can be measured are also variable, ranging from determining the ability of NP to induce death, but such studies should be enriched by the further inclusion of other endpoints such as biochemical markers of oxidative stress, genotoxicity or histology. In addition to looking at effects at the biochemical, cellular and organismal level, effects at the population level (e.g., reproduction) need also to be considered. There are a number of standard protocols published by the EPA and the OECD that should be investigated for the suitability to study NP ecotoxicity, and it is likely that minor modifications will make these useful tools in the future. Finally, in order to allow the rapid progression of NP ecotoxicology, knowledge relating to the toxicology of NP (e.g., importance of surface area and surface reactivity) will be useful when considering experimental design.

REFERENCES

1. ASTM (2006). Standard Terminology Relating to Nanotechnology. Standard E 2456–06. American Society for Testing and Materials (ASTM) International, in partnership with American Institute of Chemical Engineers (AIChE), American Society of Mechanical Engineers (ASME), Institute of Electrical and Electronics Engineers (IEEE), Japanese National Institute of Advanced Industrial Science and Technology (AIST), NSF International, Semiconductor Equipment and Materials International (SEMI).
2. Bergeron N, Archambault E. Canadian Stewardship Practices for Environmental Nanotechnology. Report prepared for Environment Canada by Science-Metrix, March 2005.
3. Biswas P, Wu CY. Nanoparticles and the environment. J Air Waste Manag Assoc 2005; 55:708–46.
4. Colvin V. The potential environmental impact of engineered nanomaterials. Nat Biotechnol 2003; 21(10):1166–70.
5. Li XY, Brown D, Smith S, MacNee W, Donaldson K. Short-term inflammatory responses following intratracheal instillation of fine and ultrafine carbon black in rats. Inhal Toxicol 1999; 11:709–31.
6. Ferin J, Oberdorster G, Penney DP. Pulmonary retention of ultrafine and fine particles in rats. Am J Respir Cell Mol Biol 1992; 6:535–42.
7. Brown DM, Wilson MR, MacNee W, Stone V, Donaldson K. Size-dependent proinflammatory effects of ultrafine polystyrene particles: a role for surface area and oxidative stress in the enhanced activity of ultrafines. Toxicol Appl Pharmacol 2001; 175:191–9.

8. Stone V, Shaw J, Brown DM, MacNee W, Faux SP, Donaldson K. The role of oxidative stress in the prolonged inhibitory effect of ultrafine carbon black on epithelial cell function. Toxicol. In Vitro 1998; 12:649–59.
9. Wilson MR, Lightbody JH, Donaldson K, Sales J, Stone V. Interactions between ultrafine particles and transition metals in vivo and in vitro. Toxicol Appl Pharmacol 2002; 184:172–9.
10. Giles GI, Jacob C. Reactive sulphur species: an emerging concept in oxidative stress. Biol Chem 2002; 3–4:375–88.
11. Donaldson K, Stone V, Gilmour PS, Brown DM, MacNee W. Ultrafine particles: mechanisms of lung injury. Phil Trans R Soc Lond 2000; 358:2741–9.
12. Donaldson K, Stone V, Borm PJ, Jimenez LA, Gilmour PS, Schins RP, Knaapen AM, Rahman I, Faux SP, Brown DM, MacNee W. Oxidative stress and calcium signaling in the adverse effects of environmental particles (PM10). Free Radic Biol Med 2003; 34:1369–82.
13. Peters A, Wichmann HE, Tuch T, Heinrich J, Heyder J. Respiratory effects are associated with the number of ultrafine particles. Am J Respir Crit Care Med 1997; 155:1376–83.
14. Duffin R, Tran CL, Clouter A, Brown DM, MacNee W, Stone V, Donaldson K. The importance of surface area and specific reactivity in the acute pulmonary inflammatory response to particles. Ann Occup Hyg 2002; 46(Suppl. 1):242–5.
15. Warheit DB, Driscoll KE, Oberdoerster G, Walker C, Kuschner M, Hesterberg TW. Contemporary issues in fiber toxicology. Fundam Appl Toxicol 1995; 25:171–83.
16. Donaldson K, Brown GM, Brown DM, Bolton RE, Davis JM. Inflammation generating potential of long and short fibre amosite asbestos samples. Br J Ind Med 1989; 46:271–6.
17. Nature. Don't believe the hype. Editorial. Nature 2003; 424:237.
18. Oberdorster G, Oberdorster E, Oberdorster J. Nanotoxicology: an emerging discipline evolving from studies of ultrafine particles. Environ Health Perspect 2005; 113:823–39.
19. Lead JR, Muirhead D, Gibson CT. Characterization of freshwater natural aquatic colloids by atomic force microscopy (AFM). Environ Sci Technol 2005; 39:6930–6.
20. Leppard GG, Mavrocordatos D, Perret D. Electron-optical characterization of nano- and micro-particles in raw and treated waters: an overview. Water Sci Technol 2004; 50:1–8.
21. Oberdorster E. Manufactured nanomaterials (Fullerenes, C_{60}) induce oxidative stress in the brain of juvenile largemouth Bass. Environ Health Perspect 2004; 112:1058–62.
22. Lovern SB, Klaper RD, Daphia magna mortality when exposed to titanium dioxide and fullerene (C60) nanoparticles. Environ Toxicol Chem 2006 25(4), 1132–1137.
23. Oberdorster E, Larkin P, Rogers J. Rapid environmental impact screening for engineered nanomaterials: A case study using microarray technology. Project on emerging technologies. Woodrow Wilson International Centre for Scholars and the Pew Charitable Trusts, 2006
24. Williams DN, Ehrman SH, Pulliam Holoman TR. Evaluation of the microbial growth response to inorganic nanoparticles. J Nanobiotechnol 2006; 4 :3(8pp).

25. Fortner JD, Lyon DY, Sayes CM, Boyd AM, Falkner JC, Hotze EM, Alemany LB, Tao YJ, Guo W, Ausman KD, Colvin VL, Hughes JB. C_{60} in water: nanocrystal formation and microbial response. Environ Sci Technol 2005; 39:4307–16.

26. Sondi I, Salopek-Sondi B. Silver nanoparticles as antimicrobial agent: a case study on *E. coli* as a model for Gram-negative bacteria. J Coll Interface Sci 2004; 275:177–82.

27. Koper O, Lucas E, Klabunde KJ. Development of reactive topical skin protectants against sulfur mustard and nerve agents. J Appl Toxicol 1999; 19 (Suppl 1):S59–70.

28. Lee S-H. Inactivation of bacterial endospores by photocatalytic nano-composites. Coll. Surface 2005; 40:93–8.

29. Watson JHP, Cressey BA, Roberts AP, Ellwood DC, Charnock JM, Soper K.. Structural and magnetic studies on heavy-metal-adsorbing iron sulphide nanoparticles produced by sulphate-reducing bacteria. J Magn Magn Mat 2000; 214:13–20.

30. Kim S-C, Lee D-K. Preparation of TiO_2-coated hollow glass beads and their application to the control of algal growth in eutrophic water. Microchemistry 2005; 80:227–32.

31. Yang L, Watts DJ. Particle surface characteristics may play an important role in phytotoxicity of alumina nanoparticles. Toxicol Lett 2005; 158:122–32.

32. Murashov V. Letter to the Editor:Comments. In: May L, Watts DJ, eds. Particle Surface Characteristics Toxicology Letters 2005; 158 :122–32. Toxicol Lett 164 2006;185–7.

33. Brant J, Lecoanet H, Hotze M, Wiesner M. Comparison of electrokinetic properties of colloidal fullerenes (n-C60) formed using two procedures. Environ Sci Technol 2005; 39:6343–51.

34. Zhu S, Oberdorster E, Haasch ML. Toxicity of an engineered nanoparticle (fullerene, C(60)) in two aquatic species, *Daphnia* and fathead minnow. Mar Environ Res 2006; 62 (Suppl. 1):S5–9.

35. Stone V, Kinloch I, Clift M, Fernandes TF, Ford A, Christofi N, Griffiths A. Donaldson K. Nanoparticle toxicology and ecotoxicology: the role of oxidative stress. In: Zhao Y, Nalwa, HS, eds, Nanotoxicology, American Scientific Publishers 2007, in press.

36. Oberdorster E, Zhu S, Blickley TM, McClellan-Green P, Haasch ML Ecotoxicology of carbon-based engineered nanoparticles: Effects of fullerene (C60) on aquatic organisms. Carbon 2006; 44:1112–20.

37. Smith C, Shaw B, Handy R. Toxicity of single walled carbon nanotubes on rainbow trout (*Oncorhyncos mykiss*): respiratory toxicity, organ pathologies, and other physiological effects. Aqua Toxicol 2007; 82:94–109.

38. Mato Y, Isobe T, Takada H, Kanehiro H, Ohtake C, Kaminuma T, Plastic resin pellets as a transport medium for toxic chemicals in the marine environment. Environ Sci Technol 2001; 35:318–24.

39. Biswas P, Wu CY. Nanoparticles and the environment. J Air Waste Mgmt Assoc 2005; 55:708–746.

25

Nanotechnology and Toxicology: How Do We Move Forward?

Barbara P. Karn

U.S. Environmental Protection Agency, Office of Research and Development, National Center for Environmental Research, Washington, D.C., U.S.A.

BACKGROUND

Research directed at the toxicology of manufactured nano materials has been increasing steadily over the past four years. In particular, the early work of Lam (1) and Warheit (2) caught the attention of the nano-technology research community by indicating the possibility of harmful effects from these new materials. While there had been earlier research on health effects of airborne ultrafine (<100 nm) materials, these results applied to a mixture of ambient particles mainly from combustion sources. Lam and Warheit's work addressed purposefully manufactured new materials (carbon nanotubes) and found adverse effects (granuloma) when instilled into rodent lungs. These results brought an awareness to the nano-technology community that there may be health risks involved with manufactured nano materials. With this awareness, there was a call for research into the possible harmful effects of manufactured nanoparticles.

In 2002, EPA launched its first solicitation for research into the implications of manufactured nano materials. Implications addressed toxicity—both human and ecosystem—exposure routes, fate and transport in the environment, and life cycle aspects. In subsequent years, NSF, NIOSH/CDC, and, later, NIEHS partnered in this solicitation for academic research. NIOSH laboratories examined airborne nano tubes, and the next year the National Toxicology Program (NTP) began its work on select manufactured nanomaterials. These research programs have precipitated the forming of a community of toxicologists that specialize in research on nanomaterials.

Current toxicology research on nanomaterials has been done in the broader context of identified environment, health and safety (EHS) research needs. Many organizations in the US and abroad, both governmental and nongovernmental, have put forth documents identifying information necessary for risk assessment and the protection of workers, the public, and the environment (3–8). Much of the research called for in these documents involves human toxicology. Areas such as toxicity evaluation, screening tests, toxicity mechanisms, theoretical studies (computational toxicology, structure activity relationships), physiological interactions, dose/response studies are listed as research needs. Also of interest to the toxicology community are the research needs addressing metrology and standards. These, along with accurate characterization of the materials, are important long-term considerations if the toxicological effects of nanomaterials are to be fully understood.

The emphasis of many discussions on possible harmful effects of nanotechnology is reminiscent of the Asilomar meeting in Monterey, California, where a group of scientists was convened in 1975 to discuss the possible implications of genetic manipulation. Several months prior to that meeting, scientists themselves called for a moratorium on the research, questioning whether it was safe to move DNA from one organism to another. At the Asilomar meeting, the scientists decided to concentrate on the safety of the science rather than ethical considerations. Their decision kept them in the realm of science rather than moving in to harder philosophical discussions. According to Harold Shapiro, what was unique about Asilomar was that "a group of scientists was convened to reflect upon how their work affected other people's lives" (9). While there have been discussions about the ethical, legal, and societal issues of nanotechnology, the vast majority of emphasis has been on environment, health, and safety issues. In this sense, the scientists who are planning for EHS research in nanotechnology are also considering how their work effects other people's lives by trying to proactively minimize risk and prevent the surprises of unintended consequences.

PRECAUTION VS. PREVENTION

Feeding on the studies that indicate toxic effects of nanomaterials, some non-governmental organizations called for a moratorium on all nanotechnology research until the materials are proved safe. Not only is this precautionary approach to a new technology unfounded, it is also impossible to carry out. The technology has been taken up by commerce and could only be stopped by massive consumer resistance.

Evidence of toxic effects in test organisms is cause for some concern; however, it does not necessarily predict toxic effects in humans or other organisms. In addition, risk involves more than just toxicity. If exposure to a material is controlled and minimized, the risk is controlled and minimized. Findings of toxic effects indicate that we should proceed with caution; they do not beg for a moratorium on research or the products of that research.

One way to proceed with caution is to take a preventive approach. The most obvious way would be a risk prevention approach that limits exposure if the nanomaterial is toxic or until its toxicity is known. A more difficult preventive approach would require an understanding of the toxicological mechanisms of the nanomaterials based on their molecular structure. Once these mechanisms are understood, then the nanomaterial's structure could be modified by designing out the toxicological effects. These preventive approaches will be based on the research generated by toxicologists and the basic research presented here in this book.

GREEN NANOTECHNOLOGY

Green nanotechnology is another preventive approach to moving forward responsibly. It has two objectives: producing nanomaterials and products without harming the environment or human health; and producing nanoproducts that provide solutions to environmental challenges. The first of these objectives deals with production in two ways. One way considers the manufacture of nanomaterials and nanoproducts "greenly." By this, we mean using principles of green chemistry, green engineering, environmentally benign manufacturing. This is an up front approach where pollution and toxicity are designed out of the end product. In a new technology, there is the opportunity not to make the old pollutants. Toxic solvents could be replaced; production energy could be lowered; solid state reactions or molecular self-assembly could be used.

The second way considers using nanomaterials and nanoproducts to make current production processes greener. For example, nanoscale catalysts can make chemical reactions more efficient and selective, thereby decreasing the amount of energy needed and decreasing the amount of wasteful and possibly toxic byproducts produced. Separations in production processes can be made more efficient by using nanoscale membranes. In both cases, pollution prevention at the source is emphasized.

The second green nanotechnology objective, producing nanoproducts that provide solutions to environmental challenges, involves both direct and indirect applications to the environment. Direct applications are those that are focused on solving environmental problems both past and present. For example, nanomaterials such as zero valent iron can be used to remediate hazardous waste sites, or nano enabled sensors can detect extremely low concentrations of heavy metal pollutants. Indirect applications were not designed specifically for the environment; however, they protect and improve the environment as they are used. For example, LED lighting is enabled by nanomaterials. In addition to providing bright light, it saves energy and thereby reduces emissions from power generating plants. Nanomaterials in composites provide the same properties that are found in heavier composites. As a result, transportation energy for the lighter nano materials results in less fuel usage, less pollution, and less material is extracted from the earth that needs to be disposed of at the end of its life.

Green nanotechnology cannot focus on just one aspect of the life cycle of a nanomaterial or nanoproduct, but must take into consideration the full system from extraction of raw materials to transport to manufacturing to use to end of life–recycle, reuse, remanufacture, ultimate disposal. The toxicology of nanomaterials is an important factor in determining the impact of a nanomaterial or product throughout its life cycle. A recent workshop of lifecycle assessment experts determined that the current methods for LCA analysis are adequate for nanotechnology; however, toxicity impact data is missing from most nanomaterials. Without the toxicology work, even estimates of lifecycle impacts are difficult.

TOXICOLOGY AND NANOTECHNOLOGY

From the above discussion and the research presented in this book, the need for more toxicology research on manufactured nanomaterials is clear. In addition to standard tests, there is a need to develop better and rapid screening methods and to move into more predictive toxicology. The former will help prevent risk by knowing where to control exposure; the latter will help prevent risk by helping with design parameters to remove toxicity by design. Of particular importance to the LCA community is the toxicity of those nanomaterials that are in production for use in large-scale products.

The challenges are great, and the new research directions are exciting. Toxicology studies are the basis for protection of human health and the environment relating to nanotechnology. It is only through addressing the issues raised by toxicological studies that nanotechnology will be able to realize its full potential.

REFERENCES

1. Lam CW, James JT, McCluskey R, Hunter RL. Pulmonary toxicity of single wall carbon nanotubes in mice 7 and 90 days after intratracheal instillation. Tox Sci 2004; 77:126–34.

2. Warheit DB, Laurence BR, Reed KL, Roach DH, Reynolds GAM, Webb TR. Comparative pulmonary toxicity assessment of single wall carbon nanotubes in rats. Tox Sci 2004; 77:117–25.
3. U.S. Environmental Protection Agency Nanotechnology White Paper. (EPA100/B-071001) 2007; http://es.epa.gov/ncer/nano/publications/whitepaper12022005.pdf.
4. The Royal Society, Nanoscience and Nanotechnologies: opportunities and uncertainties, Royal Academy of Engineering 2004; www.nanotec.org.uk/finalReport.htm.
5. Chemical Industry Vision2020 Technology Partnership. Joint NNI-Chl CBAN and SRC CWG5 nanotechnology needs recommendations 2005; www.chemicalvision2020.org/pdfs/chem-semi%20ESH%20recommendations.pdf.
6. European Commission; Communication from the commission to the council, the European parliament, and the economic and social committee. Nanoscience and nanotechnologies: an action plan for Europee 2005–2009, 2005. http://ec.europa.eu/research/industrial_technologies/pdf/nano_action_plan_en.pdf.
7. Maynard, A, Nanotechnology: a research strategy for addressing risk. Project on emerging nanotexhnologies July 2006; www.nanotechproject.org.
8. National Nanotechnology Initiative. Environmental, health, and safety research needs for engineered nanoscale materials 2006; www.nano.gov/NNI_EHS_research_needs.pdf.
9. Barinaga, M, Asilomar revisited: lessons for today? Science 2000; 287(5458): 1584 –5.

Index